Frederick Hollick

The marriage guide, or,

Natural history of generation : a private instructor for married persons and those

about to marry, both male and female, in every thing concerning the physiology

and relations of the sexual system and the production or prevent

Frederick Hollick

The marriage guide, or,
Natural history of generation : a private instructor for married persons and those about to marry, both male and female, in every thing concerning the physiology and relations of the sexual system and the production or prevent

ISBN/EAN: 9783337775445

Printed in Europe, USA, Canada, Australia, Japan

Cover: Foto ©ninafisch / pixelio.de

More available books at **www.hansebooks.com**

THE
MARRIAGE GUIDE,

OR

NATURAL HISTORY OF GENERATION;

A PRIVATE INSTRUCTOR

FOR MARRIED PERSONS AND THOSE ABOUT TO MARRY,

BOTH MALE AND FEMALE;

IN EVERY THING CONCERNING THE PHYSIOLOGY AND RELATIONS
OF THE SEXUAL SYSTEM, AND THE PRODUCTION OR
PREVENTION OF OFFSPRING; INCLUDING ALL
NEW DISCOVERIES, NEVER BEFORE GIVEN
IN THE ENGLISH LANGUAGE.

BY FREDERICK HOLLICK, M. D.,

AUTHOR AND LECTURER UPON THE PHYSIOLOGY AND DISEASES OF
THE GENERATIVE ORGANS.

With numerous Engravings and Colored Plates.

200th EDITION
*MUCH ENLARGED AND IMPROVED, AND BROUGHT
DOWN TO THE PRESENT DAY.*

New York:
T. W. STRONG, 599 BROADWAY.

Entered according to Act of Congress in the year 1860,
By FREDERICK HOLLICK, M. D.,
In the Clerk's Office of the District Court of the United States
for the Southern District of New York.

HISTORICAL AND EXPLANATORY

INTRODUCTION

TO THE TWO–HUNDREDTH EDITION.

————◆◆◆————

A FEW years ago I commenced the first complete popular Lectures on Sexual Physiology, to Ladies and Gentlemen, separately, ever delivered in the United States. They
were illustrated by Anatomical Models, and Diagrams, and
in every respect were scientific and practically useful. At
their commencement, from the novelty of such an attempt,
many people regarded them with distrust, but as their real
character became gradually known, they were regarded
with increasing interest daily, and received an amount of
patronage far greater than was ever anticipated. In fact,
few novel enterprises ever succeeded so well, considering
the prejudice and misconception that had to be overcome.
For a long time " *Dr. Hollick's Lectures* " were the principal topics of conversation in New York, and also in Boston and Philadelphia! (See Notices.

My object in delivering these Lectures was to familiarize
the public mind with the discussion of such matters, in a
proper manner, and to point out the real source of numerous physical and moral evils under which society labors.
Having succeeded past my hopes in arousing the public
mind, I soon saw, as I had anticipated, numerous co-labor-
ers start up on the same field of action. Lecturers on
Anatomy and Physiology, with *Manikins*, soon became

common every where, and have since been steadily increasing in number.

As soon as this result was obtained, I turned my attention to another matter, *namely*, the preparation of a popular and scientific *Book*, on the same plan as the Lectures, so serve as a *manual*, and for the instruction of those who ould not attend the Lectures. The first publication of the kind which I issued was called "THE ORIGIN OF LIFE!" It had a most extraordinary run of popularity, and soon became regarded as *the Book* on such matters. The public needed something different from the old, obsolete, *unpractical*, and mostly indecent publications on such matters, which alone had previously existed, and "The Origin" was every where welcomed as being *just what was wanted!*

An absurd and bungling attempt was spitefully made by the Medical *Old Fogies* in Philadelphia, to prevent the sale of this Book, and also the delivery of my Lectures. As might have been anticipated however, such an attempt not only *failed*, most completely, but also increased the popularity of both Books and Lectures a hundred-fold, while the would-be-monopolists of knowledge became truly pitiable objects of public scorn and contempt.

In a short time I found my audiences making other demands upon me for more extended information. The *Ladies* desired a book on the *female system*, and the Gentlemen one exclusively on the *male system*, and all its derangements. I therefore published "*The Diseases of Women*"— and the "*Matron's Manual of Midwifery*," and soon after '*The Male Generative Organs*," all of which at once attained an immense circulation, which is constantly and steadily increasing. It was soon apparent also, that the scope and matter of the original work, "*The Origin of Life*," required extending, in accordance with the advance made in the public mind. I therefore re-wrote it entirely, making it a complete *Cyclopedia* of everything relating to sexual matters that could possibly interest adult persons of either sex, or be of use to them. To express more fully its objects and uses, the name was also changed to "*The Marriage Guide*," or Natural History of Generation, &c. This work has been more popular even than any of the former ones, and is now daily printed in increasing numbers.

All these books had to be written in the few moments I could occasionally steal from my professional duties, which became constantly more and more burthensome. At present I am so much occupied with my practice, that I can only overlook the new Editions of each work, and keep them all, in every respect, fully up to the times, by inserting all the new discoveries, and giving the latest views. For eighteen months I published a popular journal, called *The People's Monthly Medical Journal*," but finding it utterly impossible to spare sufficient time each month to compile it, I was compelled to suspend the issue, though I trust by and by to resume it in another form. At present my professional calls leave me hardly leisure enough to keep perfect the works I have already published, but in time I hope to issue others, on different but kindred topics. The general scope and objects of each Book will be partly gathered from its Title, but it may be as well to state them more fully.

The *Diseases of Women* is expressly for females' own use giving the causes, cure, and prevention, of every derangement to which their systems are liable, from infancy to old age.

The *Matron's Manual* of MIDWIFERY is intended to explain the nature and whole art of childbirth and delivery, in such a way, that any one may learn from it what to do

in case of emergency, and how to do it. From the sim
plicity and practical nature of the explanations, aided by
numerous engravings, it is suited to make this matter clear
even to the most ordinary intelligence, at the same time
that it is perfect enough for medical students or professional men.

The Male Generative Organs, is intended for Gentlemen
the same as the Diseases of Woman is for Ladies. It gives
the causes, prevention, and cure of every disease and derangement to which the Male Generative Organs are liable.
Many of the most important of these derangements were
scarcely known, even to the majority of *Medical men,* before
the publication of this Book. This was the case especially
with that most serious of all Male Generative derangements, *Urinary loss of Semen!* This fatal disease, which
consigns thousands to imbecility, and untimely death, with
out their ever suspecting even the cause of their ruin, was
never properly explained till this Book was written. It
should be observed that this is not a *venereal* work, but
treats only on these derangements to which all are liable.

Venereal Diseases are fully treated upon, in a special
work, called "*A Popular Treatise on Venereal Diseases,*"
&c. written in the same way as the other books.

The Marriage Guide has been already spoken of sufficiently to give a tolerable idea of its contents. It should be
remarked, that no other book in the English language is at
all like it, nor can the information it contains be found any
where else, except in recent French and German Medical
publications. The new discoveries on Generation especially
excite the surprise of all who first read them, the old ideas
on these matters are totally upset, and practical results
are arrived at regarding *Conception,* and kindred phenomena, as new as they are astonishing

PREFACE

TO THE FIRST EDITION

ALTHOUGH there have been many works published professedly upon the Physiology of Generation and upon Diseases of the Reproductive System, in both sexes, but few of them have been calculated to be of any service to the public. They have mostly been written either for medical men only, or else for the merely ignorant and curious, but, with very few exceptions, none have been both scientific and practically useful, and at the same time *popular.* But among them all there has never been one *specially intended to give advice and information to married persons or those about to marry;* and yet every one knows that such a work, if properly written, would be of incalculable service. Married persons, and those who are thinking of marriage, always need information upon a variety of topics both interesting and important to them, but which they have no means of gaining. It is not always agreeable to ask medical men in regard to such matters, particularly for females; and, besides, many medical men are not disposed to answer questions of the kind, and others even are not competent to do so, because they are not familiar with the subjects inquired about. The consequence is, that people generally are compelled to remain in ignorance against their inclinations, and are constantly falling into error and being subject to numerous misfor-

tunes in consequence. I have no doubt but that a
very large portion of the *disease,* and *unhappiness,*
which many married persons suffer under, arises
directly from their forced ignorance, and nothing
can be more useful, or more generally acceptable
than a book to which all can refer, either before
marriage or after, for any information they may
require. For this especial purpose *The Marriage
Guide* has been written, and such a reliable refer
ence I trust it will always be found.

Having been now engaged for many years in delivering public lectures on the Anatomy and Phy
siology of the Reproductive Organs, in both sexes,
and my practice having been almost exclusively
devoted to their disabilities and diseases, I have become fully conversant with the wants and wishes
of the public, generally, in regard to information
on these subjects. The old absurd notion being
pretty much exploded, that ignorance of these matters is advantageous, the people are looking in every
direction for information, but, owing to the mystery
with which everything of the kind has always been
shrouded, and to the prejudice of many medical
men against popular enlightenment, but little information has been conveyed to them till lately. I believe I was the first in this country to give complete
popular and scientific lectures on these subjects,
and I also published the first scientific and popular
treatise, called " *The Origin of Life.*" Since my
first essay in this way, I have repeatedly lectured
in various parts of the Union, and have become extensively known, both as a teacher and practitioner
I have also published several other works since the
Origin of Life, as I have found time to write them.
Among these may be specially mentioned " The

Male Generative Organs," and "The Diseases of Women." These works were intended to give all the new discoveries, both physiological and medical, and all the new modes of treatment, many of which were scarcely known, even to medical men. The circulation of these books has been extraordinarily great, and, together with my lectures, have brought me a practice so extensive, that I have had less time than ever to prepare new ones. During last winter, however, I became convinced of the necessity, in justice to myself, as well as the public, of making an effort to bring out *The Marriage Guide* as early as possible. Not only was a work of the kind always inquired for by my audiences, but also by numbers of letters from all parts of the country, and especially by those who had been deceived into purchasing the useless, unscientific and indecent books on such subjects, that everywhere abound. Scarcely any of these books are written by medical men, and those that are so, are in no way adapted to be of the slightest service. They are either mere obscene compilations, made to sell, or else mere reprints of old physiological theories and speculations, exploded half a century ago among scientific men. Until now, there has not been a single popular work, relating to marriage, that was at the same time both scientific and practically useful, although such a work has been urgently required. At the present time, this want is more urgent than ever, *owing to the great interest and importance of certain new discoveries respecting Conception !*

These discoveries were first announced by the German and French physiologists, but they were so strange, that few were disposed to believe them.

My own observation had led me to adopt similar views, before the works of *Pouchet* or *Negrier* were published ; but to make sure of their correctness, I commenced a regular series of experiments, dissec- tions, and observations, especially to test them. Some of them I have only just concluded, and the result of them has been to confirm all that I had previously surmised. From time to time I have given brief explanations of these new discoveries. in my lectures, and in my books, in order to famil- iarize the public mind with them, and to partly gratify curiosity, till they could be given in a more perfect form. These brief announcements, however. led to an evil, which nothing but the early publica- tion of the " Guide " could correct. From the very first delivery of my lectures, various other persons started in the same path, which I expected of course, and which I should have been very glad to see, if they had pursued a similar plan ; but few of them did so. Some few really honest and scientific men. attempted the work, but, not making their discourses *popular*, they failed in creating sufficient interest to induce them to continue. Others were not suffi- ciently familiar with these particular subjects, though well acquainted with Physiology in general, and very often they found themselves distanced, in re- gard to new discoveries, even by some of their au- dience. Eventually, all these fell off, one by one, and I was left alone in the field again ; but, then, a new class of competitors appeared—mere adven- turers, knowing nothing more of these important matters than they had gathered from reading my books, and attending my lectures. These men had never practised dissection, nor made regular expe- riments and extended observations, but merely re-

tailed, at second-hand, what they had learned from
others, often very imperfectly indeed. Their only
object being the making of money by the *lectures*,
they degraded them to the level of mere exhibitions
and entertainments, interspersing them with loose
anecdotes, and delivering them in such a way as to
attract a wondering crowd, who were neither instructed nor improved by what they saw or heard.
My endeavor was always to keep the lectures as secret and unobtrusive as possible, so as to call around
me the *thinkers*, and those who possessed influence,
first, leaving the mass to come in by degrees, not
from vulgar curiosity, but from a gradually awakened and enlightened interest. I took especial
care to give my lectures a high moral tone, and to
make them practically useful. I found, however,
that others, professing to lecture on the same subjects, had not been so particular, but had adopted
an improper tone of levity in their discourses, and
omitted, altogether, to show the utility of what was
attempted to be explained. Besides which, they had
picked up, from my lectures and books, some faint
notions of the *new discoveries* I have referred to,
and knowing that they would interest their audiences, they made them their chief topics. Not
being perfectly acquainted with them, however,
their explanations were generally erroneous, and
always imperfect, so that the people who listened
were misled thereby, and often to their great disad
vantage. This was especially the case in regard
to the *time* and manner of conception. Not knowing, practically, the laws which regulate this process, and having heard only very partial explanations, they both confused themselves and misinformed
their audiences. Many, who had heard me pre-

iously, soon discovered this, and immediately
urged that it was my duty instantly to publish a
book that would give a full and proper explanation
of the whole subject.   I saw myself the necessity
of doing so at once, under the circumstances, and
also of repeating my lectures as frequently as possible.   Accordingly I collected together my notes
and manuscripts, completed my experiments and
observations, and put "The Guide" to press.

In regard to the work itself, I feel fully justified
in saying that it is the most complete and practically
useful of the kind that ever was written.   In fact,
so far as I have seen, it is the only one adapted for
popular use.   I have taken especial care in its preparation, and bestowed more labor upon it than any
one, not conversant with such an undertaking,
would suppose requisite.   Not only has it been re
quisite to consult all the most celebrated authors
upon such subjects, especially the modern ones,
and to continue regularly to peruse the various
medical periodicals, but also to compare and tabu-
late the notes of my own observations, made for
many years past, and to study and collect the reports of various public institutions.   In addition to
which, it was also necessary to dissect extensively,
to experiment upon animals, and to compare different races and individuals together.   There are
many questions, of great interest and importance,
connected with marriage, which can be decided
only by a most careful observation of *numerous
cases* which it may take years to bring under one
man's notice, and which can never be decided correctly by any limited experience.   This is particularly true of *the causes of the difference in sex, the
time and duration of pregnancy,* and the nature of

parental influence before birth. This work I have been engaged upon many years, and, in every particular, I have fully satisfied myself, before professing to give any explanation. My intention being to make it so complete, that, for information respecting the subjects upon which it treats, u other need be referred to, and that any one consulting it, may be certain to find a correct explanation of everything in which he or she may be interested.

It has appeared to me, upon a full consideration of the subject, that if this work were confined altogether to the human being, in its physiological explanations, it would be imperfect, and would not so well fulfil the purpose for which it was intended. There is so much to be learned by comparison and analogy, among different beings, which cannot be learned in any other way that it is impossible to have a clear and comprehensive idea of the wonderful phenomena of generation, if one class only is studied. And, independent of this, the deep intrinsic interest and importance of the subject, must make every one desirous of knowing all the details and variations of the several functions explained, some of which are most perfectly performed in one class, and others in another.

I have, therefore, given copious explanations of the Generative Organs and acts in all the different classes of animals and in plants, so that everything relating to them may be found in this book, which is, in fact, a *Clyclopedia* of the Physiology of Reproduction, as well as a " *Guide* " to Human Marriage.

It will be seen that many of the most ordinary processes become, in some animals both complicated and curious, and that the form and action of the or-

gans varies in the most singular manner. **Many**
of the recent important discoveries, it will also **be**
observed, have resulted from observations upon the
lower animals, and could never have been made in
any other way

In regard to the *propriety* and *utility* of such a
work as this, but few words are requisite. When
I published my first book, it had great prejudice
and misapprehension to encounter, but that has
now been, in a great measure, overcome, and the
true character and influence of such publications
is generally acknowledged. There are but few
people now, of even ordinary intelligence. but what
perceive and admit the benefits of popular information on these matters, providing it be properly imparted, and I flatter myself that my name is now
so well known, in connection with undertakings of
this kind, that it will be accounted sufficient guar-
rantee for the present one.

My professional communication with married
persons, and the numerous questions they have pro-
pounded to me, both at the lectures and by letters,
have shown me upon what subjects they most frequently and urgently require instruction, and these
have been especially attended to. " *The Guide*" is,
in short, intended to supply the place of *a medical
adviser and physiological instructor*, with the advantage of being always at hand, perfectly reliable on
all points, and certain not to withhold any information, from prejudice or mistaken interest.

F. HOLLICK, M. D.,
NEW YORK.

Box 3606,
Post Office, New York City.

CONTENTS

PART I.

CHAPTER I.

CHAPTER II.

PART II.

CHAPTER I

CHAPTER II.

CHAPTER III.

CHAPTER IV.

PART III.

MISCELLANEOUS "CASES."

CONCLUDING PART.

ILLUSTRATIONS:

DESCRIPTION OF COLORED PLATE OF THE MALE PELVIS, ON Page 112.

ON Page 112.

SECTION OF THE MALE PELVIS TO SHOW THE SITUATION OF THE DIFFERENT PARTS.

A. the Bladder. *B.* The Rectum, or end of the large intestine. *C.* The lower part of the back bone, or sacrum. *d.d.* The small Intestines. *f.* One of the Kidneys. *g.g.* The Ureter, or Tube which conveys the Urine from the Kidneys into the Bladder. *h.* The Pubic or Frontal Bone of the Pelvis.

1. The left Testicle. 2.2. The Vas Deferens, or Tube which conveys the Semen from the Testicle. 3. The left Seminal Vesicle, with which the Vas Deferens is connected. 4. The Ejaculatory Canal, into which the Semen next passes. 5. The Prostate Gland, with which the Ejaculatory Canal connects, and through which the Semen passes into the Urethra, or Urinary passage from the Bladder, (7). 6. The Veru Montanum, or small protuberance which partly closes the neck of the Bladder. 7. 7. The Urethra, or passage by which the Urine escapes from the Bladder down the Penis. 8. The upper part of the Penis, or Corpus Cavernosum. 9. The lower part, or Corpus Spongiosum. 10. The Glans, or Head of the Penis. 11. One of Cowper's Glands.

The course of the Semen is from the Testes along the Vas Deferens to the Seminal Vesicle, then along the Ejaculatory Canal and through the Prostate Gland into the Urethra, which it enters by the lower part of the Veru Montanum, at the part indicated by the two black dots. It then escapes from the body in the same way as the Urine does.

NOTICE

ANY persons wishing to communicate with Dr H by Letters, can address to

"Dr. F. HOLLICK,

Box, **3606**, Post Office,

New York City, N. Y."

and they will be promptly replied to.

All Letters asking an opinion, or advice, must be full and plain in their descriptions, so that a correct judgment can be formed, and they must always contain the customary fee of *Five Dollars*, or they cannot be attended to.

N. B.—Persons visiting New York, can always hear respecting Dr. H. by calling on T. W. STRONG, 599 Broadway, his publisher, who will know if he is then in town or not, and will give the address of his office. In the changes constantly occurring in New York, removals frequently occur, which makes this precaution advisable Dr. Hollick's present Office is 348 Broadway.

F. H

THE MARRIAGE GUIDE.

PART I.

GENERATION IN GENERAL.

BEFORE treating upon the specialities of Marriage, i. is requisite to explain the Philosophy and Physiology of Generation in general, both in man and in other beings. This will therefore be the subject of the first *Part* of our work.

CHAPTER 1.

GENERAL VIEW OF THE REPRODUCTIVE FUNCTIONS.

THE Reproductive Organs are organically distinct and separate from all the other organs, forming, in fact, a complete system by themselves, so that their action or inaction has no effect except sympathetically and indirectly upon any other part. Nevertheless, they exert a most wonderful and mysterious influence upon the whole organization, as will be shown further on, and every thing else is more or less imperfect if they happen to be so.

The manner in which Reproduction is effected, is the same in all kinds of beings, both animal and vegetable, at least in the general plan, though there may be variations in unimportant details. The general plan is this,—there is provided, in connection with the physical systems of all beings, two peculiar substances, which are called the *sexual principles*, or the *male* and *female* principles, the union of which, under certain circumstances, results in the growth of a new being, but neither of them, alone, has any power of development whatever. These two principles, in some form or other universally exist, though under various conditions, and are always united, though in many different ways. Thus, in those beings in which we are most familiar, as our own kind for instance, the two principles are always disunited, or placed in separate individuals, whom we call, in consequence, male and female—the male forming what is called the Sperm, Semen, or Seed, and the female forming the Ovum or Egg, which are the two rudiments of all living beings whatever. In some of the inferior classes, however, an opposite arrangement exists, the two principles being united in each individual, which is, therefore, both male and female, or more properly, *Hermaphrodite*. Examples of this arrangement are found in the common earth-worm, the leech, and in many insects and moluscous animals. Some of these are so perfectly Hermaphrodite that they can connect with themselves, and bring forth their own eggs or young without the concurrence of any other individual ; but others, as the leech, for instance, though they have both principles and both sets of Organs, yet have them so disposed in the body that they cannot effect self-impregnation. There must, therefore, always be a union of two of these individuals, but each performs the double act, being impregnated by the other and impregnating it in return. In the leech and earth-worm, the double union, at two distinct points, may often be observed.

In all the most perfectly organized beings, there is no such thing as hermaphrodism, but in the inferior ones referred to it is the natural arrangement, and no other is ever seen. Where the separate arrangement prevails, there are many singular variations, both in the disposition of the principles and also in the manner in which their union is effected. Thus in most fishes, which are very inferiorly organized, there is no act of sexual union, the female depositing the Ovum or Egg in the water, and the male being directed, by a peculiar instinct, to deposit his semen upon them, or so that it will reach them, so that they are united without the male and female being required to come in contact. In some few fishes there is, it is true, a kind of imperfect connection, but, generally, there is not even that. In birds, on the contrary, who are a stage higher in the scale of organization, the two individuals always connect, though very imperfectly, and the two principles are thus united, or, in other words, the egg is impregnated *within* the body of the female. Here, therefore, we have *internal* impregnation, while in the first it was external. But even in the bird the egg is expelled from the body, after its impregnation, to be developed, so that, though the impregnation is internal, yet the development is external. They are, therefore, called *Oviparous*, o. egg-producing. In all of the more perfect beings, on the contrary, as in our species for instance, not only are the two principles united within the body of the female, but after their union they remain and develop there into the new being, so that we have both internal impregnation and internal development also. Such beings are, therefore, called *Viviparous*, because they bring forth their young alive instead of the egg merely.

Under all these circumstances, however, the process is essentially the same. There are always the two principles, the male semen and the female ovum or egg, and their union in what is called the act of *Impregnation* must always occur before the new being can commence to develop ; but the impregnation and development may be either internal or external.

In some beings there is a union of the two modes

the egg being hatched while it is passing from the body, so that the young being is really born alive, though it is produced from the egg as it is externally in the birds. These are, therefore, called *Ovi-viparous*, to denote the union of the two modes.

There are others, again, in whom the young is formed internally, as in the more perfect being, but expelled before its development is perfected, and it has, therefore, to be permanently attached to the body for awhile, externally, till sufficiently grown, to live independently. These are called *Marsupial* Animals, because the imperfect being is placed in a kind of pouch or pocket, adjoining the Teats, to which the young are fastened when first expelled. The Oppossum is an example of the Marsupial Animals, which evidently connect the Viviparous with those that are below them.

From this general sketch, it will be readily seen what organs are really essential to the generative system, in both sexes. In the Female there must, of necessity, be an Organ to produce the Ova, or Egg, and which is called the *Ovary*, or egg producer. This, in fact, constitutes a female, *though all the other parts*, usually found in that sex, should be absent, and without it, no individual can be female, though all the other parts should be present. There are also usually found certain accessory organs, by which the egg is either conveyed out of the body, when ripe, or by which the male semen is conveyed to effect its impregnation. In those also that bring forth their young alive, there is another organ, peculiar to the Viviparous Animals, which is called the *Uterus*, or *Womb*. This is a hollow organ, into which the egg is passed when fully ripe, and in which it undergoes its complete

development after impregnation. There are also certain organs of minor importance, which connect the
Uterus with the Ovary, and by means of which the
egg is conveyed from the one to the other. In the
Marsupial Animals, the Uterus is imperfect, so that
the young cannot undergo their full development
therein, which is the reason why they are expelled
and perfected externally.

In the Male system, the essential organ is, of
course, that which produces the male principle, or
Semen ; it is called the *Testicle.* In connection
with this, there are also other organs of minor importance, for the transmission and direction of the
fecundating fluid. All these accessory parts, however, may be absent, and yet the body be truly
male, if the Testicle is present, but without that,
all the others do not make it so. No being, among
the superior classes, has ever yet been found, possessing both the Ovary and the Testicle so perfect
as for both to perform their special functions, although, in some of the inferior orders, as before
shown, such an organization always exists.

In the human being, both male and female, we
find, of course, the most perfect and complicated
form of Sexual Organization, the details of which
will now be readily understood.

PLATE I.

Section of the Female Body.

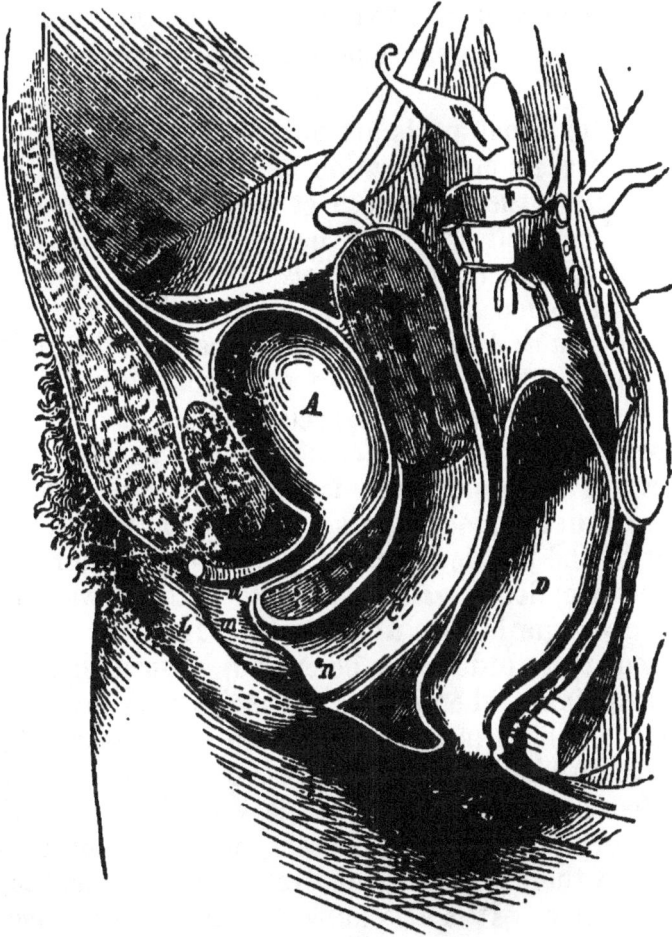

A The Bladder.—B. The Womb.—C. The Vagina.—D. The Rectum.—
L. The Large Lip.—m. The Small Lip.—h. The Mouth of the Bladder.—g. The Mouth of the Womb.—q The Clitoris.

CHAPTER II.

DESCRIPTION OF THE EXTERNAL GENERATIVE ORGANS OF THE HUMAN FEMALE.

THE external parts are not necessarily concerned in the process of generation, but still it is advisable to describe them, because certain modifications in their form and size, may be of consequence, connected with marriage, and, also, because it is necessary, on various accounts, to refer to them.

The *Pubic* bone, at the lower part of the abdomen, in front, is covered, in the female, by a thick layer of fatty matter, especially after the age of puberty, when it is also covered, more or less, with hair. This prominence is called *Mons Veneris*, and its development gives a peculiar outline to this part of the female form. The covering of hair was formerly called *Tressoria*, and its absence was universally regarded as a reproach. In fact, it was customary to order it to be cut off, in open court, in ancient times, when a female was detected the third time in illicit intercourse, as we find stated by Chitty, in his Practical Treatise on Medical Jurisprudence. In some cases it is very slightly developed, or even altogether absent, and is never seen at all in those who have no ovaries, or in whom they are inactive. It is also liable to fall off after certain diseases, or after taking powerful drugs, and will even turn color after fright, or severe agitation, the same as the hair on the head. In some individuals it becomes troublesome, from excessive devel-

opment, and will occasionally extend itself far over
the rest of the body.   In some young persons, the
growth of the *Mons Veneris* and its *Tressoria* is
very rapid, at the age of puberty, so that the ap
pearance of the body is completely changed in that
respect in a few weeks.   It is customary for parents, and even for some physicians, to regard the
appearance of the *Tressoria* as the certain and invariable sign of womanhood, and they are guided
by its absence or presence in their treatment and
communications.   This sign, however, is not always to be relied upon, for I have known young
persons, of not more than *nine* or *ten* years of age,
upon whom it was very fully grown, and the Mons
largely developed, though they did not menstruate
till several years after ; and I have known others,
at eighteen years of age, with scarcely an appearance of it, who had menstruated from the time they
were fourteen.   As a sign of puberty, therefore, it
cannot always be implicitly depended upon, though
generally it may.   I once saw an infant, of *four*
years, on whom quite a large growth of the *Tressoria* existed ; and I have known females pass the
turn of life, who had scarcely ever had any at all.

Immediately below the Mons are two large lips,
called the *Labia Pudendi*, the *Labia Majora*, or
external lips, which are formed by a fold of the
skin, made round and full by a thick deposit of
fatty matter underneath.   The outer surface of these
lips is covered by the *Tressoria*, but the inner surface is smooth, and studded with a number of little
glands or follicles, which exude a peculiar fluid,
with a characteristic odor.   The external lips commence at the frontal or pubic bone, and they descend underneath to within an inch and a half of

the fundament.   They are united together, both above and below, but perfectly separated in the middle, where they are also the largest and most prominent.   Their union below is called the *fourchette* or *fork*.   Sometimes they are very large and prominent, and at other times are very small, and with little elasticity, which makes them liable to injury during parturition.   In some young females they grow together, from inflammation, and if not separated before marriage, great distress and injury may ensue.   The removal of this disability is, however, a very simple matter, and it is fully explained in my "Diseases of Woman."

Immediately within the external lips, and lying on their two sides, are the smaller ones, like folds, which are called the *Labia Minora*, or *inner lips*, or the *Nymphæ*.   These two inner lips do not extend so far, either up or down, as the larger ones, nor are they so round and full.   In infants, the Nymphæ project out farthest, and are seen in front, but at puberty, the external lips develop more fully, so as to close together, and thus shut the Nymphæ in, and conceal them.   This is always the case in virgins, but after childbirth, the external lips become more flaccid, and separate, and the Nymphæ again project, and are seen externally.   In the females of some countries—particularly in the eastern parts of the Old World—the Nymphæ often grow to an extraordinary size, so as to partly close the passage, and it becomes necessary to remove them.   I have even sometimes found this necessary in my own practice, not only from their immense growth, but also from their peculiar condition. They are, in many persons, singularly sensitive, and appear to be the principal parts in which sexual excitement is felt, and when they are more than usually large, or irritable, that excitement becomes so great and overpowering, that it cannot be controlled, but is really a species of furor, or madness, which irresistibly impels the individual to seek gratification, in some form or other, regardless of consequences. The operation of removing them is comparatively simple, and unattended with the slightest danger.

In some of the Hottentot females, the Nymphæ are singularly enlarged, at that part where they join together above, the enlargement hanging down in front of the passage, like a veil. This is called the *Apron*, and seems to be peculiar to certain tribes, like the *tail* among the men of the *Ghilares*. It was formerly thought that this Apron was a growth produced by artificial means, but it is now generally conceded to be natural. Several of these females have been examined at various times by medical men and travellers, and their accounts pretty much conform with each other. I had an opportunity myself, when in England, of seeing a *Hottentot Venus*, as she was called, who posessed this Apron, and I was convinced that it was nothing more than an extension of the Nymphæ. In these females, in fact, the whole of the external organs, differ much from those of white females ; the *Mons Veneris* being less prominent, the external lips smaller, and the passage itself much larger. while the mouth of the opening is more underneath, *or farther back*, so that, when stooping forward, it is nearly in the same position as in some animals. The length of this apron, in the case which I saw, was about three inches and a half, but they have been observed four or five inches long ; and *L*.

Vaillant says, in his journey into the interior of Africa, even *nine* inches. Whether this singular apron serves any specific purpose, it is difficult to tell, but it certainly is a hindrance to connection, unless placed aside at the time, because it hangs down between the limbs, immediately in front. One of these females deceived the French physician who examined her very much, by concealing the apron *in a peculiar situation*, so that they could not see it, and some, in consequence, even doubted of its existence ; but the deception was afterwards discovered.

In many of the Oriental nations the enlargement of the nymphæ is so general that their incision i quite a common operation, like circumcision among the men. This is especially the case in Abyssinia and in the country of Ancient Judea. Many of the Mohammedans remove the nymphæ in most of their young girls, in order, as they say, to prevent deformity, but in reality to make them have *less sexual feeling*, so that they may not be disposed, when women, to desire more indulgence than may fall to their lot n common with many other wives. It is, therefore, the tyranny and jealousy of polygamy that leads to this shameful mutilation. A medical friend of mine, who had resided some time in these countries, informed me that he had even known them to close the two lips together, in young female slaves, with a kind of lock, so that association was impossible until it was opened, and the manner of opening it was known only to her master. In *Sonnini's Travels* in Upper and Lower Egypt much curious information can be found in regard to such customs. He tells us that, in many of the cities, there is a class of persons who make the removal of the nymphæ in young girls a trade, and that they go about the streets crying out, "Here's a good circumciser." And a more ancient traveller, Leo Africanus, informs us that they also call out, "Who is she that wisnes to be cut?" The only instrument employed by these operators is a rude species of razor, and they astringe the wound by dusting it with ashes.

It is probable that this custom of female circumcision may not have originated altogether from jealousy but partly from convenience, because when the nymphæ are large, the secretions of the parts are apt to accumulate under them, and cause great irritation, as is often the case in negresses, and occasionally even among whites, instances of which will be found in my book on *The Diseases of Women.* Sonnini also tells us that the lascivious Turks have another reason for removing the inner lips, and that is that the vulva, or mouth of the passage, may be perfectly smooth, and sexual congress more easy in consequence.

It is desirable that the condition of these parts, as well as of the External Organs generally, should be known previous to marriage, for I have known many instances in which great distress and unhappiness has arisen from something unusual connected with them. They may be too large, or exceedingly sensitive, or grow together, or even be ulcerated, and though the trouble may be readily removed, yet its existence is not desirable at such a time.

At the upper junction of the two nymphæ they project over in a kind of round arch, immediately within which is a small firm body about the size of a large pea, which is called the *Clitoris.* This organ is a most important and interesting one in many respects. It has many points of resemblance to the male Penis, both in its structure and functions, being composed of a similar sponge-like substance, capable of being engorged or becoming *erect*, and is highly sensitive. It is, in fact, the principal seat of sensation in most persons, and the intensity of the sexual orgasm apparently depends upon the perfection of its nervous organization. When it is unduly developed or excitable, the sexual propensity often becomes irresistible, causing *Nymphomania* or *Furor Uterinus*, and leading to moral delinquency, which arises more frequently from mere physical causes than is usually supposed According to Chitty, if a female, in ancient time, was detected the fourth time in illicit intercourse, the *Clitoris* was amputated in open court—a fact which shows that the law-makers of that period were aware of its influence.

In the early stages of fœtal existence it is often difficult to discover the sex of the child, because the clitoris so much resembles the penis ; and even at birth it is relatively much larger than in adult life. In some persons it attains an unusual size. so as to resemble the male organ very much, and can even be used in the same way with another female though, of course, imperfectly. This fact I can state positively, for I have seen an instance in which the clitoris was fully as large as the penis is in most boys of nine or ten years of age, and capable also of becoming quite firm and erect. It is cases like these that are supposed to be of both sexes as will be seen in the article on Hermaphrodites. The clitoris, however, has naturally no passage down it leading from the bladder, the urethra being in its proper position ; but in some few cases the passage has been found to exist although the urine did not flow down it.

In some females this organ is so exquisitely sensitive that it is scarcely possible for them to prevent its becoming excited, and creating sexual desires. Whenever the clothes touch it, or even when it comes in contact with the lips in walking, it be comes congested, and excites both the uterus and the brain. In these cases it is sheer nonsense to say that the strong sexual desire experienced arises merely from *depravity*, or that it can be overcome by *moral* efforts alone. We might just as reasonably conclude that the hunger of an empty stomach arises merely from unruly appetite, and that it also may be overcome by moral effort. In making these remarks I, of course, do not intend to deny the great power of a determined will over the feelings, under most circumstances, nor to discourage such efforts ; on the contrary, they are most important, and often highly effective, but I wish to draw attention to the obvious fact that *they alone* cannot always succeed. It is unquestionable that in many females, and especially about the age of puberty, the excitability of the nymphæ and clitoris is so great that they *cannot* overcome or escape from the feelings and desires that this excitability creates ; and, beyond doubt, it is from this cause alone that many seek improper indulgence, and become depraved. With these persons, therefore, it is not moral suasion alone, or threats, or the fear of consequences, that can be depended upon to effect a reformation, but the state of the body must also be ascertained, and the *physical* causes of the unnatural excitement removed. The timely advice of a judicious physician would, in many of these cases, remove all oc casion for moral exhortation or coercion, and effectually prevent any future evil, because licentiousness is fully as often a result of the bodily condition as it is of the mental disposition, or probably even more so. It should never be forgotten, when reasoning upon these subjects, that some persons *cannot prevent* sexual desire—though good moral training may enable them to struggle against it— while others *can never experience it*, even if they wish and desire to do so. (See my book on the *Diseases of Women.*)

A proper attention to bathing and diet will usually overcome any undue excitability in these parts ; and mothers especially ought to know when this attention is required, both for their own peace and for the welfare of their children. Sometimes these parts are preternaturally sensitive before puberty, even at a very early age, leading to vicious habits and improper conduct, for which the young person is only blamed and reprimanded, while a want of proper information prevents a removal of the cause.

When the Clitoris is too large, it can readily be amputated, more or less, as may be required, and its excitability reduced. This operation I have frequently performed with entire success, at various ages. On the other hand, when it is too small, and not sufficiently sensitive, means may be taken to make it enlarge, and to increase its excitability. This is often required to be done in cases of barrenness, and when the temperament is too cold.

The Clitoris is present in most Mammiferous Animals, even in the whale, and in the imperfect kangaroo. In the rat, the rabbit, the ape, and most Carnivorous Animals, it is especially developed, and frequently contains a small bone, like the Penis, as we see in the bear, and the otter. In one peculiar class of monkeys, called the *Spider Monkey*, the Clitoris is very much like a Penis, being three or four inches long, provided with a perfect Glans and Prepuce, and also with a Urethra, like a groove, down which the urine flows from the bladder. In the kangaroo and oppossum, the Clitoris is split, like the Glans in the male, and in the *Lemming* and some few others, it even has an interior passage, or Urethra, which makes it almost identical with the Penis.

The Preputial Glands are often much developed in the lower animals, which is the reason they emit such a powerful odor, and sometimes even Cowper's Glands are found, as they have also been in the human female, though they were formerly thought to belong only to the Male Organs.

There are never any *Nymphæ*, or inner lips, in the lower animals, nor *Mons Veneris*, not even in the monkey, and the external lips are also small and thin, and without a *Tressoria*, while the mouth of the Vagina is *round*, instead of *oval*, as in the human being. In the *Mare*, and some few others, there is a small Tube on each side of the Vagina, called the Vaginal Canal, leading to the broad ligaments of the Womb, the use of which is unknown.

These parts, namely, the *Mons Veneris*, the two *External Lips*, and the two inner lips, or *Nymphæ*, constitute the external genitals in all females, but their form and situation occasionally varies in different individuals and races, as already shown.

The opening between the lips, or the external mouth, is called the *Vulva* or *Fossa* Magna, and it is also liable to vary much in different persons. As a general rule, the Vulva or external opening, is

higher up, or more in front, in white females, than
it is in the colored races, and the Vagina is shorter
and smaller, while the external lips are more rounded and firmer. There is also a less abundant *Tressoria* ir the white female, and the Clitoris is not so
large on the average. These differences I have
taken great trouble myself to ascertain, especially
during a recent visit to the South, and I consider
them of considerable importance. The form of the
external lips alters considerably after pregnancy,
and even to some extent after association only.
The color of the interior surface also changes, from
the same causes, being a perfect *pink* in virgins,
but becoming slightly tinged with *violet*, or brown,
immediately after marriage. The lips also become
less firm then, and hang lower, and separate further. These alterations are often quite sufficient,
with a practised person, to decide whether association has been practised or not. It is, perhaps, necessary to remark, however, that other practices,
besides actual coition, may cause similar changes.

On separating the external lips, and the Nymphæ, there will be seen, at the lower part of the
opening, by the *fourchette*, the entrance to the *Vagina*, which is nearly oval, and in virgins is usually more or less completely closed by a membrane, or skin, which grows over it. This is called
the Hymen, and it is popularly, but erroneously
upposed to be always present during maidenhood.
The space below, between the lowest point of the
Vulva, or the fourchette, and the Anus, is called
the *Perineum*, and the space between the upper
part of the mouth of the Vagina and the Clitoris, is
called the *Vestibulum*, in the middle of which is
situated the *Meatus Urinarius* or mouth of the pas

sage by which the urine flows from the bladder. This passage from the bladder, scientifically called the *Urethra*, is supposed by many uninformed persons, to be the same as the Vagina, or passage from the Womb, but it will be seen that they are perfectly distinct, although, in some cases of doubtful sex, the Urethra has been found so large as to be mistaken for the Vagina, and, after violent deliveries, they are often torn into one.

The *Hymen* has probably given rise to more misapprehension than any other of the external parts, and there are more popular fallacies and prejudices connected with it. In most young virgins the external opening of the vagina is always more or less closed by a membrane of this kind, which has to be broken in the first sexual congress, but in many it never exists at all, not even in childhood. The idea that a young female is certainly not a virgin if the hymen be absent, is, therefore, erroneous, though it usually does exist. Besides being naturally absent, it is also liable to be destroyed in many ways. Thus in some it is broken by the first rush of the menses, and in others it may be ruptured by various violent accidents, such as falls or extreme separation of the limbs. I have even known it to be ruptured and flooding brought on by the action of powerful cathartic medicines, which, it is well known, will even cause miscarriage during pregnancy. A long continuance of certain debilitating diseases will also relax the parts so much that no resistance whatever is made by the hymen, even if it remain, which is the reason why those who marry late have seldom any trace of it, because if they escape all the various accidents referred to, they seldom escape sickness and debility. It should be borne in mind that the membrane is often *very thin*, and that it may be broken while using the bath or the napkin, as I believe is often the case with children in the hands of their nurses, and with young persons during their periods, especially if they use those articles too large or too firmly bound against the person. Sometimes, also, the hymen is destroyed by young persons themselves in various thoughtless or improper practices, and sometimes it is destroyed during various necessary operations and examinations by the medical man. The old Jewish custom, therefore, as stated in the Bible, of examining the *bridal sheets* for the blood stains, as proofs of virginity, was absurd and unjust. When the hymen is perfect, it is true, there is usually more or less blood lost when it is first broken, but not always even then, as I have witnessed during examinations, and sometimes blood will flow from the vagina at such times when there is a physicial disproportion between the parties, though the hymen may not exist. In some females these parts are naturally small, and disposed to contract when left to themselves, so that even widows, in a second marriage, will exhibit all the usual indications of virginity. There are even means of creating this condition of the parts *artificially*, and the deception has been so complete in some of these cases, that it has been thought the female had never had association when she, in reality, had even been a mother! In short, though there is usually more or less pain and difficulty attending the first act of coition, yet there are many exceptions, and from various causes · and it is seldom that much of either is experienced if the first act is delayed till after the twentieth year.

In nearly every case the hymen has an opening

through it at the lower part, by which the menses escape, but occasionally it is without such an opening, or *imperforate*, and the menses being, of necessity, retained, the health suffers very much. In such cases, constant suffering, insanity, or even death, is not an unfrequent result if relief is not speedily obtained. All that is required in such obstructions is to *puncture* the hymen, an operation neither difficult nor dangerous in proper hands, as will be seen from the cases recorded in my *Diseases of Woman*. It is more to our present purpose to remark, that the hymen is occasionally not only imperforate, but also *unusually* strong, so that it is difficult or even impossible for the husband to break it. I have had such cases come under my notice in which the marriage could not be consummated, and neither knowing the real cause of the difficulty, their distress was extreme. The treatment of this peculiar trouble is obvious; the surgeon's knife must first open the callous hymen, and then, if further treatment is needed, the opening must be dilated with appropriate instruments. I have known this membrane to be as hard as if it were ossified, or bony, and so unyielding that it had to be removed almost totally before association could be practised. After the destruction of the hymen, its fragments often remain round the external mouth in the form of little protuberances like pimples, which are sometimes highly sensitive; they are called the *carunculæ myrtiformæ*

PLATE II.

External Female Organs, Showing one half.

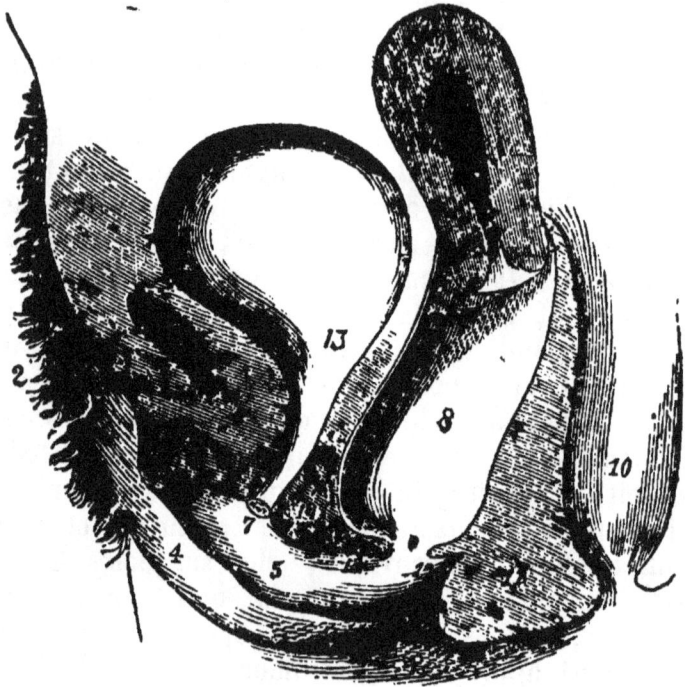

1 The Mons Veneris.—2. The Tressoria.—3. The Pubic Bone.—4 The large lip.—5. The smaller lip.—6. The Clitoris.—7. The Meatus Urinarius.—8. The Vagina.—9. The Womb.—10. The Rectum.—11. The Perineum.—12. The Hymen, through which is seen the small opening at *e.*—13. The Bladder.

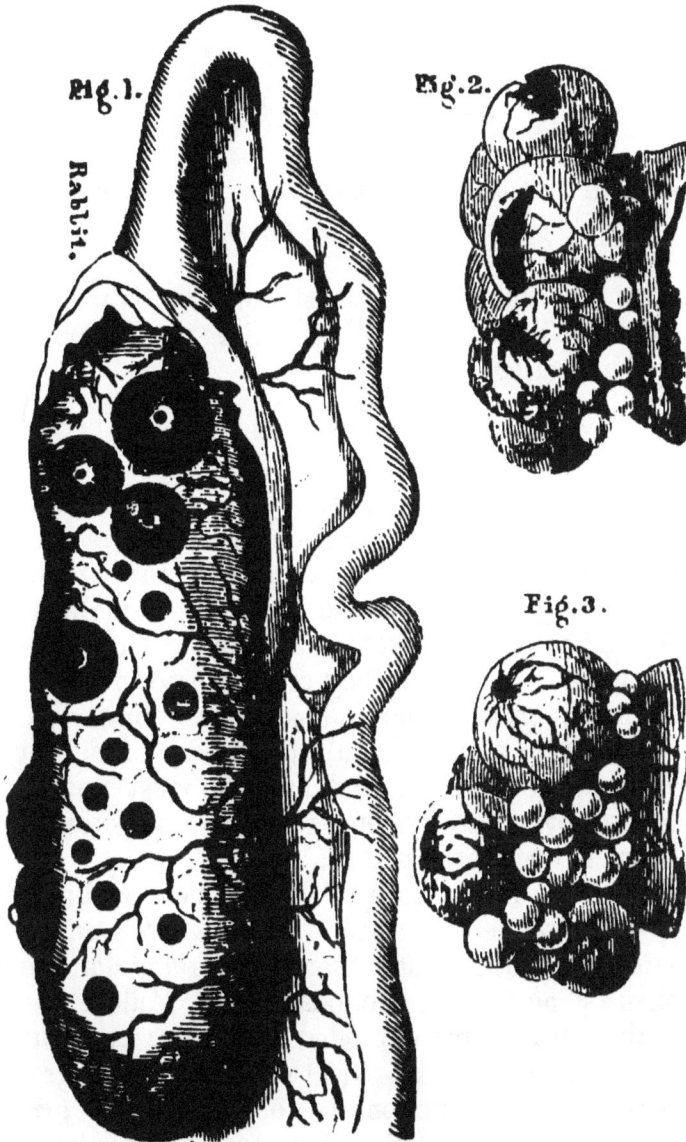

Fig. 1.

Rabbit.

Fig. 2.

Fig. 3.

In Figs. 1 and 2, the Grafian Vesicles are mostly burst open, the egg having escaped. In Fig. 3, the vesicles are just pointing and preparing to break.

CHAPTER III.

DESCRIPTION OF THE INTERNAL GENERATIVE ORGANS OF THE HUMAN FEMALE.

THE internal Organs consist of the Ovaries, the Fallopian Tubes, the Womb and its Ligaments, and the Vagina.

§ THE OVARIES.

These are two bodies placed one on each side of the Pelvis, immediately within the lower edge of the hip-bone, and just underneath the external walls. They are about the size of the male Testicle, and in shape, resemble an almond nut. Their color is pale red, and they are covered over with little protuberances and indentations. In early life they are quite small, but, about the age of puberty, they begin to enlarge, and exert a most powerful influence over the system generally, as shown in the article on Menstruation.

Before the real nature of the Ovaries was known, they were frequently called the *Female Testes*, from a mistaken notion that they were glandular, and formed something analogous to the Male Semen. But this idea is now exploded, and their true functions are known. The part they play in the grand process of Reproduction, is to produce the *germs* called, scientifically, the *Ova*, or, commonly, the *Eggs*, as explained in the article on Reproduction in general, and from which all living beings ori ginate, the human being equally with others. This is why they are called Ovaries, or *egg vessels*.

On cutting open one of these Organs, it is found to contain about twenty or thirty little vesicles, or cells, about the size of a small pea, called the *Graafian Vesicles*. These are filled with a whitish fluid, in the midst of which is seen an *egg*, or ovum, about the size of the point of a pin, or barely discernible with the naked eye. Usually there are from twenty to thirty of these vesicles, containing eggs visible at once ; but there are many others, that are rudimentary, and which are only seen as they develop. The actual number it is, of course, impossible to know, but, in all probability, there are many more than are usually suspected, and there is good reason for supposing that none are formed in adult life, but that the germs of *all* are contained in the Ovaries from the very first formation of those organs. Neither the Vesicles nor the included eggs are equally matured when we see them, but some are more perfect than the others, and *one* usually much more so than all the rest. In fact, they ripen or develop in succession one after another, commencing at the age of puberty, and continuing to do so till the *turn of life*, when all have been developed. As soon as each one is fully ripened, it is expelled from the Ovary, and lodged in the *Womb*, where it remains a short time, and if impregnation is not effected, it is thrown out of the body and lost, but if impregnation ensues, it remains, and develops into the new being.

This development of the egg, therefore, takes place independently of sexual excitement or connection, and occurs in all females alike, after the age of puberty, both married and virgin. But the egg it must be remembered, is imperfect by itself or not capable of further development alone. It is only *one* of the *two* generative principles, the other, the male *Semen*, being necessary to vivify it, before the development of the new being can commence. The female, therefore, forms the egg, independent of the Male, as he does the Semen, independent of the female, but *both united together*, are needed to form the new being.

This periodical development of the egg is precisely the same as is seen in all other beings, in some form or other. Thus female birds will commence to lay their eggs, and continue to do so, without ever having had any communication with the male whatever, but the eggs so produced, not being impregnated by the male principle, are infecund, and cannot be hatched. It is the same with all the Mammalia likewise, although there are great differences, as to the frequency of the development, and in some of the minor phenomena attending it. Thus, for instance, in the Lion and Elephant, only one egg is ripened in two or three years, while in most horned cattle, one or more are ripened every year, and in the Rabbit, quite a large number are ripened several times a year Each animal, therefore, has its appropriate period, and it is, of course, only at that particular time that it can conceive, because there can be no impregnation only when the egg is fully developed, and passed into the Womb. If no connection occurs with the other sex at that time, or, in other words, not till after the ripened egg has left the body, there can be no conception till another period returns again. Nature, however, has so arranged, in the lower animals that connection is desired *only at that time*, and then very strongly. In them, the maturation of the egg, and its passage into the Womb, is always attended with great irritation and inflammation of the whole generative apparatus, which causes the peculiar excitement we term *sexual* or *amorous*, and makes them desire association with the other sex. This is what is called the *Rut*, or *Heat*, or, scientifically, the *Œstrum*, and, it is well known, that the males and females of the lower animals have no inclination whatever for each other, except at those times, and if connection were to occur between them at any other period, no conception could ensue, because there would be no egg ripened and ready to receive the Semen. In the human being we see precisely the same phenomena, with slight variation. Thus the development of the egg in the human female is *monthly*, one coming to perfection, as a general rule, every twenty-eight days, and continuing to do so regularly, from puberty till the turn of life. This is why conception is not confined, in our species, to any particular part of the year, as it is in many others, but can occur much more frequently. Even in the human female, however, the same as in every other, there is a time— a certain part of each month—when she *cannot* conceive, and that is after one ripened egg has left the Womb, and before the other has reached it. This will, however, be more fully explained in the article on *Conception*.

The monthly ripening of the egg in the human female is attended with similar phenomena to the annual ripening in others, only slightly different in their manifestation. Thus, in the lower animals at the time of *heat*, we have inflammation, and strong sexual excitement, with a discharge from the parts,

A a thin, almost colorless fluid, of a peculiar odor
In the human female also, at the time of the monthly
ripening, they have considerable inflammation, with
a copious discharge of blood and mucus, termed the
Menstrual or *monthly flow*, more fully explained in
another article. The sexual desire, however, is
not generally confined to that particular time, in
our species, though it is frequently much the
strongest then, and is always most readily induced.

The manner in which the egg is expelled is very
curious, and when understood, it explains many of
the attendant phenomena. If we examine the
Ovary, at about three weeks previous to one of the
monthly periods, none of the Graafian Vesicles, or
their contained Ova, appear very different from the
others, but, in about a week later, one of them is
seen to be somewhat enlarged, and is more prominent upon the surface. This enlargement continues
to be more manifest as the period is approached,
till it assumes the form of a pustule, or pimple,
with a prominent point in the centre, indicating
that it is ready to burst; and, eventually, it does
burst, and the little egg escapes through the torn
opening. This is called *ovulation*, or the laying of
the egg, and is analogous to the expulsion of the
egg from the body in the bird, but in the human
being, it is then passed into the Womb, to remain
there for a time.

The manner in which the egg is transmitted to
the Womb, is very curious, and can be understood
fully only by referring to a view of the parts.
Each of the two Ovaries are connected with the
Womb by a short, firm cord, or ligament, down
which there is a passage. Immediately above each
Ovary is an Organ, called " *The Fallopian Tube,*"

which is much longer than the ovarian ligament, and is in shape like a Trumpet, the large end, which is loose, being close by the Ovaries, while the other end is connected with the Womb. The open end of this Tube, by the Ovary, is as large as a half dime, and is divided into a number of little finger-like prolongations, called its Frimbriæ. From this wide opening a small passage extends, down the interior of the Tube, into the Womb, between which and the Ovary, a communication is thus established.

At the time when the egg is expelled from the Vesicle, in the manner already explained, the open end of the Tube is directed over that part of the Ovary where it lies, and the finger-like ends, or frimbriæ, cling round the egg, and pick it up. By these means, it is taken into the commencement of the Tube, which then contracts behind it, and thus, by continued successive contractions, it is passed owards, till it reaches the Womb.

The egg usually escapes from the Ovary just about the time when the flow ceases, though, occasionally, not till two or three days after, and it is then from two to six days in passing down the Tube. It never, therefore, reaches the Womb till the flow is fully over, and most frequently it does so about the *second* day after, but sometimes not till the fourth or fifth day. When it reaches the Womb, it is prevented from passing immediately out, by a peculiar thin membrane, or skin, called the *Decidua*, which is formed during the latter part of the flow, and which lines the whole interior cavity. As the egg passes out of the *Uterine* end of the Tube, it pushes on this thin membrane, and makes a kind of nest. or depression, in which it lies.

While this membrane remains, therefore, the egg is necessarily retained in the Womb, and can be impregnated ; but in a certain period, varying in different persons, the membrane looses, and passes out of the body, taking the egg along with it, after which, of course, there can be no conception, till another period comes round, because there is no ripe egg in the Womb to be impregnated. From which, it follows, as before remarked, that *there is only a part in each month in which Conception is possible*, and that will be stated farther on, in the article on Conception. If impregnation occurs, the egg, instead of being expelled, attaches itself to the walls of the Womb, and remains, to develop into the new being, while the decidua forms one of the Fœtal Membranes, or envelopes.

In every female, therefore, married or virgin, an egg is formed and thrown off every month, unless conception takes place, and then a new being is produced. During Pregnancy and Nursing, however, the ripening of the ova is usually suspended, for reasons given in the article on Menstruation ; and at the change of life, it ceases entirely, because all have been developed.

As a general rule, only one Vesicle is broken each month, but, occasionally, there are two, or more, in which case, if all these ova are impregnated, there may be twins, or triplets, as the case may be Probably, also, the Ovaries act alternately, generally, one one month, and the other the next ; but this is not always the case, for one will sometimes lie dormant for a length of time, or even be destroyed altogether, and yet the other will act perfectly regularly alone. Each Vesicle usually contains but one Ovum though sometimes two are seen within, and even more. Twins, therefore, or other numbers may result either from several Vesicles bursting, with an Ovum in each, or from one Vesicle containing several Ova. Probably, in those remarkable instances where we have four or five at a birth, both these unusual occurrences take place. In the lower animals, as many Vesicles burst as they have young, unless some of the Vesicles contain more than one Ovum, which is sometimes the case, and then the number of the young is greater.

The Ovaries are among the very first Organs formed, the rudiments of them being found in the bodies of little girls two or three years old, and distinct traces are to be seen even before birth. They are also plainly distinguishable in the minutest beings—in the Infusoria, for instance, though they require to be magnified thousands of times before they become visible. In fact, in many of the smaller animals, the Ovary is larger than all the rest of the body, at particular times. The body of the Queen Bee, for instance, is much enlarged when filled with ripe eggs, and in some female Ants, the Ovary attains such an enormous size, that the head and trunk are almost lost sight of. The number of eggs found in the Ovaries of some beings, is almost incredible. Thus, in a femal Sturgeon, there has been counted *Ten Millions*, and all probability, many species form even more tha this number. In most insects the depositing, of the egg is the last act they perform; it is not done till they attain the perfect stage, and then, when the reproduction of their young is provided for, they die. In the more perfect beings, however the Ovulation is repeated many times.

The immediate cause of the expulsion of the egg from the Ovary is very curious, and shows that there is a peculiar vital action in these parts, which accumulates its force at periodic intervals. On examining the Graafian Vesicles, they are found to be surrounded by several distinct membranes, or layers, *between* the two inner ones of which the egg is placed, at the bottom of the Vesicle ; the innermost of all the membranes containing the whitish fluid, formerly mentioned. The outer membrane of the two inner ones is traversed by a number of minute blood-vessels, which ordinarily are barely seen, but, about three weeks before each period, some of them are seen to be much enlarged, and engorged with blood. This engorgement continues to increase, till, eventually, some of the blood-vessels break, and the blood is thus exuded between the two membranes, and, of course, *under the egg*, which is lifted up by it, and as the effusion of blood continues, and the quantity increases, it is eventually forced up to the *top* of the Vesicle, against which it presses. The white fluid is, in the meantime, all absorbed, and its place occupied by the effused blood, which, by its constant increase, causes the enlargement of the Vesicle, and its ultimate rupture, when the egg escapes. This secretion of blood in the interior of the Graafian Vesicle is precisely analogous to the secretion of the Menstrual fluid in the Womb, which it always preceedes, and probably originates.

On examining the Ovary just when the egg is expelled, which is usually about the cessation of the flow, there will be found, somewhere on the surface of it, a small space, much inflamed, in the centre of which will be seen a minute rent, or torn place. This is the spot where the Vesicle has broken open, and the egg escaped. Sometimes, when the dissection occurs at the proper moment, the egg may be seen between the lips of the rent, or may be found on the surface of the Ovary; it is then just large enough to be visible, and appears like a minute globe of bluish-colored starch. The Vesicle itself, about the size of a small pea, may be readily opened, by enlarging the rent, and will be found filled with dark-colored blood, with the walls sometimes shrunken together. Occasionally, a portion of the blood, in the form of a dark clot, passes out with the egg, and both may be found together. This may be as readily seen in any of the lower animals as in the human being, about the commencement of the *Rut* or *Heat;* especially in Rabbits, or Pigs, and, better still, in larger animals.

After the expulsion of the egg, the empty Vesicle gradually shrinks up, by the contraction of its walls, and eventually appears like a mere scar, of a yellowish-brown color. This scar is called the *Corpus Luteum*, or yellow body, and it was formerly thought to result only from Conception. Until recently, every anatomist regarded the presence of a Corpus Luteum on the Ovary as a proof of previous Conception. It was known that they were produced by the expulsion of an egg, but it was thought—as it is now, by many persons—that the egg was expelled *only* when it was impregnated and that, consequently the Corpus Luteum was a proof of Conception. It is now known, however, that the eggs are formed just the same when there is no conception, as when there is, and that consequently the Corpus Luteum is only an indication of ordinary ovulation, and is not necessarily

PLATE III.

The Human Female Ovaries.

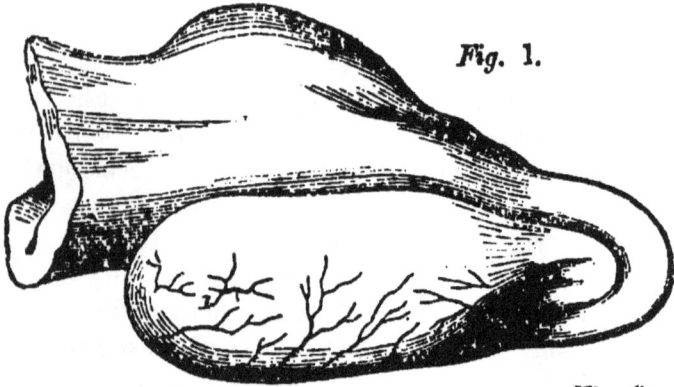

Fig. 1.

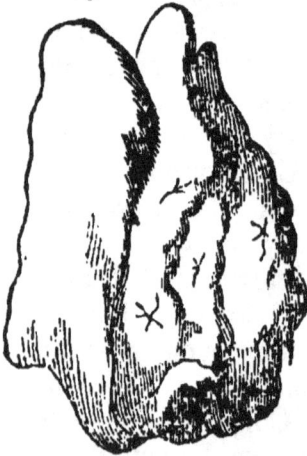

Fig. 2.

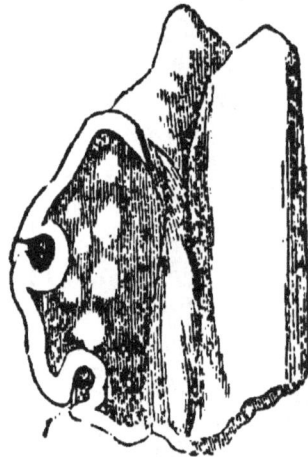

Fig. 3.

The dark scar marked 1, on *Fig.* 1 , is a Corpyus Luteum, or place where the egg has been expelled.   The Cavities marked 1, 1, in *Fig.* 3. are Granfian vesicles, from which eggs have been expelled. *Fig.* 2, is marked all over with scars, or Corpora Lutea.

connected with impregnation. This mistake, how
ever, was universal, and has had its influence in
Medical Jurisprudence. On examining the bodies
of females, for instance, in connection with certain
criminal trials, if any of these Scars were found
on the Ovaries, it was at once decided that Concep
tion must have taken place, sometime or other, and
such testimony might have a most important bearing
on the case. Suppose there should be a charge of
seduction, it might be important to the defendant, to
prove that the female had not been virtuous, and if
medical men testified, from these signs, that she
had formerly conceived, that object would be accomplished. In fact, many such cases are on record, and, no doubt, many young women have thus
had their characters unjustly aspersed, after death,
and many guilty persons have escaped punishment
in consequence of this error. This fact may be
important for *Lawyers* to bear in mind, as well as
Medical Men, more especially as they will find no
reference to it in the works on Medical Jurisprudence in ordinary use. Haller, the celebrated anatomist, used to dissect animals extensively, and, on
asking the dealers to bring him *Heifers*, frequently
accused them of deceiving him, because he sometimes found Corpora Lutea upon their Ovaries. No
matter how strongly the men affirmed that the animal had never known the male, so firmly was he
convinced of the truth of his notion, that all they
could say was disbelieved. In 1808, a Miss An-
gus died in Liverpool, under circumstances that
excited suspicions against her master, and an examination of her body being deemed requisite, the
Ovaries were seen by many of the most celebrated
anatomists in England, the greater part of whom

decided that she had been a mother, because a perfect Corpus Luteum was found. Some anatomists even now, who are not practically acquainted with these subjects, conceive that, though a Scar may be found at each month, yet. that the one formed at Conception, is larger and somewhat different ; but this is altogether erroneous, there being no difference whatever in them, let them be formed when they may.

From what has been stated, it follows that a Corpus Luteum is formed every month, and it might be supposed, therefore, that there would always be just as many as the individual had had Menstruations. This, however, is not the case, because they gradually fade away and disappear, so that only three or four are seen at most, and frequently only one. I have seen traces of a larger number under the microscope, however, and, possibly, in some persons, they endure longer than in others. As the turn of life is approached, they become more lasting, probably from the weakened power of the Ovaries to absorb them ; and, after the change has fully taken place, the whole surface of the Organ is often covered by them, and in many old persons, the Ovary is one mass of wrinkles, and shrunken very much in size ; in fact, it sometimes almost totally disappears. The old physiologists, who thought that a Corpus Luteum was formed only when a conception occurred, used to say, that by counting the number of these scars, they could tell how many children a female had borne. The fallacy of this, however, will be apparent, after the above explanation, and, indeed, many of the physiologists had begun to suspect it was not correct themselves, from the fact, that sometimes four or five Corpora Lutea would be found in the Ovaries of a young person o. *fifteen* or *sixteen*.

In most instances the Ova go on developing regularly, those on the surface coming forward first, and those in the centre working their way out wards, to succeed them till all have been ripened, and then the Ovaries shrink up and waste away But, sometimes, one or more of the Vesicles and Ova will either be buried so deeply, or be so very rudimentary, that they do not attain nearly their full development at the turn of life, and are, consequently, left in the Ovary in an imperfect state In such cases, if the Organ remains healthy, these delayed Ova may develop many years after, and may even be impregnated. This accounts for those curious instances of old females sometimes Menstruating a second time, at sixty or seventy years of age, and also of some of them bearing children when very old, as I knew one at *sixty-two*. In such cases, there have simply been one or more of the eggs left imperfect, at the turn of life, and afterwards developed.

In some persons the Ovaries are organically weak, and in others they are diseased, so that they either cannot develop the eggs at all, or else they do so imperfectly. Such persons are always irregular in their Menstrual periods, and disposed to flooding, from the debilitated state of the Organs, If the Ova are not formed at all, they are also barren, of course, and even if they are merely imperfect, Conception is not likely to occur, because the germ is deficient in vitality It has been conjectured farther, that deformity in the child may also arise from imperfect ova, there being merely vital force enough to allow of impregnation taking place, be not sufficient to insure a perfect development afterwards. I once had a patient who had borne five children, all deformed or imperfect, as I surmised, from diseased and weakened Ovaries, who had two others subsequently, quite perfect after proper means had been used to stimulate and strengthen those Organs, and to regulate their action. Those who have ever observed what imperfect *plants* are usually produced from diseased and imperfect *seed*, will readily understand the philosophy of this, and will see the necessity of a healthy condition of the Ovaries, to ensure both Conception and perfect offspring.

It must not be supposed, however, that the state of the Ova alone influences the quality of the offspring, or affects the liability to Conception, it being equally important that the *male* Organs, and the male *principle*, too, should be perfect, as will be shown farther on. The ripening of the egg in the Ovary is, in many respects, analogous to the ripening of a fruit upon a tree. It remains in the Vesicle till it has attained a certain size, and exhausted all the nutriment provided, and then leaves it, or is cast off, like a foreign body. This is the reason why eggs cannot be impregnated if they are taken from the Ovary, because they are not perfect till they leave it spontaneously, but when found in the Uterus and Fallopian Tubes, they may be impregnated.

Although, as before explained, neither the female egg nor the male Semen can develop into a new human being alone, yet, under certain peculiar circumstances, the egg will occasionally develop into a partial and imperfect likeness of a child itself, without any impregnation. What the conditions are upon which this unusual power depends, **are** unknown, but such occurrences have, undoubtedly, been observed. Possibly, the power of the Ovary may be much exalted during a state of *inflammation*, as the power of other organs frequently is. Thus, for instance, in many cases of inflamed **eyes** the power of vision is so preternaturally increased that the patient can see in the *dark*, or, rather, in what is darkness to healthy eyes. In what is commonly termed darkness, there are always *some few* **rays** of light, and the diseased eye can see with those few, though it is blinded by a full light. In the same manner, though the healthy Ovary can only develop the germ into the Ovum or egg, yet, when inflamed, it may be capable of partially developing it into an organized being. The celebrated Hufeland gives us a remarkable instance of this kind, in which there was found in a girl of thirteen years, the rudiments of an imperfect fœtus very distinct, contained in a sac in one of the Ovaries, which was diseased. Some few such cases I have also noticed myself, and it was not at all unusual, under such circumstances, to find detached bones, hair, teeth, and single limbs, as if the Ovary had not power enough to organize them together, though it could originate them individually. These occur in undoubted virgins—even in children, and the fact is both interesting and important. There are many circumstances under which such diseased growths might be found, that would seriously affect the individual's reputation, and originate most unjust suspicions.

This shows one use of *sexual excitement*. It is true, that this peculiar sensation is not *necessary* neither to the formation of the Ova, nor to Conception, but it is also equally true, that it may often conduce to both. There is no question but what Amative enjoyment stimulates the Ovaries very much, and in many cold and torpid systems, nothing else succeed so well in doing so, which is the reason why marriage is often recommended for young females who are irregular or deficient. On the other hand, there are others whose ardor it is necessary to moderate, because their over-indulgence excites the Ovaries too much, and they form the Ova too often. I have often found that producing the sexual feeling in females who had their periods too seldom, and who were cold in their temperaments, led immediately to a more frequent and regular Menstruation, although *medical* treatment had utterly failed in doing so. In like manner, I have known Conception to result from the same change, after every other means had been resorted to in vain. Blumenbach tells us, as a singular confirmation of this principle, that he has seen some kinds of Birds practice a species of Masturbation, or excite themselves with their bills, and that immediately afterwards they always laid an egg, even though there was only a half-formed one in the body to be expelled.

The condition in which beings live has a great influence over the action of the Ovaries, so as to completely change it in many respects. Thus for instance, the Wild Turkey lays but one lot of eggs in the year, and, probably, most other species of fowls do the same in a state of nature, but when domesticated, regularly and well fed, and sheltered, they will lay many more ; sometimes even they will continue to do so almost constantly. This is owing to the influence of rich and plentiful food, with the absence of privation and exposure, which allows more nutriment, and more vital power to be expended upon the Ovaries. It is probable that all Cattle, when wild, have their *Œstrum*, or heat, at some particular season of the year, but whenever they are domesticated, it occurs in them irregularly and more frequently.

Among human beings, however, the manners and customs of society have more influence perhaps than any other causes, because the sexual instinct in them can be awakened and exalted through the medium of the imagination, and because the action of the Ovaries is so frequent as to keep the whole system more or less constantly under their influence. In the human being, *Love* is a compound feeling, embracing a variety of propensities and desires, domestic and social, besides the *animal* propensity, so that it is awakened in very many different ways, while in the Animal it is only called forth by one impulse. In the article on Menstruation, the effects of social condition are made apparent, and the early amative manifestations of young persons, in all places, when their intercourse is unrestricted, it also affords abundant proof.

Too high feeding often impairs the Generative power, by unnaturally stimulating the formation of *fat*, owing to which, the functions of the Ovaries, in common with those of many other organs, are then in a great measure suspended, because all vital power is concentrated on the one absorbing process of Nutrition. On the other hand, a meagre and poor diet is also apt to impair the vigor of the sexual organs, or if it does not do so, the other organs suffer, because there is not nutrition enough to maintain them *all* in full action. In the human

being, however, as already remarked, there are
so many other causes operating upon the sexual
system, that the physical condition is not of such
paramount importance as it is in the lower animals Thus we often see whole classes of people,
who live in the most wretched manner, and are
half starved, who, nevertheless, are remarkably
prolific, and much disposed to amative indulgence.
In all these cases, however, it will be found that
the intercourse of the sexes is entirely unrestrained, there being no considerations of prudence, no
calculation of means or consequences, but a perfect abandonment to the mere sexual impulse. Consequently, marriages occur early, and there is no
motive whatever for restraint afterwards.   In these
people, however, the Virile power does not endure
so *long* as in those who are better circumstanced,
and its exercise being one of the few indulgences
left them, they are apt to abuse it.

At the present time, we know of many means by
which the power of the Ovaries can be either increased or decreased, as may be most advisable,
and by which also the egg itself can be made more
perfect. Some of these are described in my work
on *The Diseases of Woman*, and others will be
eventually further on.

§ THE FALLOPIAN TUBES.

The Fallopian Tubes, as already explained, fo·
the only means of communication between the
Ovaries and the Womb, and it is into them that the
ripe eggs are passed when they leave the Ovary
The structure of these Organs is very peculiar
and they are of great importance to *health*, besides

PLATE IV.

The Internal Organs cut through

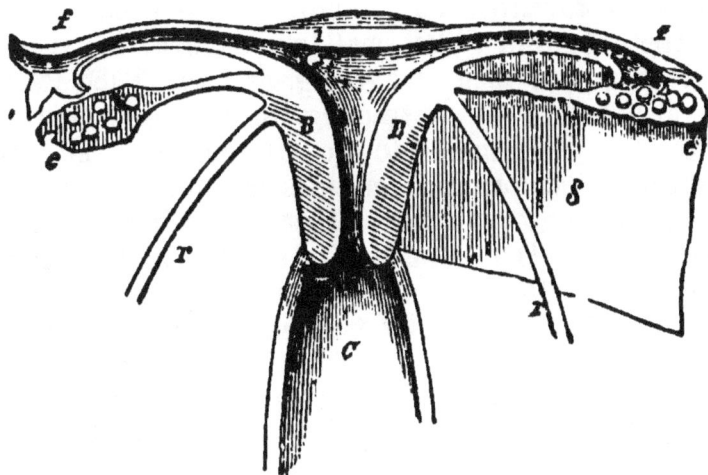

B, B. The Womb cut through.—*C.* The Vagina.—*g.* The Mouth of the Womb.—*f, f.* The Fallopian Tubes.—*e, e.* The Ovaries.—*r, r.* The Round Ligaments.—*S.* One of the Broad Ligaments. On one side, marked 2, the egg is just entering the Tube from the Ovary, and on the other at 1, it is just passed into the Womb.

being essential to generation. In dissecting them, the interior passage is found to be covered with a number of Cilia, or hair-like threads, which are directed towards the Womb. These Cilia are in perpetual motion, like small worms, drawing themselves up and then elongating, and the Tube itself is also constantly contracting, in successive waves, from the Ovarian end to the Uterine end. The result of these combined motions is, that, so long as they continue, any object, of proportionate size, can enter at the Ovarian end of the Tube, and be conveyed *down* to the Womb, but nothing can enter at the Uterine end, nor be conveyed *up* to the Ovary. The Ovarian end of the Tube is also expanded, so as to embrace or cover any object, and is provided with Fimbriæ, or fingers, to grasp, but nothing of the kind exists at the Uterine end. It is evident, therefore, that, except under peculiar and unusual circumstances, to be explained further on, nothing can pass *from the Womb to the Ovary*, but only in the opposite direction. The great use of the Tubes is, undoubtedly, to transmit the ripe eggs to the Womb, after they are ejected from the Ovary; but, besides this use, they also serve another purpose, of great consequence to female health. The continual excitement to which the Ovaries are subject, causes them to be always secreting various fluids and other substances, which, if not expelled from the body, are apt to cause many evils. Now, the only mode of escape for these secretions is down the Fallopian Tubes, which are consequently perpetually embracing the Ovaries, by their expanded terminations, to allow of this escape taking place. A large portion of those discharges therefore, occurring at ordinary times from the Vagina, are really the secretions of the Ovaries, transmitted down the Tubes into the Womb, and thence to the lower passage. If the Tubes are obstructed, or paralyzed, as is sometimes the case, this transmission cannot take place, and the Ovarian secretions are retained. When this occurs, they either cause continued irritation, by their contact with the interior surfaces, or acute inflammation, by being absorbed. And in this way often arises Inflammation of the Ovaries, Dropsy of the Ovaries, Tumors and Abscesses.

There are many causes that tend to weaken the action of the Fallopian Tubes, and which, therefore, dispose to the above diseases, and also lessen the liability to Conception. In some persons they are almost totally torpid, *from want of sexual feeling*, the production of which puts them in vivid motion almost invariably. It follows, therefore, that this peculiar excitement—which many uninformed persons affect to despise and totally condemn—is really, in many instances, a preventive of disease, and its experience becomes essential to the preservation of health. On the other hand, *excessive* amorous indulgence will so weaken the Tubes, by the incessant excitement to which it subjects them, that they will almost lose their power of contraction, and then the individual will be liable both to disease and sterility. This is, in fact, the chief reason why Prostitutes do not conceive so frequently as married females ; the continued and excessive excitement which they experience, causes a paralysis of the Tubes

In several instances, proof has been obtained that, at the moment when the egg passes from the Vesicle, the Tube *erects*, and its fimbriæ grasp round the Ovary, so as to include the Ovum within the open end. It is probable also that, at the same time, the body of the Uterus expands, while its mouth closes, owing to the excitement experienced, and thus there is a powerful *suction*, by which the egg is drawn into the first part of the opening. In some females the motion and erection of the Tubes can be distinctly *felt*, and it is occasionally so energetic, that it may be *seen* externally. It is always very readily excited, by external treatment, and is often all that is required to remove many diseases, in their incipent stages.

A perfect Paralysis of the Tubes, or closure of the passages down them, of course, necessarily causes sterility, because the egg cannot reach the Womb. This fact is sometimes of practical value in preventing breeding in female animals. Instead of *Spaying*, or removing the Ovaries, which is the common operation, a ligature is tied round each Tube, which, by closing its passage, and preventing the passage of the egg, effectually prevents any future conception also. In some females the action of the Tubes is very slow, and the egg becomes decayed and spoiled before they convey it to the Womb. The sterility arising from this cause may always be cured by quickening the action of the Tubes. In ordinary cases, the egg is conveyed down them in about two days, and it first passes into them immediately it is expelled from the Ovary which is just about the cessation of the flow. The egg, therefore, reaches the Womb, as a general rule, about the second day after Menstruation is over, and then commences the liability of Conception. It may, however, pass down in one day, or less, and may be as long as five or six days. It is probable that sexual excitement, just at the termination of the flow, hastens the passage of the egg, and thus makes conception so much earlier.

It is probable that many cases of *Hydatids*, and other living bodies, and also Polypi, are caused by eggs being retained, through the inaction of the Tubes. This retention first causes inflammation of the Ovaries, and then the inflammation causes the Ova to imperfectly develop, as already explained.

At the present time, barrenness from want of passage in the Fallopian Tubes, can be cured, an operation being performed, by which they are opened. This consists is passing a silver tube, properly made, into the Womb, till the end of it touches the opening of the Fallopian Tube, and then a very small probe is thrust out of it, and pushed along the passage, so as to open it, or remove any obstructions ; with proper instruments, and using due care, this apparently difficult operation becomes quite feasible, and its results are often as acceptible as they were unexpected. I have known barrenness, of many years' standing, cured by this practice— Conception occuring in a few weeks after.

The usual length of the Tube is about three inches, but I have seen them four, and even five inches. Sometimes they are too short, and cannot reach the Ovary, which is, of course, another cause of sterility, and an incurable one.

§ THE WOMB.

The Uterus, or Womb, called also the *Matrix*, was formerly thought to be the most essential of the Generative Organs, but is now known to be merely a receptacle, in which the ripe egg is placed for a

PLATE V.

Section of the Womb, Natural Size.

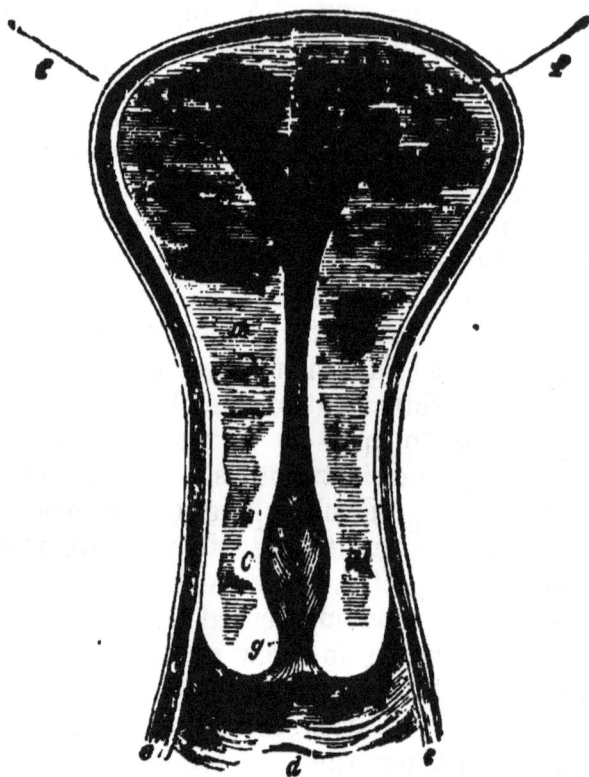

EXPLANATION.

a, a. Are its Thick Walls.—*b.* Is the Cavity in its upper part, or *body* —*c.* Is the Cavity in the lower part, or *Neck.*—*d.* Is the Vagina.— *e, e.* The edges of the Walls of the Vagina, cut through.—*f, f.* Two threads, passing through the openings of the Fallopian Tubes, and appearing in the inside.—*g.* Is the Mouth of the Womb, or Os Tincæ opening into the Vagina.

This view being of the *full size,* will give an idea of the astonishing change this organ has to undergo in the process of Gestation.

short time after its ejection from the Ovary, and in
which it develops into the new being if Conception
occurs. There is no Uterus, therefore, in those animals that do not bring forth their young alive, the egg
in them being expelled and developed externally.

The situation of this Organ in the body will be
readily understood by the explanations already
given. It is placed midway between the lower
edges of the two hip-bones. and its upper part lies
immediately upon the Bladder, which is in front of
it, while behind it is the Rectum, or lower part of
the large Intestine. The Womb does not extend
downwards but about two inches, or little more, and
immediately below, connected with it externally, is
the pipe or tube called the *Vagina*, which leads up
to the Womb, and opens externally at the Vulva,
between the Labia. When viewed externally, the
Womb and Vagina seem to form but one Organ, but
internally, the distinction between them is easily
seen.

The form of the Womb is nearly that of a Pear.
the larger end being at the top. It is not round but
flattened, being widest across the body from side to
side, and it is slightly curved, or bent, the con-
cave part being towards the back bone. The lower
part of it, called the *Neck*, hangs down into the Vagina, the walls of which are attached to the exterior of the Womb, some distance above. At each
one of the upper corners of the Womb is one of
the Fallopian Tubes, and the Ovary underneath,
the Tubes being about three or four inches in length,
and the ovarian ligament about two or three inches.
Underneath these, some little distance down the sides
of the Womb there are also attached two round
cords, one on each side, very firm and strong, which

are called the *Round Cords*, or Ligaments of the
Womb. These are about five inches long, curved
round, and by their other ends firmly attached to
the pubic or front bone. These act like stays, and
keep the Womb in the centre of the body, on the
rounded top of the bladder. Without them it would
be constantly liable to displacement, but as each of
the ligaments acts with equal force, and in an opposite direction to the other, they necessarily maintain the Organ in the centre. Besides the round
Ligaments there are also the *Broad Ligaments*,
which consist of two broad sheets of strong membrane, one on each side, which extend from the top
of the Womb, nearly the whole length down, en-
closing the round ligament, Tubes, and ovarian
ligaments in their substance. These grow fast to
the sides of the Pelvis, and assist in maintaining
the uterus, the Ovaries and Tubes, in their proper
situations. There are also two ligaments that connect the Womb with the bladder in front, called the
anterior ligaments; and two others which connect
it with the Rectum behind, called the *posterior ligaments.* All these, however, do but little towards
actually *supporting* the womb, which is really kept
in its place more by the firmness and density of its
own substance, and that of the Vagina below, and
by the tension of the muscles in the Perineum than
by any thing else. When these parts become weak
from debility or disease, the ligaments stretch, the
Perineal Muscles relax, and the walls of the Womb
and Vagina soften till all fall down together, and
then we have *Prolapsus Uteri*, or Falling of the
Womb, the causes, symptoms, and treatment of
which are fully given in my book on "The Diseases
of Woman."

The length of the Uterus is about two inches and a half, its breadth at the top about one inch and a half, and at the lower end a little less than an inch; its thickness also, through the flat way, is a little less than one inch. The walls being very thick the interior cavity is necessarily small, and it is different in form to the exterior. In the upper part the cavity is shaped like a Triangle, the Fallopian Tubes entering at the two upper angles; in the lower part it is continued downwards like a Tube which swells out considerably a little more than half way down, and at its termination opens by what is called the *Os Tincæ, Os Uteri,* or mouth of the Womb, into the Vagina. This opening, or mouth of the Womb, is like a cleft, placed cross-wise, on the prominent Neck of the Womb, and is readily felt at the top of the Vagina in manual examinations. The two lips formed by this cleft are perfectly smooth and round in those that have not borne children, but are apt to be torn and covered with scars in those who have. The anterior lip, or the one in front, is considerably thicker than the other, so that the cleft, which is about a quarter of an inch long, is not quite in the centre. In virgins the internal cavity is very small, the walls nearly touching each other, and the Mouth of the Womb, or cleft, is so narrow and its lips so firmly closed, that it can scarcely be ascertained. In young persons in fact, the neck feels precisely like the end of the nose, the Os Tincæ merely giving the impression of a slight hollow between the lips. In those that have borne children the walls of the Womb separate farther asunder, so that the cavity increases in size, and the Os, or Mouth, also enlarges and remains more or less open, so that the cleft is plainly felt. In speaking of the whole Organ it is usually divided into three parts, namely, that above the Failopion Tubes, called the *Fundus*, that between the fundus and the Neck, called the *Body*, and that which projects into the Vagina, which is called the *Neck*.—The Neck projects into the lower passage somewhat less than a quarter of an inch, and is plainly felt at the upper part, like a small firm tumor, across which is the cleft or Os Tincæ.

. In Virgins, the Womb is more straight than in those who have borne children, and it is also higher up in the body, and the neck is considerably thicker In some persons, however, the Womb is naturally much lower than it is in others, and also smaller, and all are not so much altered by child bearing even when they have had several.

. The substance of the Uterus appears to be muscular, and it is capable, in its contractions, of exerting most tremendous force. The increase in size which it undergoes, at the different periods of gestation, are most extraordinary, and its after contraction to its original dimensions are still more so. Thus at the full period of nine months it will measure over a foot in diameter, each way, in some cases, and yet in a few days after delivery will return to its original dimensions. In my work " *The Matron's Manual of Midwifery,*" all these changes are fully represented by Plates, and intructions are given by which the period of pregnancy may be ascertained by them.

Arteries, Veins and Nerves are plentifully supplied to the Womb, so that it is abundantly nutrified, and highly sensitive. Indeed there is no other Organ in the body, except the Ovaries, that has such extensive sympatnies, or that is capable of such rapid growth. The Womb, however, is altogether dependent upon the Ovaries both for its development and its functional ability. If there be no Ovaries the Womb will be found merely rudimentary, and if the Ovarian actions cease, those of the Womb cease also. The Neck of the Womb, which hangs down into the Vagina, is usually the most sensitive part of it, and is, in many persons, the principal seat of sexual feeling, even more so than the Clitoris. In fact, I believe that sexual excitement is never known in its full intensity excepting when it is experienced in the Neck of the Womb, it being always weak and partial when confined only to the Clitoris and Nymphæ. It is to this part therefore that our treatment must frequently be directed, when that peculiar condition becomes desirable.

When the Erotic excitment is intense in the female during connection, the Womb experiences a species of erection and vibration, by which it becomes engorged with blood and is drawn with considerable force and rapidity up and down the Vagina. This brings the neck into contact with the Glans of the Male Organ, which is also the most sensitive part, and their mutual pressure hastens the Orgasm in both. The fact has never been mentioned by any previous writer on Physiology, and it is one of considerable medical and moral importance. The idea which some persons entertain that the Male Organ enters the Womb is both erroneous and absurd, as a consideration of its structure will show ; neither is it true, as others think, that *always* when conception ensues the Semen is thrown *into* the Womb. It is true, that during a perfect Orgasm, much as referred to above, the *Os Tincæ* opens when the Womb descends to meet the Male Organ, and if the Semen is admitted at that time also it will pass directly into the mouth. This is the reason why conception is *more likely* when the Orgasm is mutual and simultaneous, but still it is not absolutely necessary in either.

Sometimes the Womb is very small and imperfect, so that the egg is not retained, and barrenness of course results, and occasionally it is *absent altogether*. A remarkable case of this kind is given in my Diseases of Woman, in which a young person who had never Menstruated, was married, and it was afterwards discovered that she had *no Womb*, though in every other respect quite perfect. This smallness and imperfection of the Womb is very likely to be found in those who are late in Menstruating, or who have been irregular.

In many Quadrupeds the Womb is forked, or like two horns, and it has been found *double* in the human being, in some very rare cases.

The form of the Uterus varies much in different beings, so much, in fact, that it scarcely appears to be the same Organ. It is sometimes round, oval, and even triangular, and not unfrequently divides into two horns, as in the Cow, Pig, Horse, and hale, in which we also find the Fallopian Tubes very long and contorted. In most of the Carnicereus Animals, and in the Rodentia, as the Rat and Squirrel, the Uterus is very short, and divides at the lower end into two parts, communicating with two short and·straight tubes. In the greater part of the Rodentia, in fact, as in the Hare and Mouse, the Womb is really double, there being a separate one in connection with each Fallopian Tube, and consequently two mouths, both of which can be distinctly seen in the Vagina. In the Marsupial Animals, as the Opossum and Kangaroo, there is no Uterus, properly speaking, but the end of each Fallopian Tube, when it opens into the Vagina, is expanded, and made to answer the purpose of one. In these imperfect wombs, the young are retained but a short time, and are then expelled, and placed in the pouch outside, as before explained, in which they are gradually perfected. The Vagina, also, is double in these animals, one communicating with each Tube. Occasionally the Vagina is partly closed, previous to connection, by a species of Hymen, as in the Mare, the Cow, and Ape, but it is never so perfect as in the human female.

In very rare cases, the Womb has been found double in the human being, each Organ being distinct and separate from each other, and opening by a separate mouth into the Vagina. In such cases, one Womb is connected with the right Ovary only, and the other with the left, so that Conception can occur in one and not in the other at the same time, though it may do so afterwards, and cause a superfœtation, or Conception in a person already pregnant. More frequently the Womb is simply divided by a partition inside, and is not properly double, though, possibly, superfœtation might take place even then.

§ THE VAGINA.

The Vagina is the passage leading from below upwards to the Womb. At its lower extremity is the *Vulva*, or external Mouth, between the lips, and at the top of it is the Neck of the Womb. The Vagina is like a pipe or tube, with very firm, thick walls, capable of dilating or contracting to a very considerable extent. The length of it is from four to six inches, though I have seen it as long as eight inches, and as short as three. The diameter varies from an inch and a half, to two inches and a half. It is not straight, but curved, the hollow part of the curve being in front, next to the bladder, while the convex part is next to the rectum, or large intestine.

The diameter of the canal of the Vagina is not uniform in its whole length, it being some little narrower in the middle than at either end. It is lined with a Mucous Membrane throughout, like the Uterus, and in virgins is not smooth, but is marked with a number of *rugæ*, or folds, which gradually disappear after connection, and especially after delivery. Under the Mucous coat is another thick one of Cellular Membrane, and under that again is another coat, called the *Corpus Spongiosum Vaginæ.* This is a true *erectile* tissue, like the Corpus Spongiosum of the Male Organ, and capable, like it, of becoming congested with blood during excitement, and of erecting and contracting. It is this power that enables the Vagina to draw down the Womb during the Orgasm, as explained in the previous article, and it also makes it *compress* the Male Organ at the same time, by thickening the walls, and contracting the passage, and thus increasing the pressure and excitement in both. The principal portion of this erectile tissue is, however, confined to the lower part of the Vagina, though it exists more or less in its whole length. And it is a knowledge of this fact that enables us to use many internal instruments advantageously, for the cure of falling of the Womb. When the instrument is once produced, the contraction of the lower part of the passage which is acted upon by the presence of the foreign body, prevents its being expelled. In some females the erectile tissue is much developed at the narrow part of the Vagina, about half-way up to the Womb, and it will contract so forcibly there, from any excitement, that a passage can scarcely be effected beyond. Those who have the erectile tissue imperfectly developed, are always liable to a lax Vagina, which leads to falling of the Womb, and also to rupture of the bladder and rectum through its walls. In all such cases, if the erectile tissue is made to act, by the excitement natural to the parts, the relaxation is much relieved, and a step is made towards permanent improvement.

At the mouth of the Vagina is a strong circular muscle, like that which closes the mouth and eyes, It is called the *Sphincter*, or *Constrictor Vaginæ*, and when it acts properly, the mouth of the Vagina is kept nearly closed by it. This Muscle is of great importance in maintaining the parts above, by drawing the lower walls of the Vagina together, and making them more firm. It also co-operates along with the Erectile Tissue, in increasing the pressure during coition. In some females it acts so powerfully as to close the passage completely, and, so strongly, that an entrance can scarcely be obtained. This is often the case in those who have an irritable Clitoris, or Nymphæ, and every act is as difficult with them as the first, though not painful. When this Constriction of the Sphincter is conjoined with great engorgement of the Erectile Tissue, the difficulty is of course still greater, but in all such cases the intensity of the *Orgasm* is also proportionably increased

The relaxation of the Sphincter Muscle, which is very common, is a serious evil, as it disposes all the parts above to displacement, and much impairs the sensibility of the parts. The lower part of the Erectile Tissue, round the base of the Nymphæ, exhibits a curious net-work of Veins, called the *Plexus Retiformis*, which during excitement are singularly enlarged. They are apt sometimes to become obstructed, and swell, causing *varicose veins*, and enlargement of the lips.

The *Hymen*, which partly closes the mouth of the Vagina in Virgins, has already been explained. The opening in it is usually crescent-shaped, and is thought to have originated the symbol of *Diana*, and Goddess of Chastity, which was a *half moon*, or crescent.

Immediately within the Vagina, on each side, are certain little openings called the *Glands of Duverney*. These secrete a thickish gray-colored fluid, of a peculiar odor, which is often discharged in great quantities during connection, and was formerly thought, by uninformed persons, to be a kind of Semen. The situation of these Glands causes them to be compressed by the Constrictor Muscle, which is the reason why they discharge most during the strongest excitement. In some persons the quantity of fluid amounts to several ounces.

In addittion to the Glands of Duverney, there are also a number of Mucous Follicles, both in the Vagina and on the inner surface of the lips, which also discharge freely under similar circumstances.

The Vagina, like the other parts, is liable to various malformations. Thus in some it is too small, and in others it is closed by the inner walls or external lips growing together. In others, again, it is

annaturally large, so that the Womb continually
falls down to the lower part of it.   Many of those
cases in which the Vagina is closed, are not discovered till marriage, and then great distress and
suffering result.   Many such instances are given in
my book on the Diseases of Woman, and also the
means of remedying the defect, which can be often
done without medical assistance.   When the canal
is too short, great distress may often ensue in marriage, unless certain precautions are observed. ·

Most of these difficulties appear much worse than
they really are, it merely requiring time and skilful
appliances to remedy the worst of them, as the cases
in my book will show.

In rare cases, the Vagina has been found *double*,
like the Womb, sometimes with two Uteri, and at
others with only one.   I once saw a case of this
kind myself, in which. connection could be effected
perfectly in either of the two passages, each having
a perfect external mouth and Sphincter Muscle of
its own, one being below the other

Expulsion of the Egg.

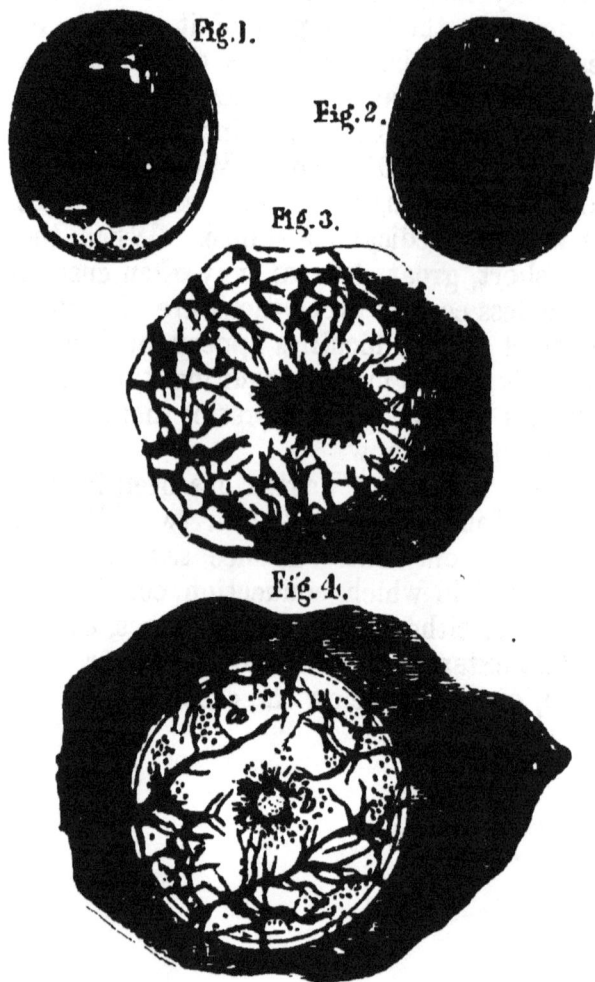

Fig. 1. The Egg, *a*, at the bottom of the Vesicle.
Fig. 2. The Egg, *a*, carried to the top by the Vesicle filling with blood.
Fig. 3. The Vesicle just breaking open, and the Egg, *a*, passing out.
Fig. 4. The Egg, *a*, as it appears when attached to the membrane, *b*, in the Germinal Vesicle.

CHAPTER IV.

THE FEMALE EGG, OR OVUM.

Having now described all the Organs of the female system, and shown how the egg is formed, we will next proceed to describe its structure and changes.

It has always been remarked that the egg of the human female does not differ, in any essential particular, from that of any other being. On examining it with the microscope, it is found to be composed principally of a mass of yellow grains, constituting what is called the *Vitellus*, which is analogous to the yolk of a bird's egg. Around this is a thin layer of *Albumen*, or white, and in the interior of the yellow grains is seen a small round, greenish-colored body, called the *Germinal Vesicle*. The different parts are also held together, and separated from each other, by various enclosures or membranes, and these several parts constitute the whole *Ovum*. At its fullest development in the human being, it is not larger than the point of a pin so that it can scarcely be seen with the naked eye, and yet from this mere atom emerges *a living human being*. In the case of the bird, the young has to develop away from the mother's body, and the germ has therefore to be surrounded by a mass of nutritive matter, to afford it the material for its development, which is the reason why the bird's egg appears proportionately so large. In the human being, on the contrary, the germ is, from the very moment of conception, attached to the mother's body, and takes its nutriment from thence, so that it does not need any surrounding material.

The Germinal Vesicle is the same thing as the white opaque spot, or *Cicatricula*, that is seen on the surface of the egg of the bird, and which is erroneously supposed to be the male principle. The Vesicle is placed first in the centre of the Vitellus, but afterwards changes its position, as will be explained further on, and in its centre may be seen a dark colored spot, called the *Germinal Dot*.

The yellow part, or *Vitellus*, is composed of little round Vesicles, or grains, which are hollow and filled with still smaller bodies, called *Granules*. The Membrane which covers each vesicle is also *granulated*, and thus we have first the round egg itself, made up of little round vesicles, and each of these made up again of still smaller bodies or granules, while the covering of each vesicle is also granulated like the interior. This is in fact, a succession of vesicles, or spheres, one set included within another, as far as we can observe.

The *Germinal Vesicle*, which is larger than the Vitelline Vesicles, among which it is placed, is also composed of granules, and is covered with a granulated membrane. The granules in the centre of it being much condensed, or crushed together, so as to be opaque, and thus form the *Germinal Dot*.

The Vitellus, or Yellow, is the material from which the new being is first formed, and it is found in the egg of the Virgin precisely the same as in that of a married person. In fact, the perfect formation of the vitellus constitutes the *ripening of the Ovum*, which escapes from the Ovary immediately it is formed. Many singular and interesting changes takes place in this substance, after the egg enters the Tube, some of which throw great light on the manner of the first commencement of the new being. On examining the Vitelline Vesicles immediately on the escape of the Ovum from the Ovary the enclosed granules are seen to be in rapid motion, round a number of different centres, and this motion continues till the primary arrangement of the Ves icles is entirely broken up. They then re-arrange themselves in a different order, and begin to form the principal Vital Organs of the new being. This however will be more fully explained further on.

Another remarkable change which takes place, soon after the egg enters the Tube, is the escape of the Germinal Vesicle. This is first placed, as before remarked, in the centre of the Yellow Vitellus, where it is readily distinguishable by its greenish color, and by the darker dot in the centre. Just at the time when the egg escapes, however, the Germinal Vesicle mounts to the upper part of the Vitellus, the Membrane surrounding which then tears open and allows it to pass out. This leaves *an open passage* into the interior of the Ovum, which it will be seen further on, is essential to impregnation. The Germinal Vesicle always escapes in this way immediately, so that we can never find it in the egg except at the moment when that is leaving the Ovary ; after that event we merely discover the rent through which it passed. This is the reason why many Microscopical observers never found the Germinal Vesicle, because they only examined an Ovum taken from the Tubes, or Uterus, and from all those it had, of course, escaped. The reader will see from this, what a singular analogy there is between this event and the Ovarian expulsion of the

Ovum. As soon as the Vitellus is fully formed the egg is expelled from the *Graafian* Vesicle, and immediately afterwards the Germinal Vesicle is expelled from the Vitellus in a similar way.

The Yellow Vesicles forming the Vitellus, are disposed so closely that they press upon one another, which makes them not round, but many sided, like the cells in a honey-comb. In the spaces between the larger Vesicles smaller are seen, so that the whole substance is very dense. This may be seen very perfectly in the yolk of a bird's egg, when boiled hard and broken across. The Vesicles, like small round grains, can be readily distinguished with an ordinary glass.

Sometimes one or more of the Vesicles will burst while we are examining them, and the contained granules will flow out. In such cases they always pass in a steady current, and it takes some ten minutes or more before the Vesicle is completely emptied.

To discover all these curious formations and changes requires, of course, numerous and careful observations, with the most perfect instruments, which is the reason why they have not been made before. They are, however, of the greatest value, and until we were acquainted with them, many of the most important generative processes could not be explained.

There is good reason to suppose that the outline of the future being, always exists in the egg even before it is impregnated, and indeed in the Ova of some beings it can be distinctly seen. Thus Haller plainly observed the form of the bird in the egg of a hen, which had never been impregnated, and the same thing has frequently been seen in the eggs

of various Amphibious animals. The bodily structure, therefore, probably exists in the egg from the
first, independent of impregnation, but the male
principle is necessary to give it life. This will explain those curious cases, formerly mentioned, in
which imperfect Fœtuses have been found in Virgins. These were simply the structures which naturally existed in the egg more than usually developed. They had grown like vegetables, but had no
life.

CHAPTER V.

MENSTRUATION.

It is wel known that in all healthy and properly developed females, after a certain age, denominated puberty, there occurs a discharge of blood and mucus from the Vagina, at certain regular periods, usually a month distant from each other, and which lasts as a general rule from two to four days. This discharge is called the *Courses,* or the Menstrual, or Monthly Discharge, and it is intimately connected both with female health and with the process of conception The real cause and nature of this singular phenomenon has always been a matter of dispute among philosophers and physiologists, and it is only in modern times that the truth has been known. Even at the present time many of the best informed people, including medical men, are not acquainted with it, and in consequence of that ignorance we have all kinds of errors and improper practices prevalent, and producing disease which medical men cannot cure, because their treatment is based on wrong principles.

Some of the most curious and important discoveries in human physiology have been made by observing the lower animals, with whom we can make experiments and observations in a more complete and methodical manner than with our own species, while the general laws which regulate their physical functions are the same with those that regulate our own. It was formerly thought that many organic actions

In the human being were totally different to any that took place in the inferior animals, but it is now known that this is an error. There is no physiological action occurring in our own systems that we cannot find the counterpart of in other beings. It is true it may vary some little in the manner of its occurrence, and in unimportant details, but still it is always essentially the same action, and serves the same purposes. Thus it was formerly thought that this very function of Menstruation was one peculiar to the human being, and that nothing analogous to it was to be observed in the lower animals, but it is now known that a corresponding phenomenon occurs in nearly all, in some form or other.

To understand how menstruation is produced we must here make a brief reference to *Ovulation*, and the functions of the *Ovaries*. It is only since a comparatively recent period that the existence of Eggs, or *Ova*, in the human female has been satisfactorily proved, but it is now known that they do exist the same in her as in all other females, and that they are uniformly developed according to a regular plan. The Ovaries contain the Ova or Eggs in a rudimentary state, and they begin, at the age of puberty, to ripen, or develop, as explained in the article on the Functions of the Ovaries. At the age of puberty the first Egg is ripened and expelled in the manner already explained, and the same process occurs at every monthly period afterwards till what is termed *the change of life*, usually about forty-five years of age, when the last Ovum has been expelled and the Ovaries cease their functions. Now this ripening and expulsion of the Egg every month is a very curious and important phenomenon, and exercises a powerful and peculiar influence over both body and mind, making the Female essentially different to the male in her physical requirements and capabilities, and also in her nervous sympathies.

It is undoubtedly true that the monthly ripening and expulsion of the egg in the female, and its development into the new being when Conception occurs, is *the great and principal business of her Organic System*, and that it absorbs more of her nervous power and more of her physical strength, than any other process she performs. In fact, all other processes, both nervous and nutritive, appear subservient to this, and chiefly intended to carry it on. There is nothing analogous to this *Ovulation* in the other sex, and, therefore, there is nothing to compare it with, and that is the reason why the peculiarities of the female constitution and character are so imperfectly appreciated. In man there is no periodical function that absorbs, as it were, all the rest, and to which they are merely auxiliaries, but each acts independently, and it is only in exceptional cases that any one preponderates over all the others. Thus we sometimes see cases in which—either from Organic peculiarity, or from weak indulgence, the stomach is so active, that *Digestion* is the all-absorbing process, and every other function is imperfectly performed in consequence of its preponderating requirements. The person can neither think nor perform muscular exercise, because he has no vital energy for anything but Digestion. In the same manner, others do little else than *think*, through the Brain being the overactive organ. Such instances may enable any one to conceive what follows when any one function overpowers, as it were, all the others, and to see how they must necessarily be subservient to it. But, it must be remembered, that such cases as these are merely exceptional and unnatural ones, and that they are not of the same character as the peculiar function referred to, though a consideration of them may enable any one to better understand its influence. The monthly Ovulation of the egg in the female is not an exceptional occurrence, nor an unnatural over-excitement, but a legitimate and necessary result of her peculiar Organic action, and the consequences of which she cannot therefore escape from. From the age of puberty till the change of life, Nature is constantly laboring at this one function, and the female seems to live chiefly for this purpose. This is the true explanation of those peculiarities that are seen in the female character, especially their excessive sympathy, sensitiveness, and excitability, and also much that is peculiar in their diseases. The incessant action of the Ovaries keeps the nervous system in a constant state of irritation, and makes all the Organic functions liable to derangement, so that it is impossible for a female to preserve that equanimity of mind, and that evenness of temper and disposition which to individuals of the other sex is a comparatively easy matter. The female is, in fact, in a great measure, like a man who is constantly subject to annoyance from those around him, and who is obliged to use constant efforts to keep himself cool. Her situation is, indeed, in some respects, even worse, because the cause of her uneasiness is inherent in herself—she cannot escape from it, and knows not what it is, and those around not knowing it either, she meets with but little sympathy and consideration. There are numbers of females who are most unfortunate in this respect, some being subject to distressing depression of spirits, or the most melancholy despondency, while others are irritable or peevish, or subject to ebullitions of the most frantic gaiety ; and others, again, constantly change from one mood to another, without any apparent reason for so doing. Ignorant persons attribute these eccentricities to mere caprice, or whim, and fancy that females can avoid them if they choose. Sometimes they are blamed or scold ed for them, and are thought to be perverse or contrary, and sometimes females even accuse themselves of being ungrateful and dissatisfied, and in this way increase their distress. If, however, the true nature of their constitution was understood, it would be seen that no blame whatever should be attached to them for these peculiarities, since they cannot be avoided, but, on the contrary, every allowance should be made for their involuntary aberrations, and the fullest sympathy exhibited for the distress which they really endure. The Ovaries and the nervous system exert a reciprocal action, so that one can influence the other to a remarkable degree, which is the reason why many female diseases can be so much modified, or even produced, by certain states of the mind and feelings. It is often the case that a female suffering from indisposition is not benefitted at all by *medical* treatment, but through some pleasing impression on the *mind* or *feelings,* is relieved immediately. I have often seen females completely prostrated, with scarcely energy or ability enough to breathe, who have been restored almost instantaneously by a word of hope, an expression of sympathy, or a little kind and pleasing attention, especially if it was from some wished-for but unexpected quarter. In such cases, uninformed people are apt to suppose that there has been no real indisposition at all, because the improvement was so rapid, and without *medicine*. A proper understanding of the subject, however, would show them that these apparent caprices are as real as any other forms of disease, and that *moral* or *mental* medicine may be as active as drugs, and often much more beneficial. In short, if the nervous system is kept in a constant state of irritation, and the feelings and sympathies are habitually outraged, it is often impossible to do much good in female indisposition. The conduct of those around the patient is of more consequence than the physician's prescription, by far, and may, according to its propriety or impropriety, either accelerate or impede the cure. There are many men who habitually act in such a way, towards their female companions, as to both cause them suffering and prevent its removal, and that, too, without either desiring or intending to do so. They do not act from unkind motives, but their ignorance prevents them from seeing the consequences of their conduct. Conceiving females to be like themselves, and knowing that *they* can shake off the vapors, as they call them, and that *their* nervous systems are not easily irritated, they cannot feel a proper charity towards their sensitive companions. Females, on the other hand, feeling that they are not understood, nor their condition properly appreciated, and having no one to repose confidence in that they think can appreciate them, are apt to become morose, and retiring within themselves conceal their suffering and disquiet from every one.

This ignorance respecting the female constitution

is, therefore, a serious evil, making them Lable to suffer, and causing the other sex to withhold from them that sympathy and charitable consideration so much required, and which would be generally bestowed, if men were better informed as to its necessity and utility.

The ripening and expulsion of the egg is effected by a real *inflammation*, similar to what is seen when a splinter of wood, for instance, is expelled from the flesh by the process of *festering*, and it is this periodical inflammation that causes the sympathetic irritation above described. The inflammation is slight at the beginning of the month, but gradually increases towards the end, when the Ovaries are found to be highly congested, and the blood-vessels in them and the Uterus are much engorged. About the time when the egg is expelled from the Vesicle. the inflammation reaches its height, and to relieve it the vessels pour out a quantity of blood and mucus, in the same way that a discharge occurs after inflammation in other parts. This is the true cause of the Menstrual flow. It is a consequence of the action of the Ovaries, and is only seen in those who possess these organs perfect. Females who have no Ovaries, or in whom they are torpid. never Menstruate.

The importance of a knowledge of these facts, both to the preservation of health and also in medical science, is very great. The medical treatment of deranged or suppressed Menstruation has always been chiefly empirical, and seldom of much service, because the *real origin* and nature of the flow itself was unknown. In fact, there is no denying that, instead of doing good in these cases, medical science has led to much evil, and probably has caused more disease than ever it has cured. And yet, when properly understood, these derangements are usually *readily corrected*, and by very *simple means* as is fully shown in my book on the " *Diseases of Woman*," by following the directions in which, any female can successfully treat most of such cases herself, provided they have not been too much aggravated by improper *Medical* treatment.

In some young females this discharge occurs suddenly the first time, without any premonitory symptoms whatever, and occasionally it continues to do so at each of the succeeding periods, but more usually it is indicated by certain well-marked signs peculiar to that condition alone. Generally the female experiences considerable excitement just previous to its appearance, with a sensation of fulness in the head, slight fever, and pain in the back and abdomen. In some, these symptoms are much aggravated, so that they suffer severely, even more than at the time of parturition. There are females who are made perfectly delirious with the pain at these times, or so completely prostrated that they have scarcely strength to move. Others are more fortunate, and experience little or no inconvenience at such times; but these are the exceptions, and there are but few who are not more or less affected, particularly by lowness of spirits or irritability, and on that account considerable allowance should be made for what may appear strange or unusual in their conduct and manner. This is what is usually termed being unwell, and it is usually indicated by certain changes in the countenance, as well as by the signs mentioned above.

In the first twenty-four hours, the discharge is generally slight, and pale in color, but afterwards it becomes more profuse, and like real blood. The time it lasts is about *four days*, but varies considerably. Thus in some it endures a week, or more, and in others only a day, or even but a few hours. Some of these irregularities are natural, and must not be interfered with, but others are accidentally produced, and should be corrected. This, however, is more properly and fully explained in my book on the *Diseases of Woman.* The discharge subsides into a colorless mucous secretion, commonly termed *Leucorrhœa,* or the Whites, which when it remains constant, and too abundant, constitutes a real disease.

The quantity of fluid lost is on an average about *six ounces,* but it varies much in different persons, in some being very abundant and in others very small. I have known females to lose over a quart each time, without any apparent ill effects. To some extent it appears to be effected by climate, being more abundant in tropical countries and less so in cold ones. In some cases it is nearly or quite *colorless,* owing to there being little or no blood mixed with it, and then the individual is apt to suppose she has not menstruated when she really has. It is for this reason that such persons can never correctly estimate the proper time when conception can occur. The real period is not suspected by them to be so, because it is colorless, and then if any *flooding,* or mere discharge of blood from weakness takes place, they think that is the period, and in this way they fail in their reckoning.

It was formerly thought that the Menstrual discharge was something peculiar, and that it was possessed of certain deleterious properties, but this is now known to be a fallacy. It is nothing more than real blood mixed with the ordinary mucous secretion of the parts. Its odor is peculiar, and sometimes powerful, owing probably to its having been retained in the uterine vessels some time before its discharge, and having in consequence undergone some change, or fermentation. And this accounts for its odor being always stronger, and its color darker, when it has been retained longer than usual.

In former times Menstruation was attributed to the influence of the *moon*, and it was thought that it only took place when she was at the full, but this is well known not to be the case ; there are probably females menstruating every hour of every day in the year. It is true the usual period between the cessation of one discharge and the beginning of another, is generally equal to the time of the moons' revolution around the earth, being twenty-eight days, but they do not otherwise correspond. Indeed, in some there are not more than two or three weeks between, while in others there are five or six, or even more, and yet this may be to *them* perfectly natural and proper. The real cause of Menstruation is the ripening and expulsion of the egg, and of course it occurs whenever an egg is developed, whether that be frequently or rarely. It was found from observation that, in *one hundred females*, sixty-eight Menstruated every twenty-eight days ; twenty-eight every three weeks ; and one every second week ; while ten were irregular.

The first appearance of the Menses varies from about the *twelfth* to the *seventeenth* year, in our country, but it is effected by various circumstances. In the greater number of females it commences from fourteen to fifteen, though it is sometimes delayed till twenty or more, and occasionally is seen at *nine,* or even earlier.   I have seen a case myself in a mere infant.   Out of *four hundred and fifty* cases observed at the Manchester Lying-in Hospital, England, ten Menstruated at eleven years of age, nineteen at twelve,—fifty-three at thirteen,—eighty-five at fourteen,—ninety-seven at fifteen,—seventy-six at sixteen,—fifty-seven at seventeen,—twenty-six at eighteen,—twenty-three at nineteen,—and four at twenty years.

The time when the Menses cease, or the *turn of life* as it is called, that is when every Ovum is developed, is usually from forty to forty-five years of age, but like the commencement this is also liable to considerable variation, some females arriving at *the Turn* when they are but *thirty,* and others not till they are *fifty,* or even more.   Sometimes after it has apparently ceased, at the usual time, it, will appear again for a time or two many years after, at advanced age.   This is probably owing to one or more of the eggs having been left undeveloped in the Ovaries at the time of *the Turn,* through being imperfect, and their ripening afterwards.   In such cases *Conception* is possible at these after periods, which accounts for those instances of child-bearing in old females, which are occasionally met with, sometimes as far as the *sixtieth* year.   Of course conception is possible as long as proper menstruation continues, but never when it ceases, or has not appeared.   It is true, that in some cases females have borne children who have apparently never menstruated, but these were undoubtedly cases in which it was simply *colorless,* and *small in quantity,* so that they did not observe it, or else thought it was only the *Whites.*   The Menstruation, in some form, must always occur before pregnancy can en-

sue, but the excitement and inflammation may be so
small, in particular constitutions, that none of the
usual indications are observed. It is owing to this
that some females, who think they do not menstruate often enough, are deceived, because many periods are apt to be unobserved by them. And on the
contrary many others who fancy they have their
turns too often are equally deceived ; many of the
supposed Menstruations being mere floodings, or
discharges of blood from weakness or over fulness of
the vessel. A mere *show* of blood therefore is no
proof of Menstruation, nor is its absence any sign
to the contrary.

In one series of observations it was found that in
seventy-seven females one ceased menstruation, or
arrived at the turn of life, at thirty-five years of
age,—four at forty,—one at forty-two,—one at forty-
three,—three at forty-four,—four at forty-five,—
three at forty-seven,—ten at forty-eight—seven at
forty-nine,—twenty-six at fifty,—two at fifty-one,—
seven at fifty-two,—two at fifty-three.—two at fifty-
four,—one at fifty-seven, two at sixty ;—and one
at *seventy !*

It is commonly supposed that Menstruation commences earlier in hot countries than in cold ones,
and in consequence of the heat, but there is good
reason for doubting this. Mr. Robertson has shown
by his researches that it commences every where at
about the same average age, and that the early intercourse of the sexes which takes place in the Indies, and other warm countries, is owing more to a
depraved state of morals, and to unrestrained intercourse than to any influence of climate. He remarks that the early marriages we see there are " to
be attributed not to any peculiar precocity, but to

moral and political degradation, exhibited in ill-laws and customs, the enslavement more or less of the women, ignorance of letters; and impure or debasing systems of religion." He also thinks that if the same manners and customs prevailed in England, or America, the same effects would be seen, and this is fully borne out in those pitiable instances, occasionally seen in our large towns, of juvenile prostitution. Many of these degraded and brutal ized children at eleven or twelve years are as much women, in certain respects, as they ought to have been ·at seventeen or eighteen, and of course any other children would be the same if exposed to the same influences, unless, as fortunately is often the case, the initiation into vice caused their death.

In cities generally, on the average, Menstruation commences earlier than in the country, owing to the more exciting circumstances that surround young persons, and which awakens the sexual instinct precociously. This is particularly the case in those places where morals are bad, and familiar intercourse between the sexes is unrestrained. In the Eastern parts of the old world Marriages are often contracted while the female is very young, but it does not follow that she was fitted for it; and in all probability if those very females had been educated like our own they would have been in no respect different. We are told for instance that Mahomet consummated his Marriage with one of his wives when she was but *eight years old*. In this, however, we simply see the proof of her degradation and enslavement, and not of her natural precocity. So far as is known also there is no *difference* as to the time of the first Menstruation among the different *races* of human beings Thus, for instance, it is no earlier, *under the same circumstances*, in the Negress than in the white female.

As a general rule the earlier Menstruation commences, and the more frequently it occurs, the earlier it will cease, and to this there are but few exceptions. It is therefore of considerable importance to the future health of the female that this grand event should not be accelerated by any factitious causes, but should be brought on by the slow and unaided process of natural development. Young females should be allowed to remain as *children*, or *girls* at least, much longer than they usually do, and not be forced into *young women* too soon. For every year earlier that they become *young* women they probably become *old* ones *five* years before they otherwise would have been. It is of the utmost importance that young females should have their muscular systems well developed previous to puberty, and that they should not have their minds and feelings too much excited. Nothing tends to bring on Puberty more than a morbid excitement of the feelings and sympathies, such as results from silly romances, and over-wrought love-tales. Excessive study also is very injurious, and the too constant attention to what are called mere accomplishments. These are often pursued to the utter sacrifice of what is useful or beneficial, and result in nothing but premature development of those instincts that had better lie dormant till a later period. In fact, the education of young girls seems too often to have but one object, and that is to *force* them into women as rapidly as possible, to the utter ruin of their health and happiness.

In former times, as we find from the Bible, a **wo-man** was thought to be *unclean* while Menstruating, and was shunned as something hurtful and deleterious. According to Pliny, the Ancient Naturalist, it was thought that she would destroy grafts, or bees, and blight corn, make iron rust, and even cause madness in dogs. Nay, he even goes so far as to say that the Menstrual fluid, by its odor, will cause fruit to fall from the trees, destroy insects, and cause seeds not to grow. Many barbarous nations at the present day entertain similar notions, and at such times compel females to secrete themselves, and shun society, when they really need the most sympathy and kind companionship. M. Morcau de la Sarthe, in his *Natural History of Women*, tell us that the South Sea Islanders, and the South American Indians, always send their females to separate huts during these periods, and that the Illinois Indians formerly punished any woman with death who failed to give due notice of her being in that condition. According to history we also find that by a decree of the Council of Nice, Women were forbidden to enter the church while Menstruating. In the Laws of the Isrealites it is enacted, that "If a man shall lie with a woman having her sickness, and shall uncover her nakedness, he hath discovered her fountain, and she hath uncovered the fountain of her blood, and both of them shall be cut off from among their people."—(See Leviticus, chap. 20, v. 18.)

Such notions it will be seen are now happily to be found chiefly among barbarians, or in the records of a former ignorant age, though there are individuals who entertain them even yet. Indeed at the present time there are persons, especially among the ill-informed in England, who believe that meat will not take the salt if the process be carried on by a female who is menstruating. Others again think that bread will not rise, and that beer will sour, if a female so circumstanced have anything to do with them. It is perhaps scarcely necessary to say that all such notions are as erroneous as they are absurd, and that they are practically disproved every day, by thousands of females who pay no attention to them, and who yet conduct all the above operations as successfully as if nothing of the kind was taking place.

The first appearance of this function is an important event, and should be carefully watched for, so that nothing may be allowed to interfere with it, and also that means may be taken to bring it on if it be too long delayed. Young females ought especially to be timely informed about it, so that they may know how to conduct themselves, and may not be needlessly alarmed, as many are when it first appears. These matters, however, belong more especially to Medicine, and will be found fully explained in my book on the *Diseases of Woman.*

It is especially important to bear in mind that females are usually more irritable and unsettled at these times, and that full allowance should be made for their being so. In a young person this is more apt to be the case, from the very novelty of her situation. The strange phenomenon that is occuring in her system, the development of her person, and the new feelings and instincts that are awakened, all exert a powerful influence, which is still further increased by the mystery with which everything relating to these wonderful operations is enshrouded. In the absence of proper information, imagination is busily at work, curiosity is excited, and the mind becomes filled with strange fancies and romantic dreams, which often exert a baneful influence in after life. Proper instruction, at the proper time, with a well-regulated mind and body, would give more correct ideas of her real duties and sexual situation, and prevent much of that sickness and unhappiness of mind which is so commonly seen after marriage.

There are few objects more interesting to the philosopher and philanthropist than a young female at this period of her existence, when the body is assuming its natural beauty of form, and becoming fit for its wondrous functions, and when the expanding mind receives the first faint perception of her real destiny.

To a great extent, the development of the whole physical system depends upon the action of the Ovaries, so that if they are absent, or inactive every other part of the organization remains imperfect. The destruction of them in early life causes a similar imperfection to what follows the removal of the Testes in the male, and even at adult age, as already shown, they exert a paramount importance over the other Organs. It is apparently the effort that is required to perfect them, in fact, that makes the body grow and perfect itself so rapidly at puberty. Every one must have noticed what an astonishing change occurs in a young female at that time. The bust becomes full, the pelvis enlarges, the features change—especially in their expression—the mind takes a different turn, and the manner and conduct become altogether different, denoting the new feelings and instincts that begin to be experienced. In short, the girl is changed into the woman, and is conscious herself of the alteration. All these changes result from the action of the Ovaries, and if they are incapable of performing their functions, no such alterations take place, but on the contrary, the system either remains always as it was during girlhood, or develops in an unusual manner, similar to the male for instance. Nature seems to refuse to put forth her energies to perfect the rest of the system if she cannot first perfect the essential organs of generation, and the first Menstrual flow, or the ripening of the first egg, is, therefore, the constant and necessary prelude to womanly development.

In reference to marriage, Menstruation ought always to precede that event, and generally for a considerable time—twelve months at least—especially if it commences early. It is not always that it continues regularly from the first commencement, but ceases for some months, or even longer, and then commences again.

The proper age for marriage is, of course, variable in different individuals, some being properly developed years earlier than others, and no general rule can, therefore, be given. One necessary condition is the perfect establishment of Menstruation, as already stated ; and, perhaps, the next most essential requisite is the proper development of the body, especially of the Pelvis and Genital Organs, for if these have not attained to a certain growth before marriage, they may never do so afterwards. A ' neglect of these matters leads often to the most serious and unhappy consequences, from which there is no escape. Nevertheless, there are cases in which Marriage may be required to perfect the development of the system, and in which it will always remain imperfect without, but these are very rare, and are usually indicated in an unmistakeable manner

The proper time for marriage is *midway* between two of the ordinary periods, let the space be what it may. I have known instances of young females marrying either at the Menstrual period, or so near that nervous agitation, consequent upon the ceremony, has brought it on, and many evils have followed therefrom, to say nothing of the annoyance and distress. This was, of course, the fault of those who had these young persons under their care, and who had neglected to inform themselves upon so essential a point. Immediately after, and immediately before Menstruation, are neither so proper as the midway, the Organs and the nervous system being at both these times more or less excited and irritable. Marriage just before Menstruation has been known to arrest it, so that it never afterwards returned.

As a general rule, Menstruation does not take place during Nursing, though, occasionally, it does so, even commencing as early as the first month after delivery, and continuing on uninterruptedly. The reason why it does not take place at this time generally, is, because the blood and the vital energy which is ordinarily expended in ripening the egg, is needed during Nursing, to secrete the milk, and it would exhaust the system too much to carry on both functions at the same time. In those cases where Menstruation and Nursing do occur simultaneously, it is either because there is a superabundance of vital energy, by which both can be supported, or the Ovaries are in a state of chronic irritation, owing to which they act, when they ought to be dormant. In the first case, no injury may result from both taking place at the same time, but when there is not a real excess of energy, this double drain nearly always exhausts the strength, and impairs the health. It is not, as some suppose, necessarily improper, or injurious to the child, for nursing to be allowed while the turns continue, unless the health and strength of the mother suffers thereby. If she becomes weak, the milk is often imperfectly formed and watery, so that the child is not perfectly nourished by it, but there is nothing positively hurtful in its nature under such circumstances. It is not necessary therefore to discontinue nursing at such times, unless the mother evidently suffers from the unusual condition.

During Pregnancy the Menses do not appear, for the same reason, though in some females they are thought to do so. All the energies of the Uterus and Ovaries are then needed in developing the new being, and the Ovaries are necessarily dormant. Besides this, the interior of the Womb is covered, immediately after Conception, with the Membranes surrounding the fœtus, which effectually close the mouth of each Fallopian Tube, and of the Womb. If either an Ovum, or the Menstrual fluid were to form therefore, it could not pass away, unless these Membranes were detached, which would cause abortion.

When a discharge occurs during Pregnancy therefore, it is not a real Menstruation, though it may take place regularly at the month, from the *habit* of the system, but it is simply an escape o. blood from the vessels of the Vagina, or neck of the Womb, owing either to their weakness or over ful ness. It is really a *flooding*, therefore, which may do no harm while it is confined to the parts below, but if it extends to the *interior* of the Womb, it is nearly sure to cause miscarriage. This is one reason why much sexual excitement is improper during Pregnancy, because it is apt to excite the Ovaries to form the Ova, and thus lead to miscarriage by their expulsion.

After marriage the question is often asked of the physician, whether connection during Menstruation is improper? To this it may be answered, that, in some cases, it is both disagreeable and painful, and therefore obviously improper, but, in other cases, it is rather desired than otherwise, and is apparently not at all injurious, and then it must be objected to on other grounds than being unnatural. Perhaps there are but few persons who need any particular reason for abstaining at such times, considerations of delicacy alone being sufficient. The feelings and instincts of the female herself are all that need be consulted, and it is very seldom that they will direct her wrong. It is certain that there are persons who never experience a *desire* for association, except at such times, and we are certainly not justified, on scientific grounds at least, in saying that it should then be forbidden. The old idea that certain diseases originated from association at such times is altogether erroneous, and without the slightest foundation.

Until recently, it was thought that Menstruation occurred in human beings only, but it is now known that it occurs in most animals, though in a different form. Every being that brings forth its young alive, has a certain period in which the development of its Ova or Eggs is effected, and at those times when they are fully ripe, there occurs a function analogous to Menstruation. Thus taking most kinds of Cattle for instance, as the Wild Deer, they are capable of Conception only at one time in the

year, and will only receive the male at that time.
This is what is called the season of *Rut* or *Heat*,
and on dissecting them, the cause of it becomes obvious. They ripen an egg only once in the year,
and when that occurs it causes the excitement which
makes them desire association, and also results in
a peculiar discharge from the Genital Organs, which
is, strictly speaking, the same as human Menstrua
tion, though it is nearly colorless. A discharge of
this nature is seen in all animals at such times, and,
occasionally, as in some of the Monkeys, it is even
tinged with blood. It is, therefore, merely in its
color, quantity, and frequency of appearance that
it varies, in some taking place but once a year, in
others every two or three months, and in the human
being monthly, according to the frequency with
which the eggs are ripened. These facts have led
some physiologists to suppose that the most appropriate time for association in the human being, is
near to the monthly periods, because in the animals
above referred to, it is *only* at such times that they
desire it. In the human being, however, there are
many essential differences, in regard to the com-
merce of the sexes, and especially in the feelings
that lead to it. In the lower animals, it is, of course,
a mere amorous propensity that impels, and which
is excited only by peculiar conditions of the Genital Organs in both ; but in human beings there are
other feelings, of a higher order, which are often
more powerful than the sexual instinct itself. The
mere animal being impelled to the act only by
physical excitement, depending on a certain condition of the parts, will, of course, feel the impulse
only when those conditions exist, but the human
being may also be impelled by mental and moral

agencies, though the physical excitement may be weak, or even if it be quite extinguished. It is not always therefore solely for the indulgence of the mere sexual propensity that human beings associate, but for that conjointly with other instincts, and therefore the same rule should not apply to them. It is, perhaps, desirable, physiologically speaking, that association should never take place without both physical and moral enjoyment in both, and therefore those times should be chosen when the female organs are most disposed to these peculiar excitements. This time is not always the same, being just after the period in some, and just before it in others, and occasionally only during the flow itself. As a general rule, it is found that in the great majority of females, the inclination is strongest immediately after the flow, and it is also then that Conception is most likely to ensue. This is analogous to what is observed in the lower animals, in whom the flow has always passed its height before the heat is experienced. In medical practice, it is found that those means which we use, in cold temperaments, to produce sexual feeling, always act best just after the period is over, and this is, therefore, doubtless the most proper and favorable time for association, though there is nothing inherently wrong in it at other times.

Formerly a notion prevailed that association during the flow was wrong, because the offspring resulting therefrom would be diseased or insane; and, in fact, certain peculiar affections were thought to have originated in that way. This, is, however, altogether erroneous, because Conception cannot occur at that time, as shown in another place.

It is probable that the Menstrual flow is also made

use of by nature as a means of periodical purification, and that many matters which would be hurtful to the body, if retained, or removed by it. This accounts for the fact that females can work, without injury, at certain employments in the metals, where poisonous fumes are evolved, and which would kill men, the deleterious matter being carried off in this way. It is for this reason also that the turn of life, when the flow ceases, is so critical a period. The cessation of this periodical purification, of course, makes the body more liable to disease, and more disposed to suffer from congestions of blood, because there is now no monthly abstraction to give relief. It is, therefore, at this time, particularly necessary to attend to all the other secretions, particularly the skin and bowels, to keep them active, so as to make up for that which is suspended. This, however, is fully explained in my *Diseases of Woman.*

It may not be out of place to remark here, that the existence of this function alone makes it impossible for Woman—except in a few peculiar individual cases—to pursue the same avocations, and follow the same mode of life as Man. It makes her, of necessity, not so continuously active, nor so capable of physical toil, while, at the same time, it causes her to yearn for sympathy and support from some being that she feels is more powerful than herself.

PLATE VI.

Female Egg and Impregnation.

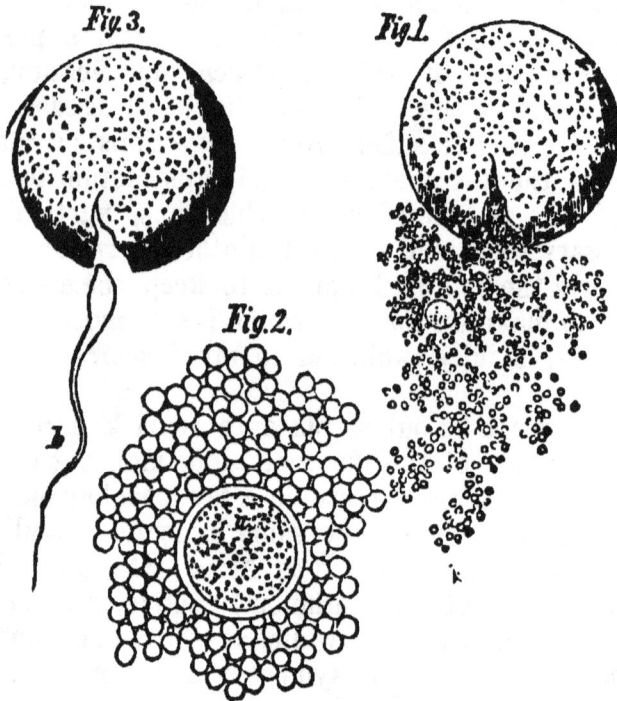

Fig. 1. Egg just burst open, the Germinal Vesicle *a*, with part of the Vitellus escaping.

Fig. 2. Germinal Vesicle with part of the Vitellus magnified.

Fig. 3. The Animalcule (*b*) entering the egg after it has been broken open by the escape of the Germinal Vesicle

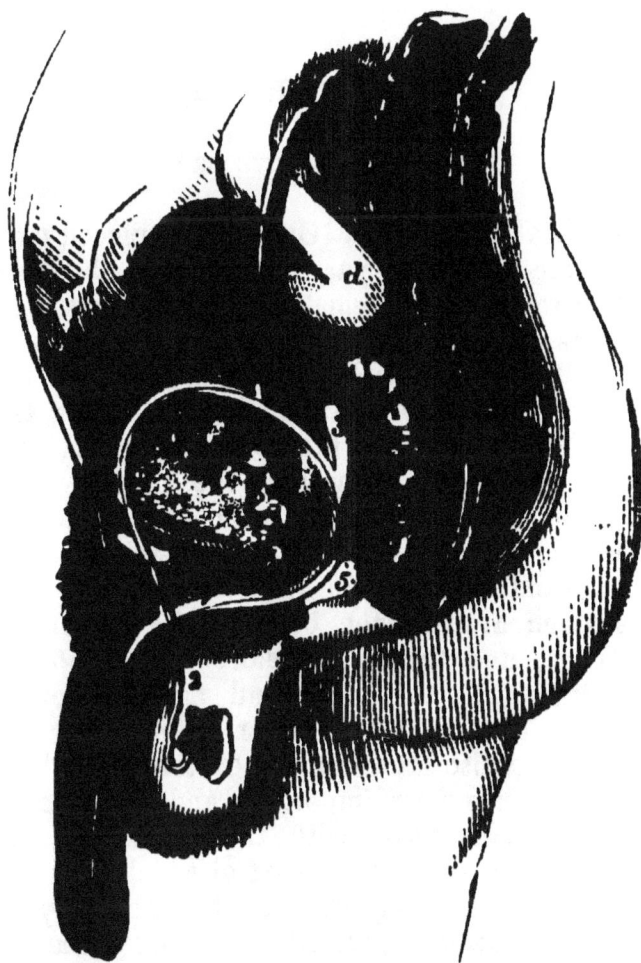

For description see page 23.

CHAPTER VI.

THE MALE GENERATIVE ORGANS.

THE Male Generative Organs are placed partly within the body and partly without, in the corresponding region to the female Organs, the most essential parts being external. They consist of two Organs called the *Testicles*, which secrete the male principle, or semen, and are analogous to the Ovaries.—Two Tubes called the *Vasa Deferentia*, which conduct the semen away from the Testicles,—and of certain accessory organs, connected with these Tubes, called the *Seminal Vesicles*, *Prostrate Glands*, and *Ejaculatory Canals*, and also other parts which are common both to the Semen and the Urine, and termed therefore the *Genito-Urinary* Organs, as the *Penis* and passage down it called the *Urethra* for instance. Respecting some of these, and also the Male Semen, there have lately been made some most important and valuable discoveries, equally novel with those concerning the Female system, the greater part of which have been so fully explained in my work on the Male System that, with some necessary additions, the account of them given therein will be precisely adapted to our present purpose.

§ THE TESTICLES.

The most essential organs in the male system are two glandular bodies, called the *Testes* or *Testicles*

which are placed, after birth, outside of the body
in an external envelop, called the scrotum, hanging
from the pubic bone. The use of these organs is
to produce the male principle, or *semen*, as the ovaries produce the female ovum or egg. The Testes,
like the Ovaries, are not capable of performing their
proper functions till a certain period of 'life, called
puberty, but unlike them, they are not liable to lose
their powers at any particular age, but may preserve them indefinitely. In the early stages of existence in the womb the testes are contained in the
abdomen, and only descend to the scrotum just before birth.

On dissecting one of the testicles, it is found to
be chiefly composed of blood-vessels and numerous
small tubes containing semen. A branch of the
spermatic artery is sent from the abdomen down to
each teste, in which it divides and subdivides into
thousands of little branches, many of which are
too small to be seen by the naked eye. It is this
artery that brings to the testes the pure blood from
which probably the semen is formed. The extreme
ends of the minute arterial branches are apparently
continuous with the commencements of the seminal
tubes, so that in examining them we gradually lose
sight of the blood and begin to find semen. The
seminal tubes are at first exceedingly minute, but
very numerous, and they gradually unite together
to form larger branches, and trunks, till eventually
the whole form but one tube, called the *Vas Deferens*, by which the semen is conveyed to the Urethra. The number of these little tubes has been
estimated at over *sixty thousand* in one testicle, and
it has been shown, that, if they were put in a straight
line, they would measure many hundreds, if not

PLATE VII.

Seminal Tubes and Appendages of the Testicles

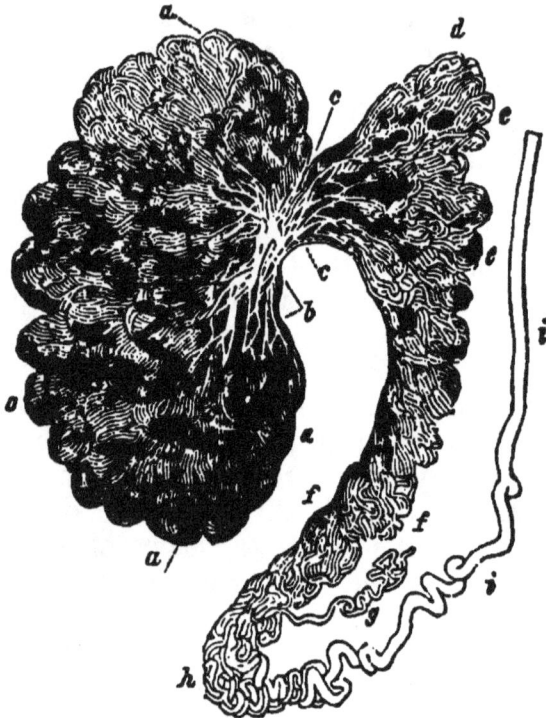

EXPLANATION.

a, a, a. Lobules of the small Seminiferous Tubes, similar to the Convolutions of the Brain.—*b.* The Rete Testis, a number of nearly straight Tubes into which the smaller ones enter.—*c.* The Vasa Efferentia, or larger Tubes, 12 or 18 in number, into which the Semen passes from the Rete Testis.—*d.* Plexuses, or conglomerations of the Vasa Efferentia, which form a kind of head, almost like a small Testicle, called the Epididymis.—*c, e.* The head of the Epididymis. —*f, f.* The body of the Epididymis.—*g.* An appendix of the Epididymis, called the *aberrans.* It is not always met with.—*h.* The Tail, or Cauda of the Epididymis.—*i, i.* The Vas Deferens, which is at first very much twisted, but becomes finally straight.

From this view it will be seen, that the small Seminal Tubes gradually merge into the large straight ones, called the *Rete Testis*, into the still larger, called the *Vasa Efferentia*, and finally they all coalesce into one Tube, the Vas Deferens.

thousands of feet. There is also a branch of the spermatic *vein* connected with each testis, which ramifies in its substance similarly to the artery. This vein is to take away the impure and refuse blood when no longer needed.

The Testicles are therefore mainly composed of three kinds of tubes, or vessels, namely, *Arteries, Veins,* and *Seminal Tubes.* In addition to which there are also numerous *nerves,* and Lymphatics, of absorbents, the whole being connected together by a cellular substance or tissue. Each one is connected with the body by what is termed the *spermatic cord,* which is a kind of sheath, or tube, about half an inch in diameter, containing the main branches of the Artery, Nerves, and Lymphatics, going *to* the Teste, with the main branch of the vein, and the Vas Deferens, coming *from* it. This spermatic cord ascends into the Abdomen, when the different vessels composing it are distributed to their respective places. Each teste is also surrounded by a distinct coat, or *tunic,* beside the scrotum, or outer skin, in which both are enclosed.

The manner in which the semen is actually made is of course unknown to us ; we can only point out the place where it originates and explain its progress towards the exterior of the body.

The Vas Deferens from each Teste, into which all its seminal tubes have poured their contents, ascends into the Abdomen through the spermatic cord, and rises nearly as high as the top of the bladder, behind which it turns, and then begins to descend till it meets near its lower part with two small organs called the *Seminal Vesicles,* with which it becomes connected. From the seminal vesicles the semen passes down a small tube called the *Ejacula-*

ory Canal, which is attached to the bladder, and which joins immediately *under* it, an organ called the *Prostate Gland*. Finally, by means of some curious openings through the Prostate Gland, the seminal fluid is passed into the *Urethra*, or passage down the Penis, by which the urine escapes from the bladder, and is thus ejected from the body.

These several parts comprise the whole male generative system, and in the act of impregnation each one has a special function to perform. The Testes secrete the semen, the Vas Deferens and Ejaculatory Canal convey it to the Urethra, and the penis deposits it in the Female Organs, while the seminal vesicles and Prostate Gland either secrete some necessary addition, or effect some modification in it.

As before remarked, the Testes are usually two in number, the one on the left side being lower and larger than that on the right. But sometimes more than two appear to exist, and at other times only one, or perhaps none. The arrangement of one being higher than the other, when there are two, prevents them from being crushed together when the limbs are crossed, by allowing one to slide over the other. The internal structure of them having already been explained, it is only requisite further to describe their envelops and attachments.

Immediately around each one is an envelop or membrane, called the Tunica *Albuginea* or *Peritestis*, which surrounds every part, and also sends branches, or leaves, into the substance of the Testicle, so as to divide it to a certain depth, into lobes, or sections, similar to the lobes of the brain, only of a triangular shape.

The outside inclosure is called the *Scrotum*, or purse, and is the same as the skin of the thighs. It is divided vertically into two parts by a small ridge, called the *Raphe*, and is usually covered with hairs at puberty. Underneath the Scrotum we next find a reddish cellular membrane, called the *Dartos*, which makes a separate sac for each of the two Testicles, which are separated from each other by a vertical membrane placed between them, called the *Septum Scroti*, which acts as a partition, and thus the two organs are perfectly unconnected with each other. The nature of the *Dartos* has been a subject of dispute among anatomists, some considering it to be merely a cellular tissue, and others thinking it to be a muscle. It is undoubtedly *partly* muscular, and consists mainly of long fibres, which cross and interlace each other in every direction. It is the contraction of these fibres of the Dartos that corrugates or wrinkles the Scrotum, as is well seen when sudden cold is applied to the external parts. Next under the Dartos comes a true muscular coat, called the *Cremaster Muscle*, or *Tunica Erythoides*, the use of which is to draw the Testicle upwards. This is derived from one of the muscles of the abdomen, and comes down through the abdominal ring, forming part of the sheath of the spermatic cord. The last coat is called the *Tunica Vaginalis*, which is a true serous membrane interlaced with blood-vessels, and comes next to the Tunica Albuginea.

In a healthy state the muscular fibres of the Scrotum are usually contracted, so as to draw the skin into folds and brace the Testes up against the Abdomen ; but during a state of debility, or from great fatigue, they become relaxed, so that the testes hang low, and pull upon the cord. It is an almost certain sign of ill health when this relaxation of the Scrotum occurs, at any period of life, and often its removal is the first indication of improvement. In old people, and in those of a bad habit of body. this relaxed state becomes permanent.

By inspecting antique statuary, it will be seen that the ancients were practically acquainted with this physiological fact, that they have accordingly accurately represented it in their works of art. The figures of all their men in health and vigor have the Scrotum invariably drawn up to the abdomen, while those of old men, or sufferers, hang pendant.

As a general rule the muscles of the Scrotum are independent of the will, or act involuntarily, but instances have been known of men who made them act as they pleased. Some boys exhibit this power before puberty, being able to draw the Testes up to the abdominal ring, and let them fall again, but it is seldom this command over them continues, though one instance is on record. This man drew the Testes up into the groin, so as to form apparent ruptures, in order to escape being impressed into the service. Being detected, however, he confessed the trick, and made an exhibition of his extraordinary power to the examining physicians. He could pull up either one alone or both together, and could also make one go up while the other was coming down; in short, he had the same command over them as over his arms, and could move them as quickly. In another instance a man, who was charged with being the father of an illegitimate child, endeavored to evade the responsibility by alleging he had no Testicles, and, therefore, could not be the father, but it was discovered that he could draw them up into the groin at pleasure. In a healthy state the scrota muscles are brought powerfully into action during coition, so as to brace the Testes tightly against the Pelvis, and one cause of partial impotence in very weak or old people, is the loss of this power, owing to which the semen is not expelled with sufficient force.   In children the relaxed or firm condition of these muscles is often a valuable indication of the state of their health.

The form of the Testes is that of a somewhat flattened oval, with one end a little larger than the other.   The average weight is about one ounce.

The Vas Deferens, or common Tube into which all the small ones are emptied, commences at the *globus minor*, or lower end of the epididymis, and then passes into the spermatic cord by which it enters the Abdomen, where its course has already been traced.   It is altogether about thirty-two feet long. The sheath of the spermatic cord is composed of two coats, the outer one of which is very firm, like cartilage, so that the tube is not easily compressed ; the inner coat is a mucous membrane, similar to that inside the Urethra.   The cord can be readily felt externally.

This description of the Testes and their envelops, combined with that before given, will be sufficient to give a clear understanding of the various diseases and derangements to which they are liable, and also of the reasons for the line of treatment laid down. It will be seen that they are so placed, without the body, as to have no direct connection with any other organs, and they may, therefore, be removed without any other part being interfered with.   This operation, termed *Castration*, is sometimes necessary in certain diseases, and sometimes it is the effect of accident, or, in some parts of the world, even of design.   The removal of the Testes, however, in what-

'ver way it may be effected, not only destroys the power of procreation, but also interferes in a remarkable manner with the growth and functions of various other parts of the system, from which it is evident that they are necessary for the perfection of the individual's own system, as well as for the purpose of bringing new beings into existence.

ANAMOLIES IN THE SIZE AND APPARENT NUMBER OF THE TESTES.

The usual size of the Testes is about that of an ordinary pigeon's egg, and their weight, as before stated, is about *one ounce*. Occasionally, however, they are seen much larger, and sometimes much smaller, and their weight may be also considerably greater or less than the average. I have seen them as large as a full-sized hen's egg, yet perfectly healthy, and as small as marbles without being in any way deficient in power. This is important to bear in mind in many cases that may come under the physician's notice. I have known men hesitate about marrying when the Testes were very small, from fear that they would be deficient in power, and it was with difficulty they could be convinced to the contrary. In one instance, of a young man aged twenty-six, they were no larger than those of a child of nine years old, yet his powers were but little, if any, inferior to those of persons generally. After a great deal of hesitation, and much persuasion, he married and became the father of a large family. It is necessary to remark, however, that in these cases all the other organs were of proper size, and that the smallness of the Testes had existed from childhood, and was therefore a natural state. If they had *decreased* in size, after having been properly developed, it would have been very different. The falling away or *wasting* of the Testes, which follows many diseases, and sometimes takes place without any assignable cause, is usually a serious matter, and is nearly certain to be followed by a loss of power. The injudicious use of certain drugs, particularly of Iodine, will frequently cause the Testes to waste, and so will the exhalations from some metals, as lead for instance, many workmen in which I have known so effected. In giving an opinion in such cases therefore, their previous history must always be known, as well as the condition of the other parts, and the physician will then have but little difficulty in coming to a proper decision. Sometimes one only will be small, and the other of average size, or one only may waste away, without injuring the other.

An unusually large size of the Testes should always excite suspicion of its being the result of disease, and a most careful examination and inquiry should therefore be made. If they have always been of that size, or nearly so, from puberty, and especially if the other organs are large also, there may be nothing to excite apprehension. The symptoms of the different diseases hereafter described should, however, be carefully studied, particularly those that cause *enlargement*, as Hydrocele and Hernia Humoralis, for instance. I have known the Testes of a youth of *fourteen* to be much larger than those of most men, and yet perfectly healthy , such cases of unusual development are not necessarily accompanied by extra power

In some instances the development of all the genital organs is very tardy, owing to the slow growth of the Testes. I have seen a youth of *nineteen* that was in every respect in the same state of these parts, as when about seven years old. He was also but very little grown in other parts of the body, having the appearance of one about twelve years old. In this case there were perfect evidences of sexual power, though slight, and all the parts were evidently healthy. It was therefore a case of torpid action, or retarded development, and I thought that in all probability nature could be aroused. I accordingly gave him directions to use stimulating lotions, with frictions and shampooing, and to have a stimulating diet, with regular warm bathing and plenty of out-door exercise. The effects of this practice was soon evident; in less than six months an evident increase had taken place, both in the size of the parts and in the intensity of the sexual feeling. The external parts, which had previously been perfectly bare and smooth, like those of a child, became covered; the voice assumed a more manly tone, the muscles were more solid, the mind more active, and manhood began to dawn. This improvement continued going on till he was twenty-one, when there was but little difference between him and other young men of that age. If this case had not been promptly and properly attended to, in all probability no further development would *ever* have taken place, and an early death would have terminated his imperfect existence. To what age and improvement of this kind is *possible* we cannot of course tell, though I feel sure it may be effected in older persons than is generally supposed, perhaps till nearly thirty. The younger, of course, the better. Several cases have been known of the Testes growing after twenty-six years old.

Sometimes there appear to be *three* Testicles, and *possibly* in *some* of these cases there may really be three, but more frequently one of the three bodies is either the epididymis, somewhat enlarged, and much separated from the Teste, or else it is a small tumor. Most of those that have been observed in dissection have been small harmless tumors, existing from birth. Three perfect Testicles, however, are occasionally found, but they are not always accompanied by any unusual sexual power.

At other times there appears but *one* Testicle, or perhaps *none*, and I have known young men in the deepest distress from this cause. In some of these instances there is really but one organ, as has been proved after birth, and yet the individual has had full average powers. It is more often the case, however, that these deficiencies are apparent rather than real. Before birth the Testes are contained in the Abdomen, and they usually descend into the Scrotum in the last month. It sometimes happens, however, that the descent of one or both does not take place, and the individual then appears so far deficient. In these cases the power of the Testes is not impaired by their unusual position, but perhaps is often increased, and this has led uninformed persons to think that men sometimes had procreative powers *without Testicles*, because they could not be found. A man once died in one of the London hospitals who had long been noted as having *no Testicles*, and yet having all the usual powers. On dissection, two perfect ones were found in the Abdomen that had never come down, and thus the wonder was solved. These cases, however, are but rare. Dr. Marshall examined *ten thousand eight hundred* young recruits, among whom he found *five* in whom the right Testicle had not come down, and six in whom the left had not; there being but one man in whom both were not descended.

It is much better for the Testes to remain totally in the Abdomen than to descend only to the groin, as they sometimes do, because in the last position they are apt to be compressed, by the other parts crowding about them in the ring, and thus waste away. The imperfect or non-descent of the Testes must, however, always be considered an imperfection, and though it *may* not cause inconvenience, or loss of power, it is nevertheless always to be feared The Teste itself is as liable to all its different diseases while in these unusual positions as when in the Scrotum, and unfortunately cannot then be reached. The neighboring parts also became affected from it, and thus life may be lost from a simple affection which could have been completely removed, if the Teste had been in its natural position.

In some instances the retained Testes descend late in life, and if they then become fast in the ring great swelling and severe inflammation may result, with ultimate wasting away of the organs. Such cases have been mistaken for ruptures, and some men, from want of information, have thought that the Testicles really grew at that time, all at once.

When there are really *no* Testicles from birth, there is always an imperfect development of the whole system, and a total absence of sexual power or feeling.

In some animals it is natural for the Testes *never* to descend, but always to remain in the Abdomen, and in others they descend only at certain seasons, that is, when they attain their periodical development, owing to the full growth of the animalcules

It is stated, on the authority of several travellers, that there is a tribe of Hottentots at the Cape of Good Hope that never have but one Testicle ; but many naturalists think that more likely it is a cus tom among them to remove one in youth. It is quite possible, however, that this deficiency may be natu ral, and it is not in any way more singular than many peculiarities observed in the genital organs of the females of those tribes. I have known two brothers, twins, one of whom had three Testes and the other but one.

In some instances the two Testes have been found *grown together*, so as apparently to form but *one*, owing to the absence of the usual septum.

The Testicles are sometimes drawn so close up against the abdomen, owing to a contraction of the cremaster muscle, that they cannot be discover- ed without close examination, and are then often thought to be absent, though they are quite perfect, and even outside of the body. Medical men have even testified that there were no Testicles, in such cases as these, which shows the necessity for a close and thorough examination of such apparent mons- trosities.

This state of things is not dangerous in itself, but had better be removed if possible, because the Tes- tes are likely to adhere to the neighboring parts and wase away, so as to cause perfect impotence. A surgical operation is necessary to liberate them, which is both difficult and somewhat dangerous. In some few dissections the Testes have been found completely absent, and without any trace of their having existed. Sometimes the Vas Deferens ex ists by itself, and sometimes with the Epididymis though at other times there are no traces of either

These cases of total congenital absence are, however, very rare, and are always indicated by deficiencies in other parts of the system.

In some rare instances the Testes have descended into the *Perineum*, instead of the Scrotum, but most probably from some imperfection in the parts about the Perineum and Scrotum.

In the course of my practice I have been consulted in many of these cases of Testicular anomalies, and have often had the pleasure of removing unfounded apprehensions, and of giving happiness and confidence to those who had previously been the victims of hopeless despair.

The Testes are liable to many different diseases and derangements, some from birth, and others that originate afterwards, many of which ought to forbid marriage altogether. A full account of every one, with directions both how to treat and avoid them, may be found in my book on the Male Organs, and if every young man was in possession of that information in time, we should see but few of these diseases compared with what we do now.

Many men are alarmed very much at any affection of these Organs—and with good reason, too, considering the inefficiency of all medical treatment in them—till very recently. Now, however, some of the worst of these affections, both organic and accidental, are cured very readily, and means are used successfully to increase their power when deficient, or restore it, in many cases, if lost. Some most extraordinary cases of this kind will be found in my book, that have been treated by myself, and I have also a number of Letters from persons who have successfully treated themselves, by following the directions given therein.

In those Animals the females of which only admit the male during one particular season of the year, that of the *rut*, a beautiful provision is found in the male, by which the two are made to correspond The Testicles of these Animals do not secrete Semen continuously, as they do in others, but only at those times when the female Ovaries act, so that both experience the sexual impulse at the same time. At all other periods the Testicles are quite small, but then they suddenly enlarge, and when the season is over they decrease again. In some Animals the Testicles descend from the body only at that time, and at every other period are drawn up into the Abdomen. In many, the enlargement of these Organs during connection is very evident, and in some of the lower animals, and Insects, there is only sufficient Semen secreted for one single act.

According to recent observations, it appears that the Semeniferous Tubes are about *one two-hundredth part of an inch in diameter*, and that the Vas Deferens, in all its convolutions, is nearly *thirty-two feet* in length, while the whole of the Tubes are, probably, full *five thousand feet*.

The condition and mode of action of the Testes exert a similar influence over the male to that which is exerted over the female by the Ovaries, the secretion of the Semen being strictly analogous to the maturation of the Ova. The development of the body is also totally dependent upon their growth, and both intellectual power and moral disposition are, to an immense extent, influenced by them.

The form of the Testicles varies among the different Mammiferous Animals, equally with the other Organs, being sometimes round, at others oval, and at others again long and slender, as in the Whale. It is seldom, however, that they are contained in a *Scrotum*, as in Man, except among the Carnivori, the Ape, the Horse, and the cud-chewing beasts. In the Beaver, the Testicles are contained in the Perineum, and in some similar animals, in the abdomen, while in the Bat, and some others, they always glide back into the belly during the Rut. The Whale, Kangaroo, Opossum, Elephant and some others, have the Testicles fixed permanently in the Abdomen, one on each side of the Rectum. This is the case also in the Porpoise, whose Testicles at the time of heat attain an enormous size, having been found nine inches long and four wide, and weighing *two pounds each*.

In all cases the internal structure is much the same, and probably the formation of the Semen is always much the same process. The composition of it is also similar, and in every case it possesses animalcules, though they differ in form.

The Seminal Vesicles and Prostate Gland also vary in form, though, probably, they always serve a similar purpose. Some have only one Prostate, like Man, while others appear to have several, or rather it is much divided. Cowper's Glands also, though usually present, vary much in their development, and so do the Vasa Deferentia.

§ THE PENIS.

The Penis is a hollow spongy organ down which runs the passage from the bladder, called the *Urethra*, by which the urine escapes, which also serves for the exit of the Semen, as before explained.

The Anatomical structure of this organ is not thoroughly understood by Anatomists, owing to the difficulty which necessarily exists of dissecting it in its several states Sufficient, however, is known to explain its Physiological action, which is all we now require to know.

The body of the Penis consists of two distinct parts, each of which is very porous, or rather spongy. The upper part, which is the largest, is called the *Corpus Cavernosum ;* the under part, which is much the same in its structure, is called the *Corpus Spongiosum.* Both parts extend from the Pelvic Bones to the Glans at the end. The Corpus Cavernosum is divided down the middle into two parts, by a septum, or partition, and some physiologists on that account speak of *two* Cavernous bodies, or the *Corpora Cavernosa ;* it is, however, strictly one. These two parts are rounded on the under edge, so that when they come flat together there is a groove formed underneath, and in this groove lies the Urethra. They are both firmly attached to the front bones of the Pelvis under the Perineum, by two roots called the *Crura Penis.*

The Corpus Spongiosum surrounds the Canal of the Urethra underneath, and fills up the remainder of the groove, so as to round the whole organ. It terminates posteriorly in what is called *the Bulb of the Urethra.*

The whole organ is surrounded by the skin, excepting the end, where we find a body called *the Glans Penis,* which is both different and separate from either of those described. The inner fold of the skin of the Penis is attached to the termination of the Corpus Cavernosum, while the outer fold is extended beyond, so that it only partly covers the Glans, but is not attached to it, and may be drawn back. This loose skin is called the *prepuce*, or *foreskin*, and is the part cut off in the rite of *circumcision*. In some persons it extends further over the Glans than it does in others, but generally leaves more or less of it exposed. The Glans is probably an enlargement of the peculiar erectile tissue surrounding the Urethra, and is covered by a highly sensitive and vascular skin, of an exceedingly delicate structure. It is in the form of a section of a cone, and terminates on the posterior or upper margin of an elevated ridge, called the Corona Glandis, behind which is a depression called the Cervix, or Neck. In this depression are several glands called the *Glandula Odorifera*, which produce a whitish secretion, of a peculiar odor, that sometimes accumulates in great quantities in those who neglect proper cleanliness. On the under side of the Glans, the Prepuce is attached nearly at the end, by a fold or ligament, called the *Frænum*, or *Ligamentum Præputii*. This ligament, or cord, is sometimes too short, and during erection is so pulled upon as to cause great annoyance ; occasionally, it even ruptures, or tears, causing severe pain, with loss of blood.

These parts constitute the substance of the Penis, and are therefore most essential to the performance of its proper functions.

The peculiarity of the structure of the Corpus Cavernosum, and of the Corpus Spongiosum, consists in their being full of curiously arranged blood-vessels and cells, or cavities, like those of *sponge*, all communicating with each other, and being connected with the main branches of an artery and a vein. In ordinary states these vessels, excepting the larger ones, and also the cells, are nearly or quite empty, but under appropriate excitement the blood from the artery is impelled into them and fills them up, in consequence of which the organ enlarges, like sponge when filled with water. This is called the Phenomenon of *Erection*, and it depends upon a peculiar sensibility proper to the parts, which are therefore sometimes spoken of as being composed of *Erectile Tissue*. There is no other part of the body that in any way resembles the Penis in structure, except the *Clitoris* in the female, which has a similar Tissue, and is usually capable of erection to a certain extent, in precisely the same way.

When the excitement is withdrawn, the blood ordinarily flows back by way of the cavernosus vein, and the erection subsides, but sometimes its return is prevented, and the erection then remains, though all excitement is gone. The Corpus Spongiosum is so distinct from the Corpus Cavernosum that erection will sometimes take place in one and not in the other, which necessarily curves the organ, or draws it into the form of a bow, producing what is termed a *chordee*. The erection and emission of Semen is also assisted by a number of different muscles particularly by one called the *Erector Penis*, or *Ischio Cavernosus* Muscle. Sometimes in erection the rush of blood will be so sudden and violent that the vessels will burst, and the erectile tissue be thus totally destroyed. In some persons the filling up of the blood-vessels always occurs in a very short time, while in others it is the reverse; and in like manner the erection subsides in a short time in some, while in others it will continue for a long period and subside very slowly. This depends upon some peculiarity in the vital action of the blood-vessels, not yet understood. In old age the blood generally flows in slower, and flows out much quicker than it does in youth, so that the erection is longer in taking place and goes down more rapidly.

The uses of the Penis, as before remarked, are two-fold, firstly it serves as a conduit, to convey the urine from the body, and secondly as a conductor to carry the semen into the female organs. For the first use erection is not necessary, but it is for the second, and therefore its proper occurrence is both natural and essential to the performance of one of the functions of our nature.

The form of this organ varies in different animals, for the purpose of adaption, and is sometimes very singular. In some it is covered with *spines*, so as to give great pain to the female during connection, as in the cat, while in others its structure causes that act to be much lengthened, as in the dog. In birds, the male organ is merely rudimentary, so that there is no actual union, properly speaking, but merely an *emission* into the female organs. In the human being there are occasional deviations from the ordinary development, and sometimes even peculiarities in structure. Thus instances have been known of the interior of the Corpus Cavernosum being more or less ossified, so that a distinct bone always existed in the middle of the organ This is often the case in Negroes, and in some o the lower animals it is natural. In a few rare instances the Penis has been found *double*, or rather divided into two parts, only one of which, of course, contains a urethra, though both may be capable of erection as I observed in one case in my own practice. Probably amputation of the imperfect part might have been safely effected, but as little inconvenience was experienced it was not thought necessary.

The various peculiarities of structure and development that interfere with the functions of this part will be treated under appropriate heads as we proceed.

§ ABSENCE AND MALFORMATION OF THE PENIS.

Besides being liable to be lost by several accidents, and by necessary operations, the Penis may also be deficient from birth. I have seen instances when it was not more than a quarter of an inch in length, and sometimes only a slight swelling, like the top of a small tumor. In such cases, of course, there can be no *connection*, but still such men may be *fathers* providing all the other parts are perfect, because, as before explained, the semen may impregnate if it be only shed *within the external lips*, which of course may be effected in the worst of these instances. I have known instances of married couples, with families, who never had any association, from similar causes. It is unnecessary to say, however, that marriage should *never* take place in such cases without the nature of the infirmity being first known, though I believe the law would declare any marriage binding if impregnation was possible. In giving an opinion under such circumstances, it is, however, difficult to decide this point. In general, in healthy females, the placing of the semen artificially in the vagina will induce conception, but not always. Hunter relates an instance where he advised the injection of the semen with a syringe, after its escape from the husband, and impregnation followed. There are some females, however, in whom its absorption will not take place without a certain amount of 'excitement, dependent upon actual association, so that there will always be more or less uncertainty, and much less probability than when no such deprivation exists. Independent of this, however, there are other considerations that should forbid the marrying of men so situated, unless with a full knowledge of the circumstance and its consequences by *both*. In some of these cases, especially, when a portion of the Organ is left, as after operations and accidents, the difficulty may be much remedied by an instrument, so constructed as to fit on the part remaining, and resembling that which is lost. I have known instances of conception following the use of such an instrument, when the Penis itself was not more than *a quarter of an inch* long. But then the semen was formed in great quantities, and was remarkably healthy.

In some children the Penis is tied down to the Scrotum, or some other of the neighboring parts, by bands, which never allow it to be extended, and of course prevent the performance of the functions. I saw one child of seven years in whom it grew flat on the Abdomen, causing great trouble and annoyance in urinating, from the direction in which the fluid had to flow. Nearly all such cases can be easily corrected by a slight operation at any age, the adhesion being usually only by the skin, but are better attended to early in life. The one referred to was put right very readily, and in two years' time, scarcely a trace of the operation could be seen.

Occasionally the Penis will have a wrong *direc*-

tion, being turned so much either on one side, under, or upwards, that association is impossible. If this depends upon contraction of the skin, or of the muscular fibres, it may be corrected by simply dividing them, but if t results from a tumor, or swelling, that must be removed before any alteration can be effected. Aneurisms, and swellings of the veins will sometimes bring about such deviations, and so will too long-continued erection, by rupturing some of the cells or vessels, and so causing accumulation of blood. I knew one instance of this kind in which every time erection occurred a large tumor was formed on the left side, full of blood, which of course turned the end of the organ to the right side, and thus prevented connection. This accident had been caused by numerous forcible and long-continued erections in one night, during intoxication. The tumor was as large as an egg, and when full could be distinctly felt to pulsate. It was also very painful, and appeared almost ready to burst. The remedies proposed were cold astringent lotions and wearing a thin plate of smooth horn over the part, bound on so firmly as to prevent any swelling from accumulation of blood. This plan succeeded very well in giving relief, though it is probable there will always be more or less tendency to a recurrence of the trouble.

Besides Scrofulous and other Tumors in the Penis there will sometimes be bony swellings, and accumulations like calculi or stone in the bladder. These may either compress the Urethra, and so prevent the passage of the Urine and Semen, or they may curve the organ so as to prevent its use ; in general, however, they can be removed.

Sometimes the Frænum or cord that binds down

the prepuce at the end underneath, will be so snort or contracted that during erection the point of the Glans will be pulled under. This not only prevents the Semen being thrown straight forward, but even prevents connection in many instances, either by causing severe pain, or by bending the end of the organ too much. This difficulty is easily remedied, by cutting through the cord with a pair of scissors, or a lancet. I advised a gentleman out West how to do this, in a letter, and he wrote afterwards to inform me that he had succeeded perfectly, with his *razor*. It is simply necessary to take care to cut only deep enough to *just sever the cord*, and afterwards to keep the parts stretched asunder, so that they do not grow together again ; a simple dressing of cloths dipt in *cold water* is all that is required after. I have known the cord to be eaten through with caustic, but the plan is not so good as cutting, being more tedious and painful, and leaving a larger scar. In some persons it has been broken suddenly during a violent erection, or on attempting coition, but such accidents are always painful, and are better avoided by a timely operation.

§ WANT OF DEVELOPMENT, OR CONGENITAL SMALL. SIZE OF THE PENIS.

It is sometimes difficult to say whether the Penis is *too* short or not, because there is no precise standard of limitation, and in different people the development varies very much. In some persons it never grows from the condition in which we find it in childhood, while in others it will attain a medium size, and in others again it will be nearly rudimentary. This may also be totally independent of any deficiency in the other organs, though most usually they correspond more or less. Thus I have seen a man of forty years of age in whom the Penis was only two inches long, and about as thick as the little finger, but whose Testes were of a full average size, and who had strong sexual feelings, with a full flow of Semen. Sometimes the organ can scarcely be traced at all, being merely like a wart or small tumor.

When the non-development of the Penis is dependent upon a general torpor of the Genital Organs, more especially of the Testes, their action must be aroused, and their functions fully established, in the manner pointed out in the chapter on the Testes. If this can be done, the Penis may be made to grow even to an advanced period of life, as I have there shown.

In those cases in which the Penis alone is not sufficiently developed a different treatment is required, as it is simply a local effect we wish to produce. In some of these instances the organ, though small, is capable of perfect erection, and both connection and impregnation may be effected by its means ; it is not, then, a matter of such urgent moment for any improvement to be effected, though under certain circumstances it may be desirable. More frequently, however, erection either does not take place at all, or so imperfectly, that coition is impossible, and the flow of Semen is so imperfect and irregular that impregnation can seldom be effected, even artificially. Under such circumstances it is a matter of the greatest consequence to produce an increased development, so that both these functions may be performed, and it may be both new and pleasing, to many persons, to learn that there are means by which this desirable end may be often attained, even under the most unpromising circumstances. It is proper to remark, however, that the cases now referred to are those in which the small size is *congenital*, or existing from birth, and not in those which the organ has *decreased*, from disease or excess, after having been of average development, though even in many of them, when the constitutional stamina is not too much impaired, the same means will frequently restore what has been temporarily lost.

The causes that prevent the proper development of this organ, as well as of others, are of course unknown in those cases that are congenital, because they operate before birth, but in those that become arrested during childhood or youth, we generally trace it to early masturbation, blows on the Testicles and other accidents, or to some severe disease which has impaired the vital energy very much. Some diseases are particularly apt to affect young persons in this way, as the *Mumps* for instance, which often make the Testes swell.

Scarlet Fever and Measles, when severe, I have known to seriously injure the virile power, but not so frequently as rickets or scrofula.

A similar deficiency is sometimes found in females, in some the Uterus or Ovaries being very small, though the Vagina may be large enough to allow of coition, while in others these organs will be of usual size, but the Vagina will be too small, so that marriage is not allowable. In my work on "The Diseases of Woman," I refer to such cases, and explain what can be done to relieve them.

To effect an enlargement of the Penis, in addition to every means proper to improve the general health

and impart stamina, there are certain *mechanical*
and *manual* applications, the effects of which, under
right direction, are often of the most unexpected
and pleasing character. To understand the nature
of these, and their mode of action, it is necessary
to bear in mind the anatomical structure of the
organ, and the requisites for erection. That phenomenon, it will be recollected from our previous description, depends essentially upon the filling up of
the vessels and cells of the spongy and cavernous
bodies with blood, and of course if there be any
fault in their make or mode of connection, or if the
blood does not flow into them, erection cannot take
place.   Now this is precisely the fault that is found,
to exist in most of the cases of non-development
above referred to, and is what requires to be corrected. . On dissecting such cases after death we
find that the cells and minute vessels have never
been congested or filled with blood, and consequently the organ has never been able to grow nor
become erected.   In the same way after long continued excess, or debilitating disease, the artery
seems to lose its power of transmitting the blood
with sufficient vigor, and the cells, from want of
being filled, decrease in size, and eventually grow
up more or less, causing the organ to shrink.   This
is the reason also why absolute suppression of sexual excitement, if continued too long, will make the
organ waste away, instead of increasing its power,
as many uninformed people suppose.

The object to be accomplished it will be seen is to
open these cells, and cause the blood to flow into
them, so as gradually to increase their size, and
dispose them to fill spontaneously, from natural
excitement.

In some persons, who have always shunned all *thougnts* of sexual matters, from a notion that they are improper, it is sometimes sufficient merely to encourage such thoughts to a proper extent, and the excitement this gives rise to in the parts will act favorably on their growth. In others the daily employment of a warm local both, with brisk rubbing, and the use of a stimulating ointment, which I shall hereafter describe, will be found still more efficacious ; and if this treatment be regularly persisted in, under judicious direction, combined with proper internal remedies, it will succeed in a large number of the cases ordinarily met with. It is requisite, however, that the external and internal stimulants should be exactly apportioned to the wants and capabilities of the individual's system, and that a strict watch should be kept upon the action and effects of each so as to know when to increase or decrease their power, and when to suspend their action altogether. Until over forty years of age, if the *form* of the organ is perfect, and its development not too small, a considerable change may be effected in this way, though the younger the patient is the more readily the parts are acted upon.

I once had a patient call upon me from Cuba, the son of a rich planter, who was troubled with this imperfection, and who was intensely desirous that it might be remedied so as to allow of marriage. He was about twenty-three years of age, and of a strong, robust habit of body, with excellent health. On examination the Penis was found about *two inches and a half* in length, and about as thick as the forefinger, properly formed, but with little more sensibility than any other part of the body. The Testicles were fully developed, and the sexual feeling

was quite strong. There had been frequent emi*-
sion of semen, under strong excitement, but no
erection, and consequently no connection could take
place. Upon inquiry I found that he had been
brought up to a very rigid code of morals, and had
imbibed certain notions about the necessity of not
indulging sexual desires, if the mind was wished to
become powerful, as he was very ambitious of
distinction he made a perfect anchorite of himself.
The bodily effect of such a course has been seen—
its effect on the mind was to make him wayward,
irritable and unhappy. A short time before he
came on to see me he met with a young lady with
whom he fell violently in love, and immediately
the desire for marriage arose, but with it came the
fear that he was totally incapacited. The new
desire, so strongly awakened, together with the fears
he felt, operated so intensely upon him that he became almost furiously insane. On assuring him,
however, that there was a reasonable prospect of
his attaining a more perfect state he became calmer,
and patiently submitted himself to the prescribed
treatment.

The first object was to induce as much heat as
possible in the organ, so as to promote the flow of
blood to it. This was accomplished by the use of a
hot stimulating lotion, two or three times a day, followed by brisk rubbing with flannel and soft brushes.
In three weeks the effect of this treatment became
obvious—erections occurred, partial at first, but
ultimately quite forcible, and the organ evidently
began to increase permanently in size. In addition
to this he was directed to use some stimulant drops,
and to live generously, to impart as much vigor as
possible to the Generative Organs. The flow of

semen soon became much larger than before under this treatment, and the procreative instinct much more powerful. There was still one fault, however, and that was a want of power in the *muscles* that assist in erection and coition, more especially in the Erector Penis muscle. This was remedied by frequent *shampooing*, and pressing of their fibres till they acquire volume and firmness, the same as any other muscle would do under similar treatment.

This system was rigidly pursued for six months under my own inspection, at the end of which time the Penis was four inches long, when erect, and quite firm, so that coition was possible. At this period he was desirous to return home, and as he was evidently determined to pursue the same treatment himself, I consented to his doing so, though I would have preferred for him to have staid still longer. I heard from him eleven months after his departure, and he then informed me that the improvement had still continued till he no longer thought it necessary to proceed. He was then intending to marry in about three months. The delight and gratitude of this young man were unbounded, rescued as he was from the very depths of despondency and despair, and raised, as he expressed it, " to the highest pitch of human happiness."

In the course of my practice I have had numerous similar cases, some of them resulting satisfactorily from the same treatment, and others requiring a different plan, which I will now explain.

When the means above described fail to induce a sufficient flow of blood into the Erectile Tissue an instrument is employed, called a *Congester*. It consists of a Tube, the size of which is adapted to the organ to which is fitted an exhausting Air-

Pump. The Penis being introduced into this the air is more or less exhausted, and the blood of course flows into the contained part immediately So great is the rush of blood, in fact, that if the exhaustion was continued too far, or made too suddenly, the Tissue would burst. In a short time, with care, the part begins to swell and look red, and erection, more or less complete, soon takes place This *never fails*, unless the vitality of the part be totally gone, or the structure of the Tissues completely disorganized. I have seen some of the most remarkable results follow from the use of this instrument that were perhaps ever witnessed, in a medical way. I have known patients in whom the whole organ was not *half an inch long*, and without the slightest tendency to erection, and yet the Congester has caused it to grow, and has given it power, until perfectly capable for the purposes it was intended for. Sometimes there only appears a simple protuberance, like a Tumor, while at other times the organ is long and suprisingly small, and quite flaccid, but still the Congester will impel the blood into the Tissues and produce the effect desired. Sometimes, it is true, we cannot gain so much as would be desirable, but nearly always sufficient for Nature's requirements, and very often as perfect in condition as if no imperfection had ever existed.

In conjunction with the Congester it is also requisite, in most cases, to act upon the muscles, by shampooing, as they are usually deficient in power, and without their action the Penis cannot erect, though it may become firmly congested.

This practice of shampooing the Perineal and Genital Muscles, to improve the erectile power, was originated in Asia, but has been known and practised in Europe for many years. The process is both tedious and somewhat painful, and requires both skill and knowledge in the operation. In Turkey, men make a regular business of this, and they succeed admirably. In this country it is necessary to direct the patient himself, or hired assistants, and the constant supervision of the medical man is therefore required. To perform this operation to advantage, it is best to have the parts made perfectly bare and smooth, and then lubricated with a proper ointment. The operator then presses the end of the fore-finger firmly into the muscle, passing it along backwards and forwards, in the direction of the fibres, till the muscle becomes hot and swells. This is done with all the muscles whose action is required, and it should be practised every day till the effect is manifest. At first the shampooing causes considerable pain and soreness, but this soon passes away, and then the muscle feels firm to the touch, and is found to be much stronger. There are two men in New-York whom I have had occasion to employ for this purpose with so many patients, that they have become quite expert, and I can always depend upon success from their efforts when it is possible.

It must be recollected that the various means I have described require a long period to be put fully in operation, and are such as can be commanded only by those who have plenty of both time and money at their disposal.

With those who are fortunately so situated as to have these essential requisites, the gain is certainly great, and well worth what it costs, and I have never known one, who was successfully treated, who did not say he thought no price could be dear to pay. Many a man has been saved from insanity or suicide by these means, and many a domestic hearth has been made the scene of happiness and delight, that was previously the abode of recrimination and despair.

I have treated patients of all ages, from mere youths up to mature age ; the oldest I recollect being about *fifty-two*, and in *most of them* with a success that has been as pleasing to them as it was gratifying to myself. Some of the means I have mentioned are scarcely known in this country, and are certainly not put into general practice ; the account I have given of them may, therefore, be the means of giving many sufferers the first intimation that help can be had. In some fictitious works on these subjects, pretending to be written by eminent men, but really made up only for sale, such things are partially referred to, but in such a way as to be of no real utility. In one of these an account is given of many *drugs*, said to be proper to use in cases of debility, some of which are highly dangerous, and many of which *do not exist at all.* The present book is, I believe, the only one on these subjects that is really scientific, as well as popular.

One of the most remarkable cases I ever treated was that of a young man of nineteen, who was brought to me by his father, himself a physician. In this person there was scarcely any appearance of a Penis, but only a small Tumor, not projecting more than a quarter of an inch, in the centre of which was the opening of the Urethra. It was quite sensitive, however, and seemed rather as if compressed downwards. The Testes were of average size, and the semen sereted in sufficient quan-

tity, occasionally, so that little seemed wanting but
the small organ. I at once told his father that I felt
assured much improvement could be obtained, but
that it would require much time and attention, with
great endurance on the part of the patient himself.
They were both delighted to hear this, and the
young man testified his desire that I should com
mence the treatment immediately, which I did. A
Congester was constructed specially for the case,
and applied daily. The lower part was of glass,
so that its operation could be seen, and it was observed that immediately the tube was exhausted of
air the Penis seemed to be drawn forward, and extended to full two inches. The patient complained
of great pain in the part during the operation, from
the rush of blood into the cells, and it remained
exceedingly tender for several days after. The
Congester was not applied again till this soreness
had subsided, but in the meantime the stimulating
hot lotions were used, and shampooing of the muscles
was practised. It was observed that even the first
application had evidently caused some protrusion,
and the young man remarked that the *internal* sensations were different from what he had ever before
experienced. The internal medication in his case
was of a more stimulating character than ordinary
because the sexual impulse was not very strong,
and only occasionally manifested. His diet was
directed to be as nourishing as possible, with wine
for drink, and every day he rode out on horseback
after a warm bath, followed by brisk rubbing of the
whole surface of the body After the first effect
had subsided the Congester was used daily, and fol
lowed by the shampooing, for ten weeks, by which
time a permanent advance had been made To

Penis measured full two inches in its ordinary state, and in the Congester was extended to three. Partial erections occured at times during sleep, and the procreative instinct became more active and permanent. I then directed him to return home for three months, and only continue the general treatment, so that I might see if Nature herself could complete the work. At the end of three months he came back to me with a still further improvement, though slight. He was then put under the old treatment again, and this time the effects were still more satisfactory. In two months, under the Congester, the Penis measured four inches, and in the ordinary state remained permanently at three, with firm erections and copious emissions of semen Finding, therefore, that every requirement of Nature could be fulfilled even as he was, and that further improvement would evidently take place with the growth of the system, I desisted from further treatment and sent him home *cured*. His father was as much astonished as gratified, and another physician who had seen him and pronounced him a *Hermaphrodite*, would scarcely believe it was the same being.

Another case was that of a man who had married at thirty-two, though imperfect, from a mistaken idea that marriage would effect a cure. The result may be imagined ; the misery of two human beings could scarcely be more complete. In his despair a friend brought him to me for my opinion. On examination I found the Penis not very small, nor in any way imperfect, but it had never been *erected*, and seemed incapable of being so. The semen was secreted plentifully enough, and the instinct was as strong as was desirable. I told him without any hesitation that he could be made perfect enough for his marital duties in a short time, providing he would follow strictly my directions, and submit to my treatment, which he was willing enough to do. The Congester was applied, and with the happiest results. At the third application a powerful erection was produced that did not subside for a considerable time, owing to want of perfect action in the cavernous veins. This, however, was soon remedied, and in two weeks, by the use of the Congester alone, natural erections occurred spontaneously, as perfect as could be desired. In a word he was perfectly cured, and is now the father of two children.

I have also had numerous instances of persons who had lost the power of erection from sexual and other excesses, from mental anxiety and from the effect of debilitating disease. In a great portion of these the result has also been favorable, though in many all vitality had left the organs before I saw them, and in others the structure was completely disorganized. Many young men especially, victims of Masturbation, whose organs had ceased growing, have by these means been rescued from impotency and imperfection. Many a man of mature age also, whose powers were unimpaired, but who could not exercise them, owing to this particular debility, has been restored to his former capability in the same way.

The Congester is not an instrument adapted for self treatment, and I would not advise any one to attempt its use without proper directions and supervision. I have known it to do great mischief, with inexperienced people, and fail in accomplishing any good. In one man who had it applied too forcibly and suddenly, the cells were nearly all ruptured, or broken into one another, so that severe inflammation was produced, and the power of erection was for ever lost, by any means.

There are some means, however, that all persons may use, provided they know when they are appropriate to the cause. The pressing and shampooing may be partially practised by the patient himself, though very imperfectly, but the general directions as to diet and exercise may be observed of course by all. Perhaps, however, there is no other functional disability so difficult to treat, or that requires so much skill and such unremitting attention.

In addition to the means already described, there are some others occasionally useful, but which are not so generally applicable. *Galvanism* is sometimes an excellent agent, when there is *nervous* insensibility combined with the other disabilities. A very good mode to use it is to galvanize the metallic congester, while the organ is engaged within it. The power must not be too great, however, nor the application continued too long, or there will be partial paralysis.

The French have a practice of *Flagellation* which is sometimes very efficacious, and will induce erection in a short time. It is rather severe, however, and few have courage or endurance sufficient to continue it long enough to derive full benefit. The *Flagellator* is made of six or eight small twisted thongs, about as thick as a violin string, but very flexible, and about eight inches long. To operate with it to the best advantage the parts should be made bare, and perfectly smooth, and the Flagellator must then be applied the whole length of the Penis, and on the Pubes, Perineum, and inside of the thighs, till the flesh is quite red and smarts The flogging must never be so hard, or long continued, as to make any bruises, nor leave any soreness, but merely sufficient to make it red and feel hot, with slight smarting. Usually about a quarter of an hour is sufficient, every day. After the flaggellation the parts should be well bathed in hot water, and the patient should recline.

This treatment may seem singular to those who never heard of it before, but it is undoubtedly more efficacious, in numerous cases, than any one could well believe who had not seen it practised. I have known many patients resort to it with the happiest results, who could not stay with me long enough for the usual treatment.—In some it will produce powerful erections the first time, and lead to an influx of blood to the parts that soon stimulates their growth.

Firing is another practice that may be resorted to, if others fail, for rousing the dormant energies of these parts in deficient growth.—It consists in *burning* the parts with a smooth iron button, made hot by plunging it in boiling water. The parts are first made smooth and then the button is taken out of the water and pressed suddenly on, repeating it as fast as possible, till the whole length of the organ has been operated upon. No part should be touched twice, nor should the iron remain on more than an instant. The pain is very slight, and no blister is raised, the places only turning *white* at first, and afterwards remaining red.—The firings should be repeated only at intervals of three or four days, waiting till the effects of one are gone off before another is practised.·

This process is sometimes astonishingly effective, a single application producing such a powerful effect

PLATE VIII

Section of the Penis

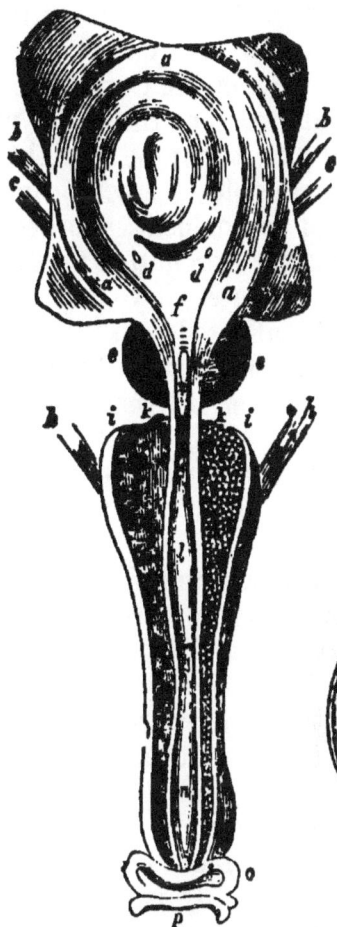

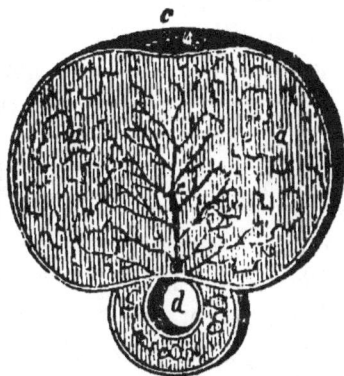

Fig. 2.

EXPLANATION.

Fig. 1.—*a.* The Bladder.—*b, b.* The Ureters.—*c, c.* Vasa Deferentia.—*d, d.* Mouths of the Ureters.—*e.* Prostate Gland.—*f.* Veru Montanum.—*g.* Seminal Ducts.—*h.* Ischio Cavernous Muscles.—*i. i.* Bulb of the Urethra.—*k, k.* Cowper's Glands.—*l.* Wide part of the Urethra.—*m.* Narrow Part.—*n.* Second wide part.—*o.* The Glans—*p.* The Prepuce.

The spongy structure of the Penis is shown on one side, and its blood vessels on the other.

Fig. 2.—*a, a.* Corpus Cavernosum.—*b.* Division or Septum —*c.* Corpus Spongiosum.—*d.* Urethra.—*e.* Great Vein.

that no further treatment is required.—Care is required, however, not to produce too much inflammation, nor to operate too near the Testes. Sometimes the development will be much less on one side of the Penis than the other, or less in the Corpus Spongiosum than the Cavernosum, so that the organ will not be straight but curved ; or it may be straight in the ordinary state but not capable of erecting in all parts alike. This state of permanent chordee is perhaps better treated by the flagellation or firing than by any other means, because they can be applied locally, and only to the affected part.

It may perhaps be as well to remark here that a modification of the congester is sometimes of great service in certain torpid states of the female organs, and that some of the other treatment is also occasionally applied to them, in a modified form, with the happiest results.

In addition to the derangements and diseases here enumerated, there are also many others to which the Penis is subject, but these are all which especially concern marriage. In my work on the Male Organs, every known affection is fully treated upon, so that if a man wishes to know about anything not spoken of here, he can be sure of finding it there.

The Penis is, perhaps, more variable in its form and situation, among the different Mammiferous Animals, than any other organ. It is only among the Bats and Apes that it hangs down from the Pubic bone, like it does in Man, being in the others always included in a sheath. In the Cat, the Rat, and some other animals it is directed *backwards*, and in the Beaver it is drawn far back into a kind of canal, like a Vagina, while in the Kangaroo it is even surrounded by the Sphincter Muscle of the

Anus.   In many animals the Prepuce is very long,
and like a sheath, and the Penis is ordinarily drawn
into it, when not erect, as in many of those above
mentioned, and as we see in the Horse ; but sometimes
the Penis is permanently so long that it cannot be
drawn into the sheath in a straight form, but has to
be bent, like the letter S, as we see in the Elephant,
and some others.

Those animals that have the Penis directed backwards, as the Cat, for instance, urinate in that
direction, but when, copulating, the organ is drawn
out of the sheath and bent forwards.   In those
species the females of which have a double Vagina, like the Kangaroo, the Penis is also double,
so that there is one for each passage, each having
a Tube to convey Semen, though there is but one
Urethra for the urine, which opens between the two
Glans.   The Alligator also has a double-headed
Penis.   The Glans on the end of the Penis is even
more variable than any other part, being seldom
soft and spongy, as in Man, but sometimes hard,
horny, and covered with sharp points, and sometimes even it scarcely exists in any form.   In some
of the Apes it is spread out like a mushroom, with
slit edges, and occasionally covered with sharp,
hard spines.   This is the case also in the Bat, and
partly so in the Shrew-Mouse, while in the Hedgehog
it is divided into three lobes.   The Hyæna has it
formed like the broad knob of a door, and in the
Bear and Dog it is like a long club.   The Glans of
the Cat is covered with horny spines directed backwards, which probably cause pain to the female, and
draw forth those horrible cries which these animals
emit during copulation.   In the Guinea Pig it is
covered with scales, and has two horny *hooks*, while

in the Hare it is drawn out to one long, thin point, and in some other animals into two points. In some it is even covered with stiff hairs, and in many has rough knobs, or Tubercles. In the Rhinoceros the Glans is *bell-shaped*, in the Horse it is bulbous, and in some of the Whales it is shaped like a Tongue, while in others it is conical. The most singular form, however, is in that curious animal, the *Ornithoryncrus*, in which it is very large, square, divided in two parts, and covered all over with spines. The *Bone* of the Penis is found in many animals, as well as in the Negro occasionally. It is very large in the Dog, but small and thin in the Cat, while in the Racoon it is crooked, like the letter S, and in some others it is formed like a hook. In the Squirrel its termination is flattened out, like a shovel.

CHAPTER VII.

THE SEMEN AND ANIMALCULES.

THE vivifying principle secreted by the male testes is a yellowishly white semi-fluid substance, having a peculiar odor.   It is slightly viscid and of a saltish savor, when fresh.   On examination it is found to consist of two distinct parts, one nearly fluid and the other like globules of half-dissolved starch, which, however, both melt together when it is exposed some time to the air.   The peculiar odor of the Semen appears to be derived from some of the parts through which it passes, for when taken from the testes it has scarcely any smell at all.

Chemical analysis shows us that the semen differs but little in its composition from other substances found in the body.   In 1000 parts there are about 900 water; 60 animal mucilage; 10 soda; and 30 of phosphate of lime, with a peculiar animal principle, the composition of which is unknown. This analysis it must be recollected is that of the semen, as it leaves the body, that is, the secretion of the Testes, Vesicles, Prostate Gland, and other parts, united together.   How far the pure semen from the testes alone differs from this is not known. By some the starchy portion only is supposed to be produced by the Testes.

The Seminal Animalculæ.—The most curious peculiarity of the semen, and in many respects the most important, is that there always exists in it, when perfect, a number of remarkable living beings, called the *Zoospermes*, or Semina Animal-culæ. These beings were discovered many years ago, but have not been accurately studied and described till very recently. The representations and descriptions given of them in old works are mostly incorrect, and sometimes very extravagant, and calculated to mislead rather than inform. Some physiologists, who saw them imperfectly, even doubted if they were living beings. The perfection of that magical instrument, the microscope, however, and the patient investigation of such men as *Pouchet* and his coadjuitors have not only corrected these old errors, but have also disclosed to us new truths, more wonderful even than the wild dreams of former times.

As far as yet investigated these Animalcules exist universally, in the Semen of all animals whatever, but have a peculiar form and development in each.

It is also ascertained that they are developed from a species of *egg*, or ovum, called the seminal granules, or vesicles. Under the microscope a number of these can always be detected, like little globules of mucus, and they are observed to undergo a regular series of changes similar to those of the female ovary. When first observed they are round and merely contain a number of small granules, which are the Animalcules, in a rudimentary state. At a further stage these granules are found to be developed into small Animalcules, while the containing vesicles have expanded and become elongated, or egg-shaped. Finally the vesicle breaks open at one end, and the Animalcules escape ; being at first very small and gradually growing afterwards to the size we ordinarily see them

The figures in the accompanying plate represent the form of the Zoospermes and the changes in the vesicles, as seen under the microscope, in the human being.

In different beings the form both of the Vesicle and the Animalculæ varies much, and occasionally the Zoospermes undergo some remarkable metamor·phoses before assuming their final form.

In the human being there are about *thirty* Zoospermes in each Vesicle, but in some beings there are more, and in others not so many. The number of vesicles varies very much, at different times, even in the same individual.

The precise size of the Zoospermes is of course difficult to ascertain, but M. Poucher estimates their *length* at about the *ten thousandth part of an ordinary hair*, and their weight at about the *hundred and forty thousand millionth part of a grain!* A spot as large as a mustard seed, he remarks, will sometimes contain *fifty thousand* of them, or more.

Notwithstanding this extreme minuteness, we are now tolerably well acquainted with their peculiarities of structure, and even with many of their *habits*, nor need this excite much surprise when it is recollected that there are beings *still smaller* that have been studied with even greater success. In Fig. 3 and 4 of the last plate, the form of the human Zoospermes is given correctly, and their internal organization is also *partly* shown by the part marked *a. a.* Fig 4, which is supposed to be the stomach. In the perfect state each one has a sucker at the larger end, represented by the white dot in Fig. 3 and 4, by which they can attach themselves to any object. They are observed to change their skins at certain periods, like snakes, and we sometimes find the loose

159

PLATE IX.

Seminal Animalcules and Vesicles.

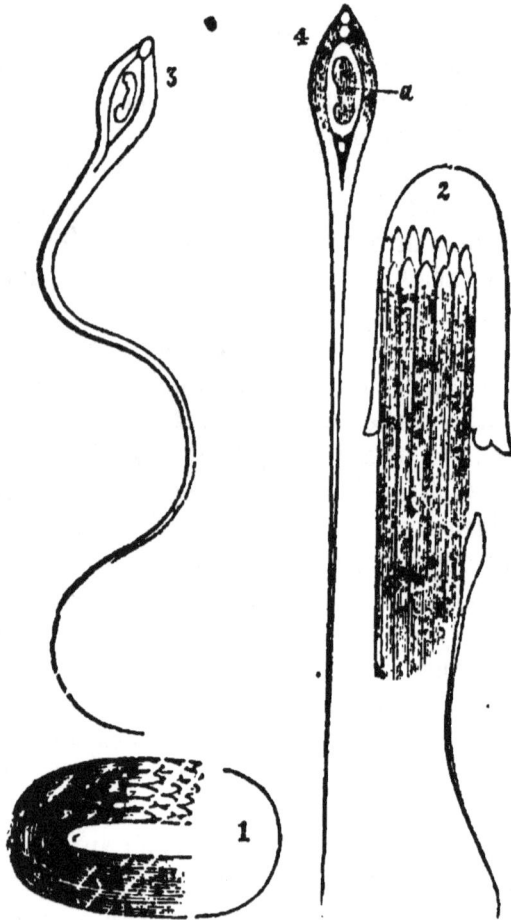

EXPLANATION.

1. One of the Vesicles, containing the Animalcules in a rudimentary state, coiled up.——2. The Vesicle broken open, and the Animalcules escaping.——3 and 4. Perfect Animalcules.—*a.* Is the stomach and intestines. The two round white spots at the top indicate the mouth and the sucker by which it attaches itself to anything. These are magnified many thousand times.

skin hanging about them in shreds ; or cast off
quite whole.   In some animals they have a number
of hairs, or cilia, by the motion of which they move
in the fluid, and some even have perfect fins.   One
Physiologist assures us that he distinctly saw they
were sexual, and that he could readily distinguish
the male and female !   They are usually lively and
active, with peculiar motions, some of which are
performed in concert and others singly, with great
perseverance and regularity ;   thus a number of
them will sometimes form into a ring, with their
heads all one way, and run round and round in a
circle for a considerable time ; or one may be seen
by itself pushing before it a large globule of mucus,
or blood, many times heavier than itself, for several
minutes together.   One peculiarity is observable in
all of them, and that is an almost invariable tendency to move only *straight forward*, and they will
seldom turn to go back even though they meet with
an obstruction, but often attach themselves to it by
the sucker and remain till they die.   Very often
they are seen to enter into combats, and a number
of them will fight till only one is left alive.   They
will live for some hours out of the body, particularly
if put in warm water, in which their motions may be
readily seen.

The Zoospermes are not found before Puberty,
nor usually in extreme old age.   Many diseases also
destroy them, and several drugs have the same
power.   In all cases where they are absent or destroyed, from whatever cause it may be, the semen
cannot impregnate, though in every other respect it
may be quite perfect, and the vigor of the patient
seem not in the least impaired.   This has been proved
by filtering them away, and by destroying them

The development of the Zoospermes it will be observed is strictly analogous to that of the ova or eggs in the females. Thus they are first found in the form of little granules, enclosed in a Vesicle which bursts as they become more perfect and allows them to escape. In some animals there is even a periodical development of them, similar to that of the ova in the female, with which it usually corresponds. In such animals the Testes are small as other times, and increase in size at these periods, because the Vesicles only attain their full growth then.

In tracing the semen from its source, we find that the animalcules are not developed till it reaches the Seminal Vesicles, and are sometimes not perfect till it has reached the Prostate Gland. In the Testicles we never find the Zoospermes themselves, but only the Vesicles containing the granules, which gradually develop as it proceeds further on.

The Testes may therefore be compared to the Ovaries, the Seminal Vessels to the Graafian Vesicles, and the Seminal Granules to the ova. Some Physiologists consider the granules to be the *ova* of the animalcules themselves, but this we cannot yet decide, though it is certain the animalcules originate from them.

The importance of these facts, in giving us a correct knowledge of the nature and proper treatment of many diseases of these organs, will be seen as we proceed, particularly when treating on Impotence and Seminal losses.

The actual process of conception is also made more clear from some of these details. For instance the tendency which the Animalcules have to move only *straight forward*, is in all probability the reason why they make their way up into the womb from the vagina, and impregnate the egg. If it were not for this tendency, combined with their great motive power, the two principles could not be brought to gether. Their power of living out of the body for some time is also necessary to impregnation, be cause they may not reach their destination imme diately. It is found that they will live in the femal organs, when these are healthy, as long as *twenty-six* hours, and of course during any part of that time conception may take place. Sometimes conception may take place in a few minutes, and at other times not till as many hours after the association of the two sexes. It has been found on dissecting an animal killed *ten hours* after connection, that the semen had not then reached the ovum, though it usually passes into the womb almost *immediately.*

It is evident from this how incorrect it is to speak of the *moment of conception,* as if it were a period certainly known. No greater mistake could be made than to suppose that it always corresponds with the moment of *connection,* because it *may* be as much as twenty hours after, or more. It is also evident from these facts why it is that conception is possible *without actual connection.* If the semen is merely deposited in the *external lips* it may impregnate, because the animalcules may make their way from thence up to the womb. It is also of littl consequence *how* the semen is deposited in the fe male organs, providing it be perfect, and this, explains why it is that conception can be effected *ar-tificially,* by merely injecting the *semen* in the female organs with a syringe, or otherwise, which has often been done. The mere presence of the male organ is in no way essential ; which is the reason

why a certain mode of attempting to *prevent* concep
tions often fails. It was also remarked, in a previous
part, that sexual *feeling* in the female was not
necessary to conception, and this will now be evident when it is recollected that the Animalculæ
move up into the womb by their own vital power.
It is probable, however, that this feeling often *conduces* to conception, by establishing certain favorable conditions of the parts, and therefore that event
is not so *likely* to occur during sleep or unconsciousness, though it is *possible* for it to do so.

The old idea that it was only the *odor* or *aura* of
the semen that ascended into the female organs and
impregnated the ovum, is too unfounded and obviously incorrect to need refutation.

The presence or absence of the Zoospermes in
the Female Organs, and other parts, is the chief
evidence sought for in cases of alleged violation,
because in such cases they may certainly be found,
if the act has been committed, for as long as twenty-
six hours after alive, and dead for almost any period
if the fluids be dried.

It is now generally considered that the Animalcule is the true rudiment or germ of the future
human being, which is supposed to be developed
from it in the same way as the plant is developed
from the seed ; or rather the human being is thought
to be one of these Zoospermes developed to a more
perfect form by the power of the egg in which it is
placed. In proof of this—we have the fact, attested
by several observers, that when the egg breaks
open, during its passage down the tube, from the
escape of the germinal vesicle, and of the Animalculæ, if then present, always creeps in. In fact
it has been seen to do so and we thus have a prob-

able explanation of the origin of human life, if we suppose this minute being is the origin of the future human being.   If they are truly sexual we may also have an explanation of the case of the difference in sex in ourselves, as this may be dependent upon ·the sex of the Animalcules from which we originate.

It is uncertain in what part the Animalcules are first produced, though, most probably, in the Testes ; nor is it clear how they are influenced by the Seminal Vesicles and Prostate, though it is well known that the Semen must pass through those parts before the Animalcules become perfect, for in no case will it impregnate when taken from the Testes, It is conjectured, in explanation of this, that the Vesicles and Prostate supply some peculiar food or nutriment, without which the Animalcules are never perfect.

There are several Drugs that will destroy the Animalcules immediately, among which may be mentioned, Opium, Prussic Acid, Iodine, and Strychnine.   The latter article even throws them into *convulsions*, precisely like those seen in human beings.   This explains the philosophy of the means which the Parisian physicians now advise *to prevent Conception*.   A preparation of one of these Drugs is so used as to *destroy all the Animalcules*, and then, of course, there can be no impregnation. Many of the ordinary means employed for this same purpose are not only ineffective but injurious to the female, and I have known many much hurt by them.   There are certain articles which, when used properly, are both certain and harmless, but it 's not necessary to mention them here.

The most curious effects are produced upon the

Animalcules by *Alcohol.* If only a drop or two be put into the warm water which contains them, they become singularly excited, and dash about as if in a perfect phrenzy. Some will whirl rapidly round and round, till they stop all at once, and are found to be dead, others become more than usually pugnacious, and they will fight with such fury, that in a short time all will be slain. Others, again, are evidently thrown into *spasms,* or attach themselves by their suckers, and vibrate the body in the most energetic manner. After a short time these effects pass off, and they become listless and dull. If a larger portion of Alcohol be used, they are killed immediately, many of them being first thrown into convulsions. I have good reason for supposing that similar effects are often produced upon them when Alcohol is taken internally, in excess, and that many inebriates are thus made impotent. I have frequently examined the Semen of impotent patients who were addicted to excessive drinking, and have often found them exhibit precisely the same peculiarities as above described. I feel confident also that the injudicious use of the drugs above mentioned, often produces impotence, by destroying the Animalcules ; and, indeed, I have proved this by direct experiment upon animals. It is well known that confirmed opium-eaters nearly always become impotent, and that Iodine will often cause the Testes to waste away, probably by preventing the development of the Animalcules. In all probability, many persons are made impotent, or, at least, have their sexual powers much impaired, by these drugs being imprudently given to them while they are children. I have seen many cases in which the Ovaries and Testes were undeveloped from this

cause ; and I am inclined to think that the evil ex
ists to a great extent.

In some instances the use of Alcohol, and other
drugs, does not absolutely destroy the Animalcules,
but prevents their full development, or makes them
imperfect, so that we find them smaller than usual,
or deformed. This is especially the case from Al
cohol and Tobacco, as shown by experiments upon
animals, and in all probability this explains why
persons who use these articles to excess, are apt to
have stunted, deformed, and diseased children, as it
is well known they often do. If the Animalcule is
the rudiment of the future child, of which there
seems little doubt, it is natural to suppose that if it
be stunted or deformed, the child will be so likewise, and thus the vices of the father entail imperfection and disease upon his offspring.

The Animalcules are often destroyed by many of
the discharges which take place from the female
organs during disease, and in this way sterility
often results. Electricity kills them immediately,
and so will sudden cold, which accounts for some
persons being able to prevent Conception by using
cold water as an injection, immediately after connection.

Before Puberty, no Animalcules can be discovered, but the Vesicles containing them usually begin
to appear about eleven or twelve years of age. In
old age, the number of them generally becomes
less, and very often none at all are found, though
the time when they cease to be found is very variable. Some men, though in good health, and robust,
become impotent when they are fifty, and others, on
the contrary, retain full possession of their powers
till over a hundred years of age. In like manner,

some children have had the Animalcules perfectly developed at ten years of age, and some young men not till they were twenty. I have known those who had no trace of them at twenty years of age, who were nevertheless perfect enough at twenty-three ; and I once was cognizant of a painful instance in which a young female of seventeen was impregnated by a Boy of *eleven*, she having improperly conducted herself with him without the slightest suspicion of there being any danger in doing so.

It is important to bear in mind that both puberty and decay may be either hastened or postponed, by proper attention to diet and general conduct.

It is a singular circumstance, that though an electrical discharge will destroy the Animalcules instantly, yet *Galvanism*, even in a very strong current, has no effect whatever upon them, which shows the impossibility of preventing Conception by the use of Galvanic instruments, as some have proposed.

Our present comparatively perfect knowledge of the Seminal Animalcules is important both to Physiologists and to the Physician, as it enables us both to discover disease, and, in many cases, to suggest a remedy. Formerly the reason could not be even surmised why certain married persons were childless, though both seemed to be in perfect health, and in the full possession of their sexual powers. It is now known, however, that in most of these cases, though the Semen is formed yet it contains no Animalcules ; from some cause or other they have not developed, and the Vesicles only are found. This condition is more or less natural to some men, and they can, therefore, never become fathers, though fully capable of association. In such cases of sterility, when no obvious imperfection existed, medical men always assumed that the fault was in the female, it being an axiom that if the male could associate and deposit Semen, he could impregnate. This, however, we have shown to be erroneous, because the Semen may be *imperfect*, though it be produced. It is wrong, therefore, to suppose, as most people do, that in cases of sterility the fault is most frequently with the female ; it is, in fact, fully as often with the male, only the principal cause of it has only just been discovered. Men who are imperfect in this way, are in the same condition as they were before Puberty, and are similar to *Mules*, many of whom secrete Semen, and can associate with the other sex, but there are no Animalcules in the Semen, and it cannot, therefore, impregnate. In these men the sexual desire is never strong, nor does it last long, and they are always incapable of exciting much ardor in the other sex. This is explained by supposing that the presence of the Animalcules is necessary to excite the organs of both, and that without them, their peculiar sensibility is not fully developed.

A number of observed facts have made it probable that the rudiments of the Animalcules are exceedingly minute, and that great numbers of them are sometimes contained in the Semen, so that a small portion of it may suffice for impregnation for a long time. Thus instances have been known in which both Men and Animals have impregnated many times though Castrated, and for a long time after. Which is explained by supposing that, when the Testicles were removed, a quantity of Semen must have been left in the Vas Deferens, Vesi-

ales, and Prostate Gland, which being mixed with the fluids of those parts formed the discharge which impregnated. There must, however, have been a large number of Animalcular Vesicles in it, and they must have been at first very rudimentary, to continue developing so long. Some Physiologists, in fact, suppose that the Semen can produce the Vesicles spontaneously, and that, consequently, they will always be found in it when perfect, no matter what part of the body it may be taken from.

One of the worst forms of Spermatorrhœa, or involuntary seminal loss, that in which it escapes with the urine only, could never be discovered if it were not for the Animalcules. In every case of this form of the disease, they can always be detected in the urine, by means of the microscope, and thus the true nature of the trouble can be ascertained beyond a doubt. Before this discovery was made, such a mode of seminal loss was unknown and unsuspected, though it is now known to be more frequent than any other, and, doubtless, thousands have died from it without either them or their medical attendants having the remotest idea what was wrong. In my book on the *Male Organs*, some most singular and instructive cases of this kind are given, which every one should read.

The form of the Animalcules varies in different animals very much, though it is always alike in all individuals of the same species, which is probably the true reason why totally different species cannot, as a general rule, breed together. The outline of the Animalcule, as will be seen by the plate of that of the human being, is almost identical with the outline of the main part of the *Nervous System*, the large part representing the brain, and the long ex tremity, the Spinal Marrow.   It is conjectured, therefore, that the Animalcule really constitutes the first rudiment of the nervous matter, while the Ovum or Egg, as already shown, forms the general organization of all the other parts.   The form of the Animaculæ must, therefore, be adapted to the form of the body produced in the egg, of which it is to become a part, and if the two be very much unlike, no union or impregnation can take place. I have ascertained, by repeated examinations, that there is a perceptible difference between the Animacule of the Negro and that of the White Man, sufficient to mark a difference in kind, though not sufficient to prevent their fruitful intercourse.   This subject, however, will be referred to again.

The delineations of the Animalcules as given in old works are nearly always false, and sometimes grossly exaggerated.   It is in fact extremely difficult to make a proper examination of them, owing to their being so transparent, and differing so little in density from the fluid in which they are contained.   It is requisite both to have good and powerful Microscopes, and to be skilled in their use.   With regard to specimens of Semen, a Physician who sees many cases of Spermatorrhœa will never be at a loss for sufficient.

In the course of my own practice I have examined these interesting beings under every variety of circumstances, and from a number of different animals, besides from our own species.   Nothing can well be conceived more absorbing than such a pursuit, and no discoveries are more suggestive of valuable and unlooked for explanations, both Medical and Physiological.

PLATE X.

Animalcules under the Microscope.

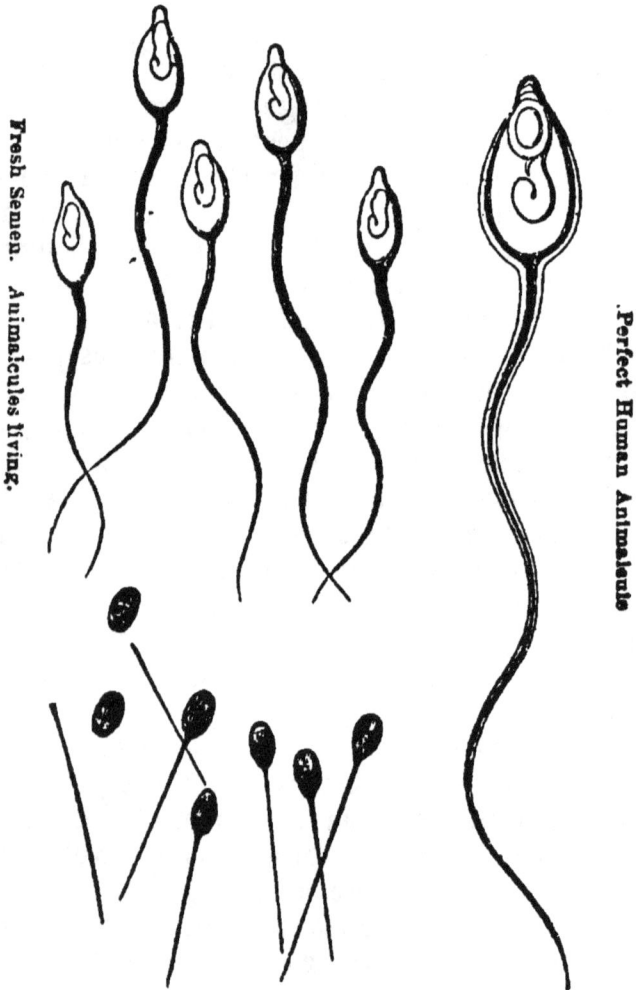

Fresh Semen. Animalcules living.

Perfect Human Animalcule.

Semen 30 hours after connection.—Animalcules dead.

CHAPTER VIII.

SEXUAL UNION, OR COPULATION.

WHEN the male principle is added to the Ovum, so that fœtal development commences, the egg is said to be *impregnated*, or in other words the female *conceives*.   Conception therefore is the union of the two principles, and fœtal development is the result of that union.

In different beings, as already explained, impregnation is effected in many different ways, being sometimes internal, by the act of Copulation, and at other times *external*, without any kind of association whatever.   In many of the lowest beings there is no copulation whatever, and frequently even no difference of sex, each individual being Hermaphrodite, or possessing both principles, but in all the higher beings a personal union, in some form or other, always takes place.   This union, or copulation, is practised, however, in many different ways, some of them exceedingly curious, and in all cases the beings are impelled to it by a peculiar and powerful instinct, the gratification of which constitutes perhaps the highest of all physical enjoyments, and leads also to other enjoyments of a superior order.

It is a remarkable circumstance, and one which shows how careful Nature has been to ensure *reproduction*, that the young of all beings, at the proper age, not only experience sexual desires but are also led, unconsciously at first, to practise those peculiar positions and modes of bodily union by which alone those desires can be properly gratified. In no instance do young animals fail in this particular, though they may have been kept carefully secluded from all others of their kind from the moment of birth. Immediately that the eggs are ripened in the female Ovary, and the Animalcules fully developed in the Male Testes, the sexual impulse is mutually experienced, and each is impelled to seek the society of the other.

The immediate causes which lead to actual personal union, between two young beings of opposite sexes in a state of nature, when neither has seen or in any way known the manner of the act, have frequently been discussed by Philosophers, and some curious experiments have been made for the purpose of ascertaining them. A careful study of the actual process of sexual union, and of the form and condition of the body at that time will, however solve the mystery to a great extent, and will show that certain physical wants and adaptions inevitably lead to certain peculiar manœuvres. The infant will seize the breast to nurse immediately it is born, and has even been known to seize the finger of the accoucher before birth, when the hand has been in the Womb during some operation. This is evidently owing to a peculiar sensitive condition of the Nerves of the Lips and Tongue, which impel the act of *suction*, and in like manner the peculiar sensibility of the nerves of the Genital Or gans, at Puberty, impels to those peculiar acts by which it is similarly relieved.

There are many circumstances connected with each sex which make them attractive to the other, and which tend to draw them together. Some of these consist in obvious excitants of the senses, while others are more mysterious in their action though their influence is equally perceptible. Among most of the lower animals, the female always emits a peculiar *odor*, at the time of heat, which when scented by the male, immediately causes in him the sexual excitement, and draws him towards ner by an irresistible impulse. Without this peculiar odor he experiences no excitement, and will not attempt to copulate, but that alone will excite him *even when the female is not present*, as experiment has proved. The *olfactory sense*, therefore, is an important agent in this process, at least among the lower beings, and perhaps it operates even in others, in some instances, more than is suspected. In those beings that are capable of reasoning and comparing, the sense of *sight* may also assist, by making differences in Organization obvious and suggesting adaptions. Besides these, however, there are certain other influences which, for want of a more *explicit* term, we will call *attractive*, the nature of which cannot be ascertained though their power is obvious. These are evidently connected with the action of the sexual organs, being experienced only when they are in perfect action, and only operating in relation to the opposite sex. It has been suggested that this mutual attraction is a species of real *Animal Magnetism*, the male being *Positive*, and the female *Negative*, so that they are drawn 'rresistibly together, like the needle and the load stone.

In the Human being there are also, at that time of life, peculiar moral sympathies and intellectual requirements which lead to mutual caresses and endearing embraces, even before the actual sexual impulse is fully awakened, and these bring about

the mode by which the novel desires may be gratified, and the peculiar sensibility of the parts relieved. It is probable that in the human being the
act of sexual union always results, in a state of
Nature, more from moral sympathy and intellect
than from the mere senses, though these undoubtedly
operate, especially *sight* and *touch.* Experiment
has shown that the Generative Organs of each sex,
when they are both in a proper state, exercise a
mutual influence one upon the other, so that their
contact can be distinguished from that of any other
part, however similar. This has been proved by
bringing various parts of the body in contact with
the Genitals, while the individual was blindfolded,
and in every instance the touch of the corresponding parts of the other sex was known instantly.
This arises in all probability from their possessing
a peculiar power of exciting each other, which
causes a species of *shock,* like that of Electricity.
It is easy to see from this how an accidental contact of these parts, during a mere caress, would suggest their mutual adaption, and would lead to
actual association.

Besides these provisions there are also others,
equally necessary, and equally curious. Thus the
nervous sensibility is placed so that it influences
certain muscles, the action of which causes peculiar motions of the body, such as are necessary during actual association. These motions are in fact
often practised, by the young, before actual connection is thought of, showing that they originate involuntarily. This is the case with both sexes, and
the motions peculiar · to each are precisely those
best adapted for favoring actual connection with
the other. Human beings however, as society is

now constituted, seldom acquire their knowledge of
this process by nature's slow and sympathetic teaching, but by the more precocious and gross medium
of instruction from others. This is perhaps unavoidable, but it is on many accounts to be regretted,
and is certainly less conducive to true morality, and
to human happiness. As the sexual impulse is now
experienced it is usually both forced and exaggerated, and is but seldom brought into play by the na
tural instincts and requirements alone.

The different Organizations of Animals makes
the act of copulation vary very much, both in its
manner and duration. In some it is a complicated
act requiring intimate internal union, and considerable time, while in others it is merely external and
effected in a very brief period. It is impetuous and
violent in some, and slow and gentle in others, but
is probably productive of intense enjoyment in all,
no matter how brief may be its duration, nor how
forcible its consummation. Some part of the Process, is however, to the females of some animals,
extremely painful, as is evinced by their cries and
efforts to escape, and by the exhaustion which they
afterwards exhibit.

The long duration of the act of Copulation in the
Dog is well known, but in some other animals it is
much longer, especially among insects, with some
of whom it continues for days, and always terminates the life of the male, while the female only
lives sufficiently long afterwards to deposit the fecundated egg and then she dies also. The long
duration of the act in the Dog is owing to two causes ; The Male Organ has a number of knots, or
swellings, towards its termination, around which the
sphincter muscle of the female Vagina closes with

such force that the two cannot separate till the parts become flaccid. So powerfully does this muscle act that even if the male be killed, or the Organ cut off, the Vagina will still retain it, till relaxation takes place. The same phenomenon is often seen in in-sects also, and the long continuance of the act is un-doubtedly owing to the semen being slowly emitted, and very gradually absorbed into the female organs.

In other animals, on the contrary, the act of copu-lation is almost instantaneous, the semen being dar-ted out in a single jet and absorbed immediately. This is the case in most birds, some of whom con-nect while on the wing. The reason for this quick-ness will be obvious on inspecting their Organs, which are not adapted for continued intercourse. In fact it can scarcely be said that birds copulate at all, except a few species. The male has no true Penis, but merely a slight protuberance, like a But-ton, which cannot enter the female organ but merely ejects the semen upon its mouth. The female also has no vagina, there being but one passage, called the *Cloaca* which is common to the excrement, the urine, and the semen. In some few birds, however, as in the Ostr h, the Penis is considerably develop-ed, and enter the Vagina, so that they really copu-late. As a general rule also the Clitoris is absent in female birds, which has led some Physiologists to conjecture that they have no pleasurable excitement during the act, but this perhaps is erroneous, as some other part may be more than usually sensitive in their case. There are a few kinds as some of the Ducks for instance, that have the Clitoris very large, and in the Ostrich and Cassowary it even has a groove, like a Urethra, so that it resembles a nis. Ducks are well known to exhibit great amative excitement, the reason for which is evidently their possessing this large and sensitive Clitoris.

In most reptiles also the act is equally imperfect, as in very few do the males have a properly developed Penis, but merely a small bulb, or protuberance. The Tortoise, and the Crocodile, however, have a single Penis, and the Alligator has a double one. In the Lizard and Serpents it is also double, and in the Rattlesnake each part is also divided again. Excepting at the time of copulation this Organ, however, is not visible, being drawn into a sheath, from which it is thrust, at the proper time, by appropriate muscles. Some Serpents copulate always at one particular season, and then great numbers assemble together and twine and interlace themselves into an immense Pyramid, with their heads directed outwards. Humboldt tells us of one of the living Pyramids which he met with in South America, and which he describes as being the most fearful and horrible sight that ever met his gaze. The whole combined mass moved slowly on over the plain, while each individual writhed its body, darted out its forked tongue, and hissed in the most horrible manner—very few females among the reptiles have anything like a Clitoris, though it is found in some, as in the Tortoise for instance.

The Frog exhibits very well the mode of impregnation without copulation, though in all probability not without mutual pleasure. At the time when the female is ready to eject the eggs the male climbs upon her back, embraces her firmly around the body with his long legs, and as the eggs are emitted he waters them with the semen. They are then left in the water by some species, and in others are fastened to the female's back for awhile, by a thick mucus, secreted for the purpose. The embrace of the male Frog is well known to be so powerful that the female seems nearly cut in two by his limbs, which contract with such force, and are so rigid, that they may even be torn off before letting go their hold. The object of this powerful compression seems to be the forcing out of the eggs, which probably could not be effected by the female herself. It is for this reason that these animals are called *accoucheurs* or *midwifes*, because they cause the female to lay their eggs.

In male Fishes we seldom find anything like a Penis, though sometimes there is an organ which partly answers the purpose of one. It is merely a cartilaginous prolongation, like the spine of a fin, which hangs down from the body. Sometimes in fact it forms part of the anal fin, though in other cases it is separate from it. Down this imperfect organ there runs a shallow grove, which serves as a conduit for the semen. In many species there is nothing like copulation, nor do the two sexes ever meet, except accidentally, but in others the male organ is applied against the female parts at the time when the eggs are emitted, and the semen is then ejected upon them. In very few there is even the slightest entrance effected. The whale it, must be remembered is *not a Fish*, though this may seem strange to some, but merely a mammiferous animal that lives in the water. Its organs, therefore, are like those of the other mammifers, and it truly copulates, the male and female standing partly erect, out of the water, when doing so.

The various forms of the sexual Organs in different beings of course necessitate different modes of connection, and probably varies much the sensa-

tions connected with it, but there is always a pow?
erful instinct, which ensures its performance, in all.
Perhaps some of the most singular modes of copulation are found among Insects, and other inferior
beings, and especially among those that are hermaphrodite. In some insects there is but one female
to many males, and no actual union ever takes place
with any, the merest touch of the female's body being
sufficient to satisfy the instinct of each. This is the
case with Bees, the males of whom will crowd
round the Queen in hundreds to touch her body.
In other species, however, the sexes are always in
equal couples, and when they copulate, the connection continues for days together uninterruptedly, the
female carrying the male about with her on her
back. Some kinds of hermaphrodite Snails exhibit
a very singular mode of mutual impregnation, each
individual being provided with a number of horny
darts, or spears, enclosed in a sheath, which they
dart at each other in turn, having first asssumed a
proper position for the amorous combat. The double
connection of the common earth-worm, which is
hermaphrodite, may be seen on any dewy morning,
when they rise out of the ground, and it will be
seen that it usually continues till the sun rises,
which would seem to intimate that the continued
union is productive of pleasure, because it can be
terminated at pleasure. In the perfect hermaphrodites, who self impregnate, it may be a question
what kind of feeling is experienced, if any at all,
because they are both male and female, but it is
certain that they are as strongly impelled to the act
as those beings that associate with an opposite sex.

A very curious study is afforded also of the various modes by which the two sexes discover each

other, at the proper time, in those species in which they do not live together. Some Insects, for instance, have a peculiar song, or cry, by which the female attracts her partner, and others are decked out in brilliant colors for the same purpose. Some, which come out only at night, have a lamp provided to light him, as we see in the Glow-Worm and Fire-Fly. The peculiar cry of the Locust, the ticking of the Death-Watch, and the chirp of the Grasshopper, are intended for this purpose, and probably also the song of the bird has, to a great extent, the same object. In fact, every animal has a peculiar cry, which only it utters when desiring the company of the other sex, and which is mutually understood.

With respect to the feelings which the act of coition produces, and the instincts or desires which lead to it, they probably vary indefinitely. In all the higher beings the desire to cohabit arises from a specific irritation of the Genital Organs, acting in conjunction with certain moral sympathies and intellectual perceptions. And when the connection occurs in a proper manner and under proper circumstances, it is always productive of intense and peculiar enjoyment to both. This is especially the case with human beings, and with all others similarly organized. The peculiar excitement which first causes coition to be desired, and which also makes it so intensely pleasurable, arises from the development of certain parts, namely, the *Clitoris* in the female, and the *Glans Penis* in the male. The perfection of either of these organs in the one sex is invariably attended by a similar perfection in the corresponding part of the other sex, so that they are mutually excitable, and generally pretty equally so. We never find a well-developed and sensitive

Glans in the male, but we also find a well-developed
and sensitive Clitoris in the female, or else there is
some other part, as the Neck of the Womb for in
stance, which acts in the same manner.   In many
of the lower beings, who have none of these parts,
it is probable that nothing like what we call *sexual
feeling* is ever experienced, but that they are im·
pelled to connection simply by the mysterious work·
ings of the *parental instinct*, which, as we well
know, leads to many actions in which no direct plea·
sure is felt.   The careful depositing of their eggs
by insects, in the most proper places, and the patient
sitting of the hen upon hers, may be adduced as in·
stances of these blind promptings of the parental
instinct, and, probably, in some beings, actual con·
nection is brought about in the same way.

The more perfect development of the Generative
Organs in the higher order of beings, and their
greater sensibility, especially in Man, is only in ac·
cordance with the greater perfection of every other
part of the system, and is doubtless intended as an
additional means of increasing their felicity.   The
higher any being is placed in the scale of creation,
the more multiplied are its means of enjoyment,
and the more intense those enjoyments become, as
we see in regard to true sexual intercourse, by an
actual union of the organs of the two sexes, or in·
tromission of the male, which is altogether confined
to the most perfectly organized.

In the lower animals, the situation of the organs
in the two sexes, and the position which they are ne·
cessarily compelled to assume during coition, is cal·
culated merely for the perfect accomplishment of
the act, and often causes both inconvenience and
pain, but in the higher animals other adaptations

are found. The position which *they* naturally assume, is not only adapted for the most perfect and
convenient performance of the act, but also for
causing enjoyment to each. With human beings
this is more obvious than with any other, because
their capability for enjoyment is greater. With
them the position is such as to call forth mutual en-
dearment and admiration, both during the act and
previous to it, and also to excite sympathy and tenderness in the more ardent and less sensitive of the
two. No other beings, at this time, can see each
other's eyes—those windows of the soul, by whose
glances ardor can be aroused and excitement subdued—nor those expressive lineaments of the face,
which can call forth pity and forbearance when
timidity conquers love. In many cases of attempted
violation, the vision of the victim's face, full of in-
tercession and reproach, and compelling deference
and admiration, has overcome the fury of amorous
lust, and driven the would-be ravisher · away in
spite of himself. Even in lawful marriage, sanc-
tioned by love and reason both, this circumstance,
though it may seem of little moment, prevents many
injuries and evils which the peculiar and delicate
organization of Woman would otherwise subject
her too. In fact, there is as much *design* and admirable contrivance exhibited in this particular, as
there is in any action connected with the human
frame, and with rational beings it is equally worthy
of attention. It is also equally proper to be understood, and its study is eminently calculated to subdue those gross and merely animal feelings with
which alone everything of the kind is usually
approached. · This portion of our physical nature
was designed and formed by the same power that

originated every other part, and was equally made perfect for its specific use ; it is, therefore, deny-ing the wisdom and goodness of that Power, to say that these organs are imperfect, or that their legiti-mate use is improper. To be ashamed of a rational and virtuous knowledge of them, is really being ashamed of the Creator, and accuses him of inde-cency and impropriety. My object is to show that all those subjects usually considered the most gross and degrading, are so merely from our ignorance, and that they can be refined and elevated in their character, till our conceptions of them become pure, moral, and worthy of rational beings.

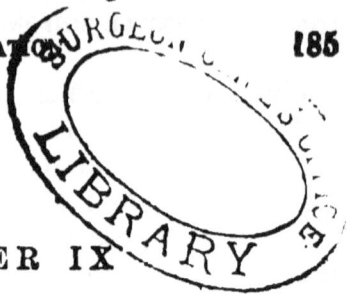

CHAPTER IX

IMPREGNATION.

THE actual process of Impregnation, or that union of the two principles from which the new being originates, has always been a physiological mystery, and a fruitful theme for philosophical speculation. It is evident, however, that the only way to clear up such a mystery, is to examine the Generative Organs and their products, under every possible variety of circumstances, and to do this with care and patience for a length of time, so that a sufficient number of observations may be made. This task has only been undertaken very recently, and consequently our knowledge of this mysterious process, until lately, has been altogether incomplete and imperfect. The investigations already referred to, and others which will be mentioned further on, have developed the laws of Fecundation, and removed that process altogether from the field of mere speculation. M. Pouchet was undoubtedly the first who clearly enunciated these laws in any publication, though others had arrived at them independently; we will, therefore, state them as he has done, and then make whatever comments and further statements may be necessary.

M. P. lays down *Ten Laws*, some of which have already been explained, but others will now come first under notice.

POUCHET'S TEN FUNDAMENTAL RULES WHICH GOVERN THE PROCESS OF FECUNDATION.

1*st. Law.* Generation is essentially the same in all beings, Mankind not excepted

2*d. Law.* In all beings, the Female Eggs exist before and independent of Conception, the same as the Male Semen does.   .

3*d. Law.* The Egg is never impregnated in the Ovary or Organ that produces it.

4*th. Law.* The Egg must always have attained a certain development before it can be impregnated, and must also have left the Ovary.

5*th. Law.* In all beings the Egg leaves the Ovary independent of Impregnation.

6*th. Law.* In all Animals the Eggs are emitted at certain regular periods, peculiar to each, at which times there also occurs a peculiar excitement of the female organs.

7*th. Law.* Conception can never occur only when the Semen is present at the same time with the perfectly developed Egg.

8*th. Law.* The Menstruation of the human female is strictly analogous to the periodical erotic excitement of other animals, sometimes termed the Rut or Heat.

9*th. Law.* Consequently Conception is necessarily connected with Menstruation. and there is, therefore, in human females, a period when impregnation can occur, and one when it cannot, *and those periods can be pointed out.*

10*th. Law.* In the human being, Impregnation always takes place either in the Womb, or in the very end of the Tube next to the Womb.

The first of these Laws has been already well illustrated in our first articles, where it has been shown that the generative process is essentially the same in Man as in all other beings, though it was formerly thought to be different. All Animals, it was there explained, are devoloped from eggs, formed in the female's body, only in some these eggs are impregnated and developed internally, and in others externally ; and in some, as the human being for instance, they are very minute, and, therefore, difficult to discover. There are four different varieties of the generative process : the *Viviparous*, or that in which the eggs are impregnated and developed into the new being within the body, as in the Human being : the *Oviparous*, or that in which the eggs are impregnated within the body, but expelled and hatched without, as in Birds ; the *Oviviparous*, or that in which the eggs are impregnated within the body, and hatched while they are passing out, as in some Insects and Reptiles ; and lastly the *Marsupial* variety, or that in which the young are half-formed within the body, and complete their growth without, as in the Kangaroo. To one or the other of these varieties the generation of every animal can be referred, though there may be some unimportant peculiarities in certain kinds.

An example of Oviviparous Generation may be seen in the common *Meat-Fly*, which does not lay eggs upon their meat, but little larvæ, or maggets, perfectly formed, their eggs being hatched while passing down the canal from its body. In some species, the young have even developed into perfect insects, and are ready to undergo their metamorphose when they pass from the body of the mother The young *Scorpion* is perfect, and begins to walk

immediately it is born, having been hatched and de
veloped within the parental body, and the same
thing is observed in the common *Aphis*, or green
plant-louse. Some insects can even generate both
ways, and produce sometimes eggs, and sometimes
perfect young, or even both together, in immense
numbers. The structure of the egg is always the
same, but in the Oviparous Animals it has added to
it a quantity of extraneous nutriment, by which
the new being is formed while in the shell, or outer
covering. The eggs of the Viviparous have nothing of the kind, because they are attached, from
the first moment of conception, to the mother's body,
and derive their nutriment from it. The large
portion of Vitellus, or yellow, which we see in the
egg of the chicken, is intended to apply nutriment
to the young, and so is the Albumen, or white,
which, with the shell, form no part of the egg
properly speaking, but are formed around it, *after it
leaves the Ovary*, and while passing from the body.

An examination of the Ovarium of the bird will
make many of these statements readily understood,
and will be found a very useful study. It consists,
during the laying period, of a large number of
Ova, of various sizes, all fastened by ligaments, or
small stems, to a central point, which is the true
Ovarium, and from which they all originate. Some
of the Ova, or eggs, are very minute, like mustar
seeds, while others are larger, and a few are near.,
as large as when expelled from the body, but none
of these have either white or shell while they
remain connected with the Ovary. As the egg en
larges, the ligament which hold it becomes less,
and, eventually, when it has attained its full growth,
the ligament breaks and the egg is dropped into

the Canal, or passage, by which it is to escape from the body. It then consists merely of the Vitellus, or yellow, and the Cicatricula, or Germinative Vesicle, but as it proceeds along the passage, the white, or Albumen, is deposited around it, and the shell forms around the whole, till it assumes the form we usually see. The shell and the Albumen, therefore, are mere extraneous matters, and not essential parts of the egg or ovum, though necessary to its protection and development when out of the body, and it is not unusual for the egg to be expelled without them, especially when the bird is diseased, or not provided with sufficient lime for the shell.

The true definition of a viviparous animal therefore is one whose egg cannot develop without being connected with its body, while the egg of an oviparous animal is capable of developing alone, merely by the application of a proper degree of heat.

The truth of the Second Law is obvious in respect to all oviparous animals, especially birds, who are known to have eggs, and to lay them, before being impregnated, but it is not so obvious in respect to viviparous animals, whose eggs are so small that they are only discovered by the microscopical anatomist. A consideration of the facts already adduced will prove, however, that in the whole class, mankind included, the law also prevails, and that eggs are formed and expelled in them also independently of impregnation. The celebrated Harvey was convinced of this proof, though he had not the proof of it, and he laid down an axiom in accordance with his conviction which can now be received without question,—" Every thing living," said he, " comes from an egg."—There are some of the

lower animals, it is true, that seem to reproduce
their young without eggs, by *Fissiparous* or *Gemiparous* Generation, but these are now known to be
only modifications of the oviparous process. In
Fissiparous Generation the parent simply splits up,
or divides spontaneously, into two or more parts,
which grow into new beings that also divide again
in their turn in the same way, and thus the species
are continued. The fresh water *Polype* is an instance of this mode of generation, and if it be cut
into pieces with a knife each part will grow into a
perfect being, which may also be divided in the
same way, apparently without limit. In *Gemiparous* Generation the original being simply gives
out little buds, or germs, from its body, which develop into perfect beings, as we see in the sponge,
and the oyster, the buds being sometimes cast off to
develop alone, and sometimes all remaining attached
to the parent till a large bed or mass of them is
formed.

These animals that propogate by the Fissiparous
process are all exceedingly simple in their organization, and many of them may be turned inside out,
like a glove, without the slightest injury or inconvenience. It is probable, therefore, that the whole
being is merely like an ovary, and that every atom
of it is a germ or egg, capable of development alone,
like the bud of a Tree. Those that propagate by
the Gemiparous process are also very inferiorly
organized, and in all probability the buds or germs
which they give of are really ova, or eggs, expelled
spontaneously. In fact many of these beings propagate by the oviparous mode as well, and their
whole substance seems to resolve itself into germs
of new organizations—The Third Law says that the

semen cannot reach the eggs, to impregnate them, while they remain in the vesicles of the ovary, and a slight consideration of the numerous obstacles interposed will show that this must be so. In the first place the action of the Fallopian tubes, and the cilia which line their interior, as before explained, is such that nothing can pass *towards* the ovary from the womb, but only in the other direction. And besides this, while the egg is in the vesicle it is surrounded by a number of different membranes, either of which would present an impassible barrier to the semen, even if it could reach the exterior of the ovary. But there is still another obstacle if these were overcome, as if nature had taken especial care that no such event should take place. The interior of the Tubes is compactly filled with a thick mucus, in which the cilia work, and through which the semen could not possibly force its way. In fact there seems to be considerable difficulty even in forcing the egg down the Tubes the right way, and it is probable that very frequently it does not pass down before its structure is broken up, so that it cannot be impregnated. This is apparently the reason why there are but few women who continue to bear children uninterruptedly, most of them having more or less interval between, frequently of years. They form the egg regularly every month, and might conceive therefore *every ten or twelve months*, but all the eggs do not reach the womb in time, a large number of them being so long in passing down the Tubes that they are spoilt before the semen can reach them. Perhaps this is an express provision, to prevent women from being debilitated by sickness, and worn down by anxiety, as most of them would certainly be if they were to

bear children continually.   With human beings
there are many considerations which make it undesirable for reproduction to be frequent, and this is
probably a natural check.   Some females it is well
known are not restricted in this way, but continue
to conceive regularly a short time after every delivery.   In such persons there is no doubt a uniform
transmission of the egg, which, therefore, always
reaches the womb in a state fit for receiving the
male semen.   In many cases of barrenness also, I
find that stimulating the Fallopian tubes, at the proper time, will remove the disability, apparently by
quickening their action, and causing the egg to
reach the womb earlier, and in a better condition
for being impregnated.

The old theory of impregnation was that the
semen was absorbed, or sucked up, into the womb
and along the Fallopian Tubes till it reached the
ovary, when it impregnated one of the eggs and so
stimulated it to commence developing.   It was then
supposed that this impregnated egg, after a time,
separated from the ovary and passed down the tube
into the womb, where it formed into the Fœtus.
The facts just mentioned, however, show the fallacy
of this theory, even if the correct process had not
been given before, but still it has been received
so long, and has become so *orthodox*, that many celebrated men hesitate to reject it even now.   I have
known Professors in our Medical Colleges retail this
exploded theory to their students, though the Medical Journals were daily giving them facts utterly
opposed to it, and with the exception of my own
work there is not a Book in the English Language
that gives a full account of the new discoveries.

Some years ago I published a work myself, *The*

Origin of Life, before these important discoveries had been made, and I was compelled then to give the old explanation of conception, because no better was known, but I was careful to give it merely as a *Theory,* which might any day be shown to be erroneous. In fact I was then engaged in making experiments for the purpose of testing it, and in the later editions the true explanation has been added in the form of a note. The present book, however, is the only one which gives all the details in full.

Abundant proof has been obtained that the thick portion of the semen must actually touch the egg itself, without any obstruction, or there can be no impregnation. Spallanzani proved this by his experiment upon the eggs of Fishes. He found that if semen from the male fish were put into the water along with the female eggs they would, after a time, begin to develop, and ultimately form into young Fishes, but not if the semen were kept away. He then filtered the semen, and tried the thin part of it, but that had no effect, though the thick part, which contained the Animalcules, impregnated immediately. Some Physiologists had concluded that it was merely the *Aura,* a kind of steam from the semen, which impregnated, and he therefore exposed some of the eggs to this steam, for various periods of time, but always with no effect. The same results have also followed experiments made upon animals, by myself, for in no case did impregnation follow from the mere aura of the semen, though it was applied directly to the mouth of the womb, as well as in the Vagina. It is therefore certain that the thick semen itself must touch the egg, and this it cannot do while the egg is in the Vesicle of the Ovary, because it cannot reach the Ovary.

The fourth Law asserts further that before the egg can be impregnated it must have acquired a certain development, and must have separated from the Ovary. Reason alone would assure us of this, because it is evident that the egg must be perfectly formed before it could be affected by the semen, and when it has attained this stage it is *ripe*, and is cast off from the Ovary like a ripe fruit from the tree.

The precise period when the egg leaves the Ovary appears to be when it has exhausted all the nutriment in the vesicle, as evidenced by the complete absorption of the white fluid, and it is detached in order to seek the means of further growth elsewhere, as the ripe seed of the plant is thrown to the ground.

In the great majority of animals the egg is not impregnated till it has passed a long way from the Ovary, which is usually deep within the body, and sometimes it even leaves the body before it is fecundated. The eggs cannot be impregnated if taken from the Ovary, as experiment has proved, but they must have left it spontaneously, and sufficiently long for the peculiar change we have before explained to take place in them. Impregnation could not take place, therefore, from the semen reaching the Ovary, even if its passage there was possible. •

In the case of the bird the egg is impregnated immediately it leaves the Ovary, before the shell is formed over it, but not while attached by its ligament. The female bird is provided with a peculiar pouch, or receptacle into which the semen is absorbed at the time of copulation, and in which it will remain unchanged for a long time. This Pouch is so placed that the egg passes by it leaving the Ovary, and in such a manner that it attaches a portion of the semen contained in it, and thus becomes impregnated. The quantity of semen thus stored up is something considerable, and as only a small portion is needed to fecundate each egg it is possible for a single copulation to impregnate all the eggs that may be laid. for a long time after, as we often see in the common fowl.

In some animals the egg is not perfect enough for impregnation even when it leaves the Ovary, but is kept for a time longer in a peculiar Organ, provided for the purpose, in which it maturates more perfectly, and is then expelled into the passage to meet the semen. This is the case with many fishes and Reptiles, and if the egg be taken before its sojourn in that peculiar Organ it cannot be fecundated.

It is evident, therefore, that the egg must have attained a certain development before it can be impregnated, and that it must also have left the Ovary for some definite time.

The fifth Law, which asserts that in all beings the eggs are formed and leave the Ovary independent of impregnation, is almost proved sufficiently by the facts already adduced, but a few additional observations will make it still more clear. With respect to birds, this Law was long known to be correct, because they frequently produce eggs without having even had any connection with the male ; and it was also equally evident in regard to most fishes, whose eggs are impregnated after they leave the body. In frogs also, as before stated, the male deposits his semen on the eggs as the female expels them from the body, which proves that their formation and expulsion is independent of impregnation, the difficulty in proving that this law appl beings, especially to the human being, arose from want of proper observation, and from the supposition that the egg in them was in some respect different to that of the Oviparii. Now that the universal similarity of the egg is proved, however, and that we know it is produced by a similar process in all it is also made evident that it is formed and emitted independent of impregnation. In fact, one essential part of the egg, the Vitellus, from which part of the new being is formed, is found in undoubted virgins, and even in children occasionally, when it could not, of course, have had its development influenced by impregnation.

Nevertheless it must be observed that sexual excitement may hasten the ripening of the eggs, because it may excite the ovaries, and expedite their functions, as our former observations have shown. In some cases it even appears that the egg will partially develop from mere excitement; without any contact with the male principle, as several instances already given have proved. In this way are produced those imperfect fœtal growths occasionally met with in the Ovaries, and which have been found even in children. And in the same way, in all probability, arises that partial development of the new being found sometimes in the unimpregnated egg of the bird, many instances of which are upon record. This appears still more probable when it is borne in mind, strange though the statement may seem, that female birds will often excite themselves with their beaks, when kept away from the male, and that they always lay eggs immediately after doing so. These facts show that though impregnation is not necessary to the maturation and expulsion of the egg, yet the excitement consequent upon copulation, or other practices, may accelerate those processes, and even imperfectly develop the egg after its expulsion. Hufeland gives us an instance of a young girl who had been addicted from infancy to masturbation, and who died in consequence at thirteen years of age, in whose left Ovary was found a sac containg hair, bones. teeth, and other fœtal remains in a most perfect condition.

In short the growth and expulsion of the egg is a process belonging to the female system alone, and no more requires the influence of the male, in any way, than he requires the influence of the female to cause the Testes to form the Semen. An inspection of the ovaries, after puberty, will show that they are constantly forming ova, at their regular periods, by an action peculiar to themselves. Just previous to the monthly crisis of one of the Graafian Vesicles will always be found ready to burst, and if carefully examined the egg will be found in its interior. After the period is over, on the contrary, the Vesicle is found torn open and filled with blood, the egg having been expelled, and *menstruation* having occurred in consequence of its expulsion. In fact many females, who possess sufficient physiological knowledge, and who have been observant of their own systems, know precisely the time when the egg leaves their body, and can readily obtain it at every monthly period. This I have known many do, and it is sometimes necessary in determining the causes of sterility, which occasionally results from the egg being imperfectly formed, and we cannot ascertain whether they are perfect or not without examining them.

The Sixth Law merely states that in all animals

the expulsion of the eggs occurs at regular inter
vals, varying in their duration in the different kinds.
In some beings there is only one expulsion during
their lives, and this usually terminates their existence, as we see in many insects. In some the
expulsion is annual, in others, biennial, and in others
again every three years, and sometimes it is as
often as daily ; in the human being it is monthly.
This regular Ovarian expulsion also occurs along
with the periodic excitement called the rut, or heat,
in the lower animals, and the monthly period, or
menstruation, in the human being. In fact, the
periodic excitement results from the periodic expulsion, and both are parts of one grand phenomenon.

This periodic excitement, especially as it appears
in the form of menstruation in the human being,
exerts a most potent influence over the rest of the
system, and makes the female in many respects
essentially different from the male, as was fully
explained in our article on Menstruation. It commences first in the Ovaries, but is propagated from
them to the whole of the generative apparatus, and
sometimes even to remote parts.

The excitement caused by the expulsion of the
egg is not, in the inferior beings, accompanied by
such a discharge as we observe from the human
female, though in nearly all there is some secretion,
and in particular species it is even colored. In all
cases, however, the excitement of the parts is obvious
enough, and is sometimes quite remarkable externally. In some of the Apes not only are the
external Genitals inflamed but also the parts around
the anus, and even the thighs, which are sometimes
covered with large Tumefactions, of a bright-red

color, during every period. In all birds the inflamed condition of the external parts, while they are laying, may be readily seen, and it is observable also in fishes. Occasionally this external excitement occurs in human beings at such times, and some females are always troubled then with swollen Labia, or eruptions on the skin.

In every instance the excitement and flow is terminated by the expulsion of the egg from the Ovary, which constitutes the crisis, and it is always immediately on their cessation that we detect it in the beginning of the Tube, in the human female. In no instance is there any excitement, or flow, in those females that have been castrated, because they can have no expulsion of Ova, but in all those whose functions are natural, the excitement occurs at regular periods, and is always accompanied by the maturation and discharge of Ova.

When animals are domesticated their periods are considerably modified, being usually hastened, but still they almost invariably observe a certain degree of regularity. Many females are also much affected by their mode of life, being made to menstruate, or flood, almost continually, by the influence of stimulating food and drink, and by too much artificial heat.

The Seventh Law enunciates a most important truth, which is the foundation of much valuable advice, and gives us the key to the true time of Conception. It states that Conception can never occur except when the male semen is deposited in the female Organs at the same time that the egg reaches them, or, in other words, for a copulation to be fruitful it must coincide with the expulsion of the egg. The truth of this will be obvious from our previous statements, for it is evident that if the semen cannot reach the egg while it is in the Ovary, and that has been shown to be impossible, it can only do so after it is expelled and brought into the Womb. In fact the egg has some further change to undergo after it leaves the Ovary before it can be fecundated, and this is the reason for its being somewhat delayed by passing down the Tubes, on leaving which the semen can operate upon it. This law is strictly in accordance with the fact before mentioned, that the expulsion of the egg takes place just when the flow is over, as that is the time when conception really occurs, and when most animals also desire association. It is not at the commencement of the Rut that female animals desire the male, but after the discharge has continued for a few days, and just when it is ceasing The Slut, for instance, will repel the Dog at first, and so will the female Rabbit repel the male, and even fight with him, until about the third day of heat, and then she submits. This is evidently because the eggs have not descended till that time, and nature has so provided that association shall only be sought when it is likely to be fruitful. If any of these animals be compelled to copulate during the first days of the excitement there will be no fecundation, as experiment has proved, because the presence of the Semen does not then coincide with the presence of the egg.

The Eighth Law is merely a distinct enunciation of a truth already abundantly proved, namely: that the menstruation of the human female is identical with the peculiar excitement observed periodically upon all other animals. and called the rut, heat, or œstrum.

According to the Ninth Law, it is possible, at least in the human being, to designate the precise time when Conception is possible, and also that in which it may take place. This law also follows naturally from the foregoing explanations, they having shown that the egg remains but a certain number of days in the womb, after which it passes from the body and is lost, and since the semen can reach the egg only while it is in the womb, it is evident that the days during which it stays there are the only ones in which Conception is possible, and that at all other times it is absolutely impossible, When we have ascertained, therefore, the precise time which the egg stays in the womb we know to a certainty the time when conception can occur, and also when it cannot. In another Article I shall point out this time accurately, and explain how it is ascertained.

The Tenth Law is important because it localizes the phenomena of fecundation. According to this Law the two principles can only meet in the Uterus, or at the Uterine ends of the Fallopian Tubes. The proofs of this are many and various, and quite sufficient to put its truth beyond a doubt. In the first place it must be borne in mind that the Semen cannot pass down the Tubes, as already shown, and consequently cannot get farther than the Womb. In fact, if animals be killed as long as twenty-six hours after connection the Semen is still in the Womb, and if killed after that time it has gone no further, but has begun to decompose. In some few cases it has been found a little way within the Fallopian Tube, and once or twice nearly as far as the middle of the Tube, but no further. In no case have the Animalcules of the Semen been found on the Ovary, nor beyond the middle of the **Tube**, though sought for in hundreds of cases. It is true that in some cases Anatomists have thought that they discovered the Animalcules upon the **Ovary**, but it is now generally admitted that they were mistaken, and their error probably originated in this way : There are often fragments of Mucus Membrane, partly organized, which much resemble the Animalcules, and without very close inspection may readily be mistaken for them. These are called *false Zoospermes*, and in all probability it was some of those that came under view. Every accurate observer has failed to detect them in any other parts than those mentioned.

§ WHEN CONCEPTION IS POSSIBLE AND IMPOSSIBLE.

Numerous observations have established the following facts respecting the time of Conception in the human being, and they may be relied upon with the utmost certainty.

The Graafian Vesicle, which contains the egg in the Ovary, enlarges while the Menstrual flow is taking place, and it bursts open, to let the egg escape, on the first, second, third, or fourth day after the flow has ceased, but most usually on the first day.

The egg is then taken hold of by the fringes at the end of the Tube and carried into the passage, down which it slowly progresses, taking from two to six days to reach the Womb.

The time, therefore in which the egg reaches the Womb, varies from one or two to ten days after the Menstrual flow has ceased.

When the egg reaches the Womb, it would---if

there were no special provision to prevent it—immediately fall down to its mouth, and escape from the body, but this is provided against. While the egg is passing down the Tubes, or during the latter part of the flow, a peculiar delicate membrane, or skin, called the *Decidua*, forms around the inner walls of the Womb, so as completely to block up its mouth. This membrane presses against the opening from the Fallopian Tubes also, so that when the egg passes out of the Tube, it presses against the membrane, and makes a hollow, or kind of nest, in which it lies. This, therefore, prevents the egg from passing immediately away, and it evidently must be retained in the Womb as long as the Decidua remains.

The time that the Decidua remains attached also varies from two to six days, but usually it is about four, and at the end of that time, unless conception occurs it looses from the walls of the Womb, passes out of its mouth, down the Vagina, and takes the egg along with it, so that both leave the body and are lost. If Impregnation takes place, however, or in other words, if the male semen reaches the egg while it is thus detained, it remains, and both it and the Decidua grow fast to the Womb. The egg then forms the rudiment of the new being, and the membrane becomes one of its coverings or envelopes.

When the egg and the Decidua have fallen, or, in other words, when the egg is thrown out of the body, there cannot, of course, be any conception till another period comes round, because there is no egg in the womb to be impregnated. After this time, therefore, Conception is *impossible*, and its maximum limits at least may be stated with certainty. From the above statements it will be seen that the egg reaches the Womb some time between the second and tenth day after the Menstrual flow has stopped, and that it then remains there from two to six days at the utmost, but after that it passes away. Consequently, *Conception is possible as long as sixteen days after every monthly flow has stopped, but after that time it is impossible!* In fact, it is hardly ever the case that it can take place so long as sixteen days after, because the egg is seldom more than two days in reaching the Womb, and if it remains six, as an extreme limit, *eight days* is probably about the average. If the truth could be ascertained, I have no doubt but that nine out of every ten pregnant females have conceived within the first *seven* days after the flow, and that impregnation would not follow connection after the *Tenth* day once out of fifty times, but still it is requisite to state the latest *possible* time, and that is *sixteen days.*

An instance illustrative of this principle is recorded in history. Henry II. of France had been long married without offspring, and had consulted various medical men as to the cause, without success, till he sent for the celebrated *Fernel*, who, upon due consideration, simply advised him to always associate with his spouse *immediately after the cessation of her periods.* This advice was acted upon, and she conceived, after being childless *eleven years.* In all probability the egg escaped in her case *very soon*, and association had never been had before till after it was lost.

Every other being also has its limited time, but it is various in different kinds. I have ascertained it in several, and invariably, if they were not allowed to associate with the male till that time was passed, they never conceived. There are signs, however, by which any intelligent and observant female can ascertain that time in her own case, and those signs we will now explain.

Some time within the first five or six days after the cessation of the flow, but usually on the first or second, all females experience a sensation of weight and uneasiness, or of slight pain in the region of the Fallopian Tubes, or across the abdomen, on a line with the lower edge of the hip-bones. This sensation may be very slight in some, but in others it is quite acute, and there are few but what can detect more or less of it if they observe. This indicates the passage of the egg down the Fallopian Tube, and is caused by its contraction. In fact, many females can distinctly feel the Tubes *drawing* together, as they express it, and sometimes the contractions may even be *seen* externally. Previous to these contractions the mucus discharged from the Vagina is usually thick and adhesive, but after they have ceased, it becomes thinner and more transparent. The passage of the egg down the Tube is indicated, therefore, by very obvious signs, which, I am confident, are but seldom absent.

The passage of the egg out of the Womb, or the fall of the Decidua, which makes conception impossible afterwards, is even more strongly and constantly marked, and can be known by nearly all females. The first indication is an increased flow of thin watery fluid from the Vagina, so abundant sometimes as to wet all the external parts, and not unfrequently to cause some little irritation. Occasionally the discharge is tinged of a pale pink, but more usually it is colorless, and like the white of an egg. This may continue only for a few hours, or

foi a day or two, and is always followed by the es
cape of a small grayish white clot, somewhat firm
and elastic. This clot is opaque, and varies from
the size of a pea to that of a small bean. It much
resembles the clots which are often coughed from
the throat in bronchial affections, and is readily detected. Just previous to this appearing, and when
the thin discharge is about ceasing, there is also
felt a slight contraction and pain in the Womb, accompanied with a feeling of weight and bearing
down, similar to what is experienced during the
Menstrual flow itself. If this clot be examined
with a microscope it will be found to consist of *the
Decidua and the egg*, which have thus been expelled. In fact, the slight pain and distress experienced are caused by the Womb contracting slightly
to effect the expulsion, the same as it does during a
miscarriage to effect the expulsion of the Fœtus.
This is, then, the phenomenon of the fall of the Decidua, or expulsion of the egg, called by the French,
the *Ponté*, or *laying,* and after it has taken place,
there can be no impregnation till after another period

In some females this expulsion of the egg is al
most as distinctly marked as the monthly period itself, and even cause as much distress. In others,
however, all the indications are very slight, but still
I believe they are always manifested sufficiently
for the time to be detected, if careful observation is
kept.

The time when the expulsion occurs also varies
in different persons, and under different circumstances. On the average, it is about the *seventh* or
eighth day, but may be as late as the *sixteenth*, as before explained. The *clot*, of course, is always present at the time, and indicates it beyond a doubt

I have known many females who have ascertained this time quite readily after the signs had been explained to them, and I believe nearly all would do so with a little trouble. Many of these nave even detected and preserved the *Clot*, which, on being placed under the microscope, has shown them the egg and its decidua most perfectly. Several of these clots I have in my Cabinet, both of the Human being and also of Animals. Every female who thus ascertains the precise period of the expulsion of the egg, of course knows when Conception in her case becomes *impossible*, because it cannot occur after the egg has escaped.

There are, however, many causes that may lead to error, and which may deceive persons very much if they are not acquainted with them. Thus some females are constantly liable to mere floodings, or discharges of blood from weakness, which they mistake for real Menstrual periods, and thus miscalculate. Others, again, have periods that are colorless, as before explained, and they, therefore, never suspect what they are when they really do occur. All females are liable at times to these unusual appearances, and are likely, therefore, to suppose that they have a period when they have not, and that they are free from it when it is actually taking place. In this way mistakes are very apt to occur, unless the individual has been sufficiently observant to detect true Menstruation by other signs than the mere color. It must be remembered that every discharge of blood is *not* a Menstrual discharge, and that many true Menstrual discharges are *perfectly colorless*. One sign can be always relied upon, however, to detect the true period, and that is the *odor* of the discharge, which is

so peculiar, that when once known it cannot bo
mistaken, there being no other discharge resembling it. In an ordinary flooding there is seldom
any particular odor, but this peculiar one is always
present at every Menstruation, though it be as thin
and colorless as water.

It is owing to these occasional deviations and unusual appearances that some females have supposed
they conceived immediately *before* the period.
They had simply experienced a flooding, and mis-
took it for Menstruation. Others have thought that
they conceived without having Menstruated, especially when nursing, but in them it had been color
less and unnoticed.

In very many cases I have made practical use of
these facts, when consulted in cases of barrenness,
and frequently with the most satisfactorily results, as
will be shown when speaking upon that disability.

In every instance—it may be confidently relied
upon—Conception takes place within *sixteen days*
after a Menstrual period, and usually within *eight
or nine days*, though it may be often difficult to ascertain the period, and another phenomenon may be
mistaken for it. At all other times Impregnation is
absolutely *impossible*, excepting possibly for a brief
period before the actual cessation, in the way that
will be explained in our next article.

§ MANNER OF IMPREGNATION.

The precise manner of impregnation, or the way
in which the two principles actually unite, can only
be understood by bearing in mind the account given
of the Semen in a former article. It was there
shown that the essential part of this principle con

sists of certain little living beings, called the *Seminal Animalcules*, which, undoubtedly, are the true impregnators If they are absent, or if their vitality be destroyed, the Semen has no effect whatever on the egg. This fact has been ascertained for some time, but it is only recently that the mode in which they operate has become known.

When speaking upon the female egg, in a former article, it was stated, that while in the Ovary, it contained a peculiar body, called the *Germinal Vesicle*, which, by a spontaneous movement, was cast out as soon as the egg entered the Tube, in such a way as to cause a rent, or torn place, in the membrane surrounding the egg. This bursting open of the Ovum had been noticed by many observers, but the object of it was long a mystery, till, fortunately, a curious discovery revealed its intention. It was found that if one of these Seminal Animalcules came in contact with an egg, which was opened in this way, it immediately *crept* in at the opening, and *buried itself in the interior.* The object, therefore, of the passing out of the Vesicle, is, evidently, to open a passage, by which the Animalcule can reach the interior of the egg, among the Vitellus, or yellow, and when there, it forms part of the rudiment of the future new being, as will be explained further on In this way, then, the two principles really unite, each being indispensable to the other, and the two together providing all the elements for the embryo —the Animalcule probably being the germ of the nervous system, or that part in which *animal life* really resides.

This also explains other circumstances formerly noticed, and shows that every peculiarity exhibited by either of the principles has its object. It was stated, for instance, respecting the Animalcules, that they had a remarkable tendency to move in a straight-forward direction, and with considerable vivacity. Now this tendency is evidently calcu·lated to carry them up into the Womb, so that they may reach the egg, and without it, they might never arrive there. The Semen is deposited, during coition, in the Vagina, and was always supposed to be *absorbed* or sucked up into the Womb, though not known to be so. It is probable that such absorption, or suction, does take place sometimes, but by no means invariably, I am convinced, and I have no doubt whatever, that conception can occur without it. Many females habitually lose most or all of the Semen after every association, and yet they conceive, though there evidently can occur but little passage of it in either of the above ways. The fact appears to·be that the Animalcules can pass up into the Womb themselves, by their own motions, and they evidently have the tendency above noticed, to move forward in one direction, given to them in order that they may reach their destination. Immediately they are deposited in the Vagina, if their vitality is perfect, all that find themselves placed in the proper direction, begin to move upwards, and they continue to do so till they reach the Uterus, as nothing seems to make them ever turn in the opposite direction. When any of them reach the interior of the Womb, if an egg be there that has been opened by the Vesicle passing out, one of them creeps in, and thus effects the impregnation. This fact has actually been seen under the microscope, and the entrance of the Animalcule within the egg is an undoubted occurrence.

It is easy to see from this, why it is that concep·

tion does not occur, as is often the case, when the male is too debilitated to form perfect Semen. The Animalcules are then too weak to pass up into the Womb, and consequently there is no impregnation. Any cause, therefore, which weakens their energy, and prevents their usual lively forward motion, is apt to prevent conception. As long as they are alive, however, provided one of them can be conveyed to the egg, impregnation may be effected, which explains why some females, whose organs act energetically, can conceive from these debilitated individuals while others cannot do so. If the Womb has great power it may draw up the Semen, and so allow the Animalcules to act, though they could not have moved up themselves, as they ordinarily do. In this way the greater energy of the female may partly make up for the exhaustion of the male, while, on the other hand, if the Animalcules be unusually vigorous, they may reach the Ovum entirely by their own unaided powers, and then impregnate when the female organs are totally powerless. From this we see why it is that conception can occur during sleep, or even during perfect unconsciousness from drugs, or blows upon the head, though most persons suppose otherwise. This has been proved, however, by numerous cases in human beings, as well as by direct experiment upon animals, and the reason will now be obvious enough. The condition of the female, though she be perfectly insensible, may not prevent conception, because the Animalcules can move up into the Womb by their own powers, and thus impregnate without any knowledge or concurrence whatever on her part. Many cases have been known in which females have conceived after having been violated but once, though people generally and even medical men have doubted it, and the possibility of their doing so will be obvious after this. It must be borne in mind, also, that in such cases the brutal violator is usually a man of strong passions, and of great sexual power, which may probably cause the Animalcules to be unusually vigorous, and thus increase the likelihood of conception. I once knew a female who became pregnant after violation, during which she was perfectly insensible, but who never became so after marriage; the reason why, it was of course not possible to ascertain with certainty but it may probably be found in the above explanation.

This also shows how erroneous it is to suppose, as most people do, that a female cannot conceive unless she experiences sexual enjoyment, or if the association be repugnant to her. There are numbers who never knew what the sexual feeling was, and some who have even suffered both pain and disgust, constantly, in association, and yet they have become pregnant. Nor will this appear extraordinary after our explanation, which shows that the female may be quite passive, so much sc, in fact, that conception may take place artificially, *without connection*. Experiments upon animals have proved that if the Semen be merely thrown into the Vagina, at the proper time, with a syringe, it will impregnate. And in some cases of malformation in married men, which prevented proper connection, the same practice has been advised, and with complete success. In fact, the presence in the female organs of the perfect male Semen, at the proper time, is all that is needed to cause conception, no matter how it may have come there, nor with what feelings its introduction may have been attended.

It should be observed, however, that though sexual feeling in the female is not absolutely necessary to conception yet, in many cases, it may much conduce to that event. Pleasurable excitement at the time of connection disposes the organs to more energetic action, and some females may possibly not conceive without it, though certainly all do not require it. We know that this excitement makes the Tubes contract more vigorously, and this causes them to bring the egg down earlier, and probably, also, it may make the womb contract, so as to draw up the semen more completely. In many cases barren females, of a cold temperament, have conceived immediately after having the sexual feeling produced.

From the foregoing statements it will be seen that Conception does not always take place at the moment of connection, nor even immediately after, and we shall soon discover that it may be delayed for a considerable time. As long as a living Animalcule remains in the female organs it is possible for it to reach the Womb, and thus effect impregnation if the egg be there. We have simply, therefore, to ascertain how long the Animalcules retain their vitality after being emitted in coition, and we shall then know the period during which impregnation may be delayed. In some females the Semen is either absorbed, or the Animalcules move up themselves, very quickly, so that they are impregnated almost at the moment of emission ; but in others there is no absorption at all, and the Animalcules may move very slowly. The actual time when the two principles unite, therefore, after a fruitful connection, is very different in different persons. It appears, according to accurate observations, that the Animalcules can remain alive in the female organs as long as *twenty-six hours* after they have been deposited there in connection, and it follows, therefore, that the impregnation may not take place till that time after. It is found that they begin to die, usually, after the second hour, and fewer of them are found alive as the time advances. At twelve hours usually half of them are dead; and at twenty hours but few are found living, though one or two have been discovered even at the twenty-sixth hour. As they die they break up, the tail separates from the body, and both parts begin to dissolve. It is possible, therefore, that the impregnation may take place *at any time within twenty-six hours after connection*, and it is manifestly absurd to talk, as some mere *book physiologists* do, about the importance of a proper state of mind at *the moment of conception*, as if that moment could be known. Perhaps the most frequent time is about two hours after connection, or when the Animalcules begin to die, but of course there will be great variation. When the Womb contracts with energy, or the Animalcules are unusually vigorous, the conception will be quick, and when otherwise, the reverse. And this makes it more likely to be quick in those of warm temperaments.

It is barely possible that the Animalcules could live through the latter part of the flow, if connection were had before it had ceased, and if so impregnation might follow such connection. Supposing the coition to occur twenty-six hours before the egg reached the Womb, some of the Animalcules might still be living when it arrived there, and of course could cause its impregnation, though unlikely. This is the only possible way in which conception can be effected before the cessation of the monthly flow. In many cases, however, the egg reaches the womb in less than twenty-six hours after the flow stops, and therefore connection may always cause conception at any early time after, even immediately. The *full time*, therefore, during which impregnation is *possible* is for the sixteen days *after* the flow has ceased, and perhaps for the twenty-six hours before it ceases, at all other times it is impossible.

It may appear to some persons, who have not bestowed full attention upon the subject, that there is danger in making such facts as these known, because, they say, young persons knowing that there are times when they can indulge with safety will be led to do so, when they would not if they feared the consequences. All this I have duly considered, and yet have come to the conclusion that there would be no advantage, in any way, in attempting to suppress such truths. In the first place, as society is now constituted, and with the means of disseminating all kinds of knowledge so complete as we have them, it is *not possible* to prevent any interesting fact from becoming generally talked of, if it be known to ever so small a number. Some idea of it is *sure* to get abroad, and most probably an erroneous one, calculated to mislead and do more harm, a thousand times over, than the truth could ever do. If only medical men could read and write, and if it were *certain* that none of them would ever speak of such things, they might be kept secrets, but such is not the case. In short it is *impossible*, even if it were advisable, to prevent such matters from becoming generally known, in some form or other, and it is far better for them to be known truly than otherwise.

It seems to me also that it is forming a very ow and degrading opinion of young persons, especially of females, to suppose that they are only kept from indulgence by fear of the consequences. If their virtue is solely dependent upon this, it is scarcely deserving of the name, and, in my opinion, is not very safe even with the *fear*. I feel certain, however, that there are not many young females who would either be disposed or persuaded to such practices, even if they were assured there was no risk. Those who think that such a disposition is *common* amongst them are very much mistaken. and judge from very imperfect experience. Persons who think so are generally of loose habits and principles themselves, though they may, from caution, disguise it, and their experience of females has usually been of the most unfortunate class, whom they have erroneously taken for correct types of the whole sex. The great majority of females are actuated by far more powerful and more desirable motives than *fear of consequences*, and it is well they are, for that alone would be a desirable dependence. I much doubt if *any one* ever remained permanently virtuous from this fear alone, for some time or other the fear would either be overcome, or means would be found of avoiding the consequences.

A very little consideration will, I feel assured, show the fallacy and injustice of this imputation, and explode the erroneous doctrine that ignorance is necessary to virtue. If it be true that young persons would practise association if they knew there was no danger, it follows, of course, that they are disposed to such indulgences, and that they are pleasing to them. Now, if this be the case, why is it that we do not find them, at the present time, taking and allowing other liberties, which would certainly be pleasing enough to make them desired, and in which they do know there is no danger? If we are to suppose, in respect to any two young persons, that the *only* reason they do not actually associate is the fear of consequences, we may justly conclude that they are, the whole time, in the habit of all other practices that can in any way gratify their propensities,* and which they know *are* safe. No one, I expect, will presume to say that such vicious practices are universal, and yet, if fear alone prevents worst practices, and these are *known* to be perfectly safe, why are they *not* universal? The truth is, as before remarked, that there are, especially in young females, other motives and sentiments of a higher order, which are the true barriers against vice, and when these are absent, fear alone is seldom any safeguard whatever. There are few adult persons, if any, who do not know that association *can* be practised without danger, by observing certain precautions, which still leave the indulgence pleasing enough; and yet, I presume, no one will contend that such a practice is pursued, though it certainly ought to be universally, if fear of consequences alone restrain, because here there is no danger.

Besides all this, there is another consideration, which should not be lost sight of. If it be contended that young people would immediately seek indulgence when they knew there was no danger, it must be admitted that they are usually in the habit of confidential communication with each other on such matters, and of discussing the chances of escape from the consequences, or else a mutual understanding could not be come to. Will any one

either contend or admit that this is the case? I
presume not ; and I am confident it is not so. With
all virtuous—or even commonly decent young persons, before marriage, such subjects are never
spoken of in a familiar manner, and any*attempt to
do so in either, would nea ly always alarm the
other, and put them on their guard. How, then,
could the subject be ever introduced between them,
so that everything relating to *times* and *periods*
could be calculated? The idea is as preposterous
as it is unjust, and cannot be admitted for a moment,
in reference to young people generally.

It is pretty evident to my mind, that any young
persons who would deliberately enter into such
calculations, and come to such a mutual understanding, merely from becoming possessed of this
piece of information, *could not have been virtuous
before.* They must have been in the habit of other
familiar practices, and, in all probability, of forming plans, or they could not see any superiority in
this.

It is time now that the people became acquainted
with one most important truth, namely, that ignorance is but a poor crutch for virtue, even when
it can be maintained, but at the present time it is
doubly worthless, from the fact that intelligence is
liable to knock it from under the moral cripple at
any moment. Knowledge and good principles are
far more worthy of confidence, for they will never
fail in the hour of need, nor can they be weakened
by any additional information fortuitously acquired
whereas with ignorance, there is constant fear.

It is true there are some people who will make
an improper use of any knowledge that can be
given them, but that is no reason why all others

should be deprived of it. These people are *Moral Lunatics*, and to withhold all knowledge from others, on their account, would be about as just and wise as to keep all in ignorance that fire will burn, because some madmen and criminals commit arson.

I have also noticed, that those who expressed such fear, that, to " *some people* " this knowledge will be dangerous, never include themselves among the number. They will not admit that it is dangerous to them, but fear that others may not be equally good.

It may also be remarked that in *practice* there are so many causes of *uncertainty, as already explained, that the number of days is not to be always relied upon, as a means of Prevention.*

CHAPTER X

GROWTH OF THE NEW BEING.

FŒTAL development, or the mode in which the new being first commences, and afterwards perfects itself, has, until recently, been imperfectly understood, especially the earliest stages. The embryo has been found of various ages, from a few days upwards, and also the Ovum soon after its impregnation ; but the first change in the egg, and the manner in which the embryo first organizes, have been the closest of mysteries. Certain observations, however, made very lately, have given some little insight into these incipent stages of our being, and the glance thus obtained has revealed so much that is both curious and useful, that more extended observations are being made every day, and, in all probability, we shall be, in a short time, as well acquainted with the organic actions of the embryo of a few hours' old, as we now are of the physiology of our own bodies.

The first changes observed in the egg, after impregnation, are very singular, and seem to indicate that the rudiment of the new organization is formed by a species of attraction, which concentrates the material of the Ovum, according to a certain plan, around a vital nucleus. If this nucleus be present, they form around it, as it were, by crytallization, but, if it is absent, they scatter and disperse.

On inspecting the egg at the various stages of its passage from the Ovary, we find that the first poable change which occurs in it, in the escape of the Germinal Vesicle, which takes place immediately it enters the Tubes. When it arrives in the Womb it is liable to be fecundated, and if one of the Animalcules be present, as before explained, it creeps in at the opening by which the Vesicle has escaped, and thus impregnates. The Vesicle itself appears to play no other part than that of bursting open the Ovum, and after accomplishing this, it disappears. The passing out of the Vesicle is, therefore, an indispensable event, and it is also a very curious one. If the egg be kept in view under the solar microscope, immediately after it has left the Ovary, this emission may be distinctly seen in all its stages. First there will be observed a point where the membrane surrounding the Vitellus, or yellow, becomes thin, and eventually opens, forming a minute mouth. Immediately after, part of a small globular body appears in the opening, and gradually progresses till it passes entirely through, when it drops down and disappears. This is the Germinal Vesicle, and, apparently, it is of no other use after its expulsion, the object of which is to open a way for the Animalcule. Its passage out is quite slow, often requiring four or five hours, and sometimes not being accomplished at all, in which case the egg could not be impregnated, and thus barrenness would result. In all probability, many females who have weak organs, are sterile from this cause, the egg not having sufficient vitality to expel the Vesicle.

Just before the Vesicle passes out, it is something like a minute bladder, partly full of a transparent liquid, and is far too small to be seen with the naked eye. In the centre, swimming in the fluid, are a number of minute granules, of a long oval figure, and of a yellowish color, which are closely compacted together, and form what is called the *Germinal Dot*. These granules are in almost constant and vivid motion, leaping and springing as if alive, but their motion ceases entirely immediately the Vesicle is fairly through the opening. There is always an *even* number of them, from twelve to twenty, and which is invariably the same in all individuals of the same species. Immediately after its escape, the Vesicle also breaks open, like the egg, and the granules escape, after which the whole dissolves, or disappears.

It will be observed that the Vesicle is first placed, in the centre of the Vitellus, and it appears to pass to the outer membrane along a kind of canal which naturally exists there, so that after its expulsion, there is a *direct opening to the centre of the egg* which, no doubt, is the path the Animalcule takes.

After the escape of the Vesicle, the egg undergoes some further change as it pursues its course along the Tubes, which are doubtless also necessary to fit it for being fecundated. It grows larger, and becomes darker in color, and the matter of the Vitellus appears to break up, in a great measure, or become intermixed, many of its Vesicles being burst and emptied of their contents.

It is supposed, as before stated, that when the egg reaches the Womb, after having been thus prepared the Animalcule creeps in at the opening made by the Germinal Vesicle in passing out, and that this is the actual fecundation, or union of the two principles. When the Animalcule has arrived in the interior of the Vitellus, it is properly situated similarly to the seed which is planted in the ground.

and finds precisely those materials and conditions favorable to its growth and further development.

The peculiar changes which the two principles undergo immediately after their union, have not been observed in the human being, from the diffi-culty of obtaining the proper specimens, but in other beings they have been studied at every stage, and judging from analogy in other processes, they are precisely the same in all alike.

In other beings, then, and no doubt in the human being also, immediately after impregnation the Vi-tellus, or yellow, forms itself into a certain *definite number* of cellules, or hollow globes, connected to-gether in a central mass. The number is *always even*, being *four*, *six*, or *eight*, but varying in differ-ent species, though always the same in any one species. If there be an *odd* number of these cel-lules formed, they will never produce a perfect being, but a *montrosity*, which shows that the per-fect organization is first formed or commenced on an even arrangement of the cellules, and if that is not effected, it is necessarily imperfect.

As soon as the primary cellules are distinctly formed, others begin to appear in the interstices be-tween them, till sixteen or twenty are formed, and the original ones increase considerably in size. All this occurs within a few hours, and in a short time after, varying from an hour or two, to a few days, according to the length of pregnancy in different beings, the first rudiments of organs begin to ap-pear. The even number of original cellules first form themselves *either into the Testicles or into the Ova-ries*, or, in some of the lower animals, into the *Liver*, and these are, therefore, the first parts developed.

While this is going on, we observe, under the

membrane which hold the original cellules together, myriads of minute granules, which are in constant and rapid motion, precisely like to that of Animalcules, which some have even thought them to be. This motion ceases soon after the first organs are formed, and the granules all grow together, so as to form a membrane, which becomes *the skin*. This, of course, surrounds the Ovaries and Testicles, the parts first formed, and all the other organs, as they appear, have to be developed underneath it.

The smallest portion of *opium* stops the action of these granules immediately, if it be placed upon them while the ovum is under the microscope, and so will some other substances. If they are made too hot also, as is sometimes the case under the solar microscope, though not dried, their motion ceases instantly. Now this fact may be more important than it first appears, and may give us the true cause of many *Organic Diseases of the Skin*, which otherwise can in no way be accounted for. It is probable that the peculiar motion of these granules is necessary to their proper *arrangement*, or to the perfect formation of the skin, and if anything checks or deranges that action the skin is in consequence organized imperfectly. This shows that we cannot commence the study of the human being *too soon*, and that those who think it is time enough after birth are greatly mistaken. When we find, by experiments like those above mentioned, that opium will arrest the action of the skin granules in the Ovum, is it not at least possible that it may have the same effect in the mother's body? and that in this way children may have the seeds of disease implanted in them before they are born, by the injudicious use of such drugs by the mother?

As soon as the primary organ is formed, which is before remarked is either the Testicle or the Ovary, and the skin is organized around them, the other parts begin to appear in succession, in the order described below. The position of many organs is distinctly marked before they are formed, by collections of granules, which are nearly always in rapid motions, as if arranging themselves. This is especially the case with the eye.—The first formation therefore is from cellules and granules, which agglomerate together round central nuclei, and much resemble the cellular structure of many vegetables, especially the Lichens, and some of the Fungi. In fact the matter of the egg seems to develop into the general Organic Structure, every part of which, bones, Muscles, and Organs, is first formed of cellular tissue. By itself, however, the egg can only develop in this way *like a vegetable*, and only to a limited extent. It apparently never originates the truly *animal* or *spiritual* part, THE NERVOUS SYSTEM! This is the part by which sentient beings think and feel, and which truly makes them above mere vegetables. Now this part, or at least the central portion of it, the *Brain* and *Spinal Marrow*, is with good reason supposed to be originated from the *Seminal Animalcule*, which is living to commence with. By noticing the form of the animalcule it will be seen that it is almost identical with the form of the great nervous centres, the largely developed upper part representing the Brain, and the long lower extremity the Spinal Marrow. Even the Embryo itself, in the earliest stages of its growth, has the same outline, the head being large, and the lower parts tapering off to a long thin extremity, which shortens as it becomes older. In fact the general resemblance of the new being to the Seminal Animalcule is obvious till the fifteenth day, and at the eighth or tenth they seem almost identical.

According to this theory therefore the whole of the bodily structure, excepting the nervous system, is formed by the egg, or rather exists in it always when it is perfectly developed independently of impregnation, but it is only like a framework, or shell, incapable of animal life. Into this Framework the living animalcule makes its way, being perfectly adapted by its form to dwell therein, and thus imparts what was wanting, namely, a *Nervous System*, which originates the *spiritual* or *animal* power. The two then grow together, become thoroughly incorporated, and eventually form the perfect human being.

There is, therefore, a definite part for each principle to play, and we see why it is that neither can form the perfect being alone. The egg by itself will sometimes form into a rude likeness of the body, as many of our cases have shown, but it is merely like the growth of a vegetable, and wanting the other principle, the living animalcule, to vivify it, can never become a human being.

It must be borne in mind, however, that though the Nervous System is supposed, according to this view, to originate altogether from the male, yet it is nevertheless modified, and influenced in its development, by the peculiar growth of the body in which it is contained, and that originates with the Female In like manner the body may also be influenced in its development by peculiarities of the nervous system, and thus each sex performs about an equal part in the process of generation.—If the Seminal Animalcule be weak or deformed in all probability the Nervous System of the new being will be the same, and if the egg be imperfect the body will be deformed or diseased, and of course the condition of either affects the other.

To Generate a perfect human being we must have from the female a perfect egg, and from the male a perfect and vigorous animalcule, and the two must come together under proper circumstances and condititions. All this requires perfect Organizations, and healty action in both, without which the new being must be imperfect in some particular, and being born so, no after cultivation can completely eradicate the defect.

I have no doubt myself but that the greater part of the diseases and deformities we see, both of body and mind, originate in this way before birth, and that in future years, when these things are better understood, they will be in a great measure, if not entirely avoided. The Moral Preacher and the bodily Physician will be but little needed, because the evils they now labor to cure, and too often in vain, will be *prevented*. *Innate sin* and *constitutiona. disease*, will be used simply as terms to describe a former state of things, but will be quite obsolete at that day.

As soon as the first outlines of the new Organization are formed another phenomenon occurs, which though we cannot explain its meaning, still appears deeply interesting as well as curious. The embryo, which much resembles the Animalcule in its form, appears to struggle violently among the fluids and membranes, by which it is surrounded, till it perfectly frees itself, and then it begins to *turn round* slowly and regularly at first, but eventually extremely rapid and irregular. This peculiar mo

tion has been observed in the embryos of many
different animals, and is evidently necessary in
some way or other to their development. It probably originates in the same way as the peculiar
motions observed among the forming granules, and
may serve a similar purpose.

The following description of the growth of the
Fœtus at the several after stages is partly taken
from my work, " *The Matron's Manual of Midwifery*," but since that description was written several
new discoveries have been made, and our knowledge
of the subject has been made more complete. Much
is contained in the present work therefore, that is
not to be found in the " Manual," on this particular topic, though many other subjects are there discussed which it is not necessary here to introduce
at all, the two works having different spheres and
uses.

At the *Twelfth Day* we first begin to see the new
Organization and its envelopes distinctly with the
naked eye. The whole is about the size of a large
pea, and the remains of the vitellus, or yellow, can
be readily seen. It is all surrounded by two mem-
branous coverings, the outer one called the *chorion*,
and the inner one the *amnion*. Between these is a
gelatinous substance, and within the amnion is a
fluid, called the liquor amnii. The two membranes,
the liquor amnii, and the inclosed ovum, are called
the *ovulum !* Immediately after conception the uterus also commences to secrete, from its inner walls,
a considerable addition to the *decidua*. This lines
the whole cavity, so that when the ovum first
passes out of the tube it is met by this lining which
seems to prevent its entrance into the womb. The
ovum, however, presses upon it and so makes a

depression, like a nest, to which it lies. This prevents its moving about, or falling to the bottom of the womb.

The weight of the entire ovulum is about one grain. The embryo commences in the germ, and may now be seen about the size of a pin's point The vitellus removes away from it, but remain connected by a small pedicle or thread-like tube, down which it is gradually absorbed as nutriment. A small white thread, scarcely perceptible, may be seen sometimes as early as this period, being the commencement of the brain and spinal marrow. The mouth is visible also from the twelfth to the twentieth day, and frequently the eyes. These are placed at first on the side of the head, like those of quadrupeds, and move round to the front afterwards.

At twenty-five days, the embryo is about the size of a large ant, which it also resembles in form. It begins to have a little more consistence, and the future bones begin to resemble cartilage, or gristle. A small groove may be seen denoting the neck, which thus indicates the separation of the head from the trunk. The weight is three or four grains.

The first month, it is about the size of a Bee, and is somewhat like a small worm bent together, the arms may be seen like two little warts; they are first formed under the skin, and shoot out like buds, growing straight from the body; afterwards they become folded together, in a curious manner, upon the breast. The head is as large as the rest of the body, and upon it we can now see distinctly the eyes, like two black dots, the mouth, like a line, and also the nose. The lower extremity is lengthened out like a tail. Weight about ten grains.

The second month. Every part has now become

much more developed, and the general form is that
of a human being.   The superior members are
much more elongated, and the inferior ones begin to
be distinguished, forming in the same manner as the
others.   The fingers are united together by a membrane, like the web on a Frog's foot.   In the ribs,
clavicles, and jaw-bones, a few points can be seen
ossified, the cartilage beginning to harden into bone.
The rudiments of the first teeth are also visible
The weight is about one drachm, and the length one
inch.

At about seventy days the eyelids are visible, the
nose becomes prominent, the mouth enlarges, and
the external ear may be seen.   The neck is well
defined.   The brain is soft and pulpy, and the heart
is perfectly developed.

Every organ is originally formed without either
blood or blood vessels.   The circulation which
afterwards takes place in them is merely for their
subsequent development.   The heart is perfect in
all its parts, and even has a slight motion, before
the blood is found in it.

Three months.   All the essential parts are well
defined.   The eyelids distinct, but firmly closed.
The lips perfect, but drawn tightly together.   The
heart beats forcibly, and in the larger vessels red
blood is seen.   The fingers and toes are confined,
and the muscles begin to be apparent.   The organs
of generation are remarkably prominent, but still it
is somewhat difficult, at first, to distinguish the sex
by these organs, notwithstanding their development
as the principal parts in both are nearly identical in
form.   It can, however, be ascertained by other cir
cumstances, as the form of the head, dorsal spine,
thorax, and abdomen   It now weighs about two

ounces and a half, and measures four or five inches in length.

Four months. The development is remarkably increased. The brain and spinal marrow becomes firmer, the muscles distinct, and a little cellular tissue is formed. The abdomen is fully covered in and the intestines are no longer visible. A little of the substance called *meconium* even collects in the intestines, the same as is found in them at birth. It now weighs seven or eight ounces, and measures six or seven inches. The bones are ossified in a great part of their extent, and the rudiments of the second set of teeth are visible, under the first.

The uterus now is so large that it can no longer remain in the lower part of the pelvis, but is compelled to rise up into the abdomen for more room. This change of position is improperly called *quickening !* Sometimes it takes place very gradually, so that it is scarcely noticed, but more frequently it rises suddenly, disturbing all the internal organs, and causing in them considerable derangement till they accommodate themselves to the change. This occurence often causes unnecessary alarm, though the sickness and other unpleasant sensations are always sufficiently annoying.

This stage corresponds with that in which the young and oviparous animals break the shell and escape. The human being, however, undergoes a remarkable change, and remains in the womb for a period longer than that already past, in order to become more perfected.

From four to nine months the development is proportionally much more rapid than during the first four months, owing to the circulation of perfect red blood, which is now found the same as in the adult and is probably derived from the mother.

Five months. Every part is considerably increased in size, and becomes more perfect. The lungs enlarge, and are even capable of being, to a certain extent, dilated. The skin becomes much stronger. The situation of the nails can be discerned. The meconium is more abundant, and lower down in the intestines. The length is now eight or ten inches, and the weight fifteen or sixteen ounces.

Six months. The nails are marked. The head becomes downy, from the first development of the hair. A little fat is formed. Length twelve inches weight from one and a half to two pounds. No indications of intellectual faculties.

Seven months. The whole being has rapidly progressed. The nails are formed, the hair is perfect, in the male the testicles descend to the scrotum, and in the female the ovaries reach the brim of the pelvis. The bones are tolerably firm, and the meconium collects in the large intestines. Length fourteen inches, weight about three pounds. Intellectual functions not yet exercised.

The two remaining months are merely devoted to further increase in size and weight. No new phenomena present themselves.

Nine months. Every function has become active. The skin becomes colored, and perspiration occurs. There are no indications of the intellectual functions, but the animal functions are remarkably active, particularly that of *taste*, which no doubt leads to the act of sucking, from the natural desire for its gratification. The child can now experience all the ordinary sensations of pain, hunger, heat, and cold, and is capable of preserving an independent existence if brought into the world.

§ FŒTAL NUTRITION.

THE manner in which the new being derives its nutriment, or the material by which it grows, is, in a great measure, unknown to us, though we certainly obtain some little information about it by a study of the apparatus employed in the process.

For the first fifteen or twenty days the substance called the *Vitellus*, which is analogous to the yolk of the ordinary egg, appears to supply most, if not all of the material that is required in the formation of the new being ; and, indeed, this substance does not totally disappear till after the third month, though we cannot suppose it to be the sole source of nutriment then. It is also supposed, by some, that the amniotic liquor, in which the fœtus floats, may afford same nutriment, either by being swallowed, or by being absorbed through the skin. It is certain that this fluid is nutritive, and there is nothing impossible in its absorption, though it is not very likely to occur to a sufficient extent. The idea that it can be swallowed, however, is erroneous, because the mouth of the Fœtus is firmly closed while in the Womb ; and besides, children have been born alive without *mouths*, and even without *heads*, and of course they could not have swallowed anything. It is now generally conceded by Physiologists that the material required by the Fœtus, for its nutrition, is obtained from the blood of the mother, through the medium of the Placenta, and the vessels in the Umbilical cord. It is, however, a matter of dispute whether the maternal blood is sent directly, in its ordinary state, into the body of the child, or whether it first undergoes a preparatory process, which most modern authors suppose it does.

.PLATE XI.

The Impregnated Womb at Five Months.

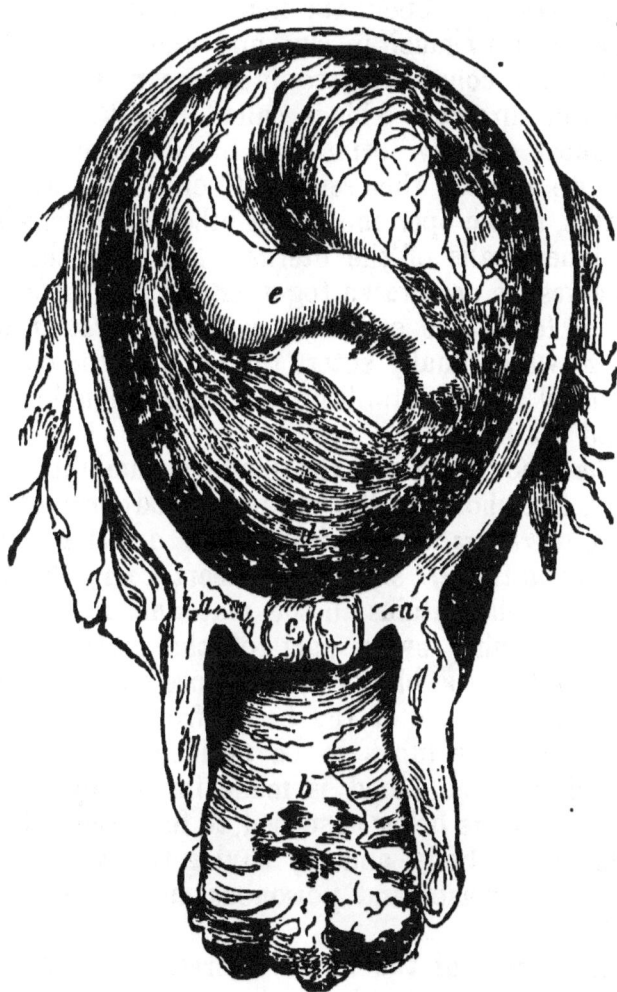

a, a. The Walls of the Womb.—*b*, The Vagina.—*c*, The Mouth of the Womb.—*d*, The Membranes —*e*, The Fœtus.

From the earliest period of gestation tho middle membrane, called the chorion, is covered, on its outer surface, with a number of small protuberances called *villosities*, which subsequently become true blood vessels. About the fourth month these have increased very much in size and number, and have all become conglomerated into one mass, in form like a mushroom. This is called the *Placenta*. It is almost entirely formed of blood vessels, which seem to attach themselves at one end, by open mouths, to the open mouths of other blood vessels on the inner walls of 'the uterus. At the other end these vessels are drawn together and lengthened out into a long tube called the *umbilical cord*, or *navel string*, which finally enters the body of the child at the navel and so establishes the connection between it and the mother.

The blood vessels in the placenta, umbilicus, and fœtus, like those in the maternal body, are of two kinds, *Arteries* and *veins*. The arteries, which come from the *left* side of the heart, carry the pure blood, which contains all the materials for forming and nourishing every part of the system. The veins contain the blood in its impure state, and take it to the *right* side of the heart, from whence it is forced into the lungs to be purified by the act of breathing. The blood is made impure by some of its constituents being absorbed, to form the different parts of the body, and by having thrown into it a quantity of waste and poisonous matter no longer needed.

The course of the blood, therefore, is from the left side of the mother's heart along her arteries till it reaches the arteries of the Uterus, from thence it passes into those of the Placenta, and thence into

those of the Umbilicus which convey it into the
body of the child. When there it circulates in its
arteries, supplies the material for its further in
crease and development, becomes in consequence
impure, and passes into its veins, the same as in the
maternal body. From these veins it passes into
those of the umbilicus and placenta, and, apparently
into those of the mother, by which it is conveyed to
the right side of her heart, and by its action to her
lungs, to be again purified when she breathes. This
explains what was previously stated, that the child
uses the mother's heart, lungs, and stomach while
in the womb, and has, therefore, no occasion to use
its own.

The diameter of the placenta is about six inches,
and its thickness about one inch and a half. The
length of the umbilical cord is from eighteen to
twenty-four inches, its diameter about half an inch
These dimentions are, however, subject to great
variation. Instances are mentioned of the cord
being five feet long, and as thick as the child's arm
I have seen one myself four feet long. Sometime.
it will be very short, not more than eight or ten
inches. It is composed of one artery and two veins,
twisted together like the strands of a cable, and of a
sheath surrounding them composed of the chorion
and amnion. Between the sheath and the vessels
is a thick gelatinous fluid called the Gelatine of
Wharton.

This explanation, it must be remembered, is in
fact, merely hypothetical. The direct passage of
the blood through the Placenta, from the mother's
vessels into these of the cord, is denied by many
Physiologists, who contend that there is an inter-
mediate set of vessels in the Placenta, in which it

first undergoes important changes. They also con
tend that the impure blood does not pass through
into the mother's veins at all, but is purified in the
Placenta, and immediately returned. Some have
even averred that the Placenta is not required at all,
to supply nourishment, but is merely a purifying
organ. It is now known, however, that it is not
absolutely essential to either process, for children
have been born alive, and perfectly formed, which
merely floated loosely in the amniotic liquor, having
neither Placenta nor cord, nor any other connection
with the mother. How they were nourished we
cannot tell. These, however, must be regarded
merely as curious exceptions, there being little
doubt but that fœtal nutrition is ordinarily effected
through the Placenta and cord, by means of the
mother's blood, somewhat in the manner we have
described.

§ PECULIARITIES OF THE FŒTAL CIRCULATION.

From the circumstance of the fœtus not using its
heart and lungs, like the adult, its circulation has
several modifications.

The engine by which the blood is forced along
its vessels is the *heart!* This is divided into two
distinct parts, each of which has two cavities, the
upper one called the *auricle,* and the lower one the
ventricle, which communicate with each other by
curious valves. In the adult the whole of the
impure blood is poured into the right auricle, that
from the lower part of the body by the *inferior vena
cava,* and that from the upper part by the *superior
vena cava.* From the right auricle it passes
into the right ventricle, which pumps into the

iungs, by way of the pulmonary artery; here it is purified by the act of respiration, and then brought, when pure, by the pulmonary veins, into the left auricle, and passes from thence into the left ventricle, which pumps it into the great aorta, and from thence into the smaller arteries all over the body.

The two sides of the heart, therefore, do not communicate directly with each other, but there is a strong partition between them. In the fœtus the arterial blood from the mother, when it leaves the umbilical artery, enters first the liver, runs through its vessels, gives off the bile found in it, and then joins the vena cava inferior. By this passage it is taken into the right auricle, along with the impure blood of the vena cava. From the right auricle it passes through a hole in the partition directly into the left auricle, instead of taking the indirect route by the lungs as in the adult. From the left auricle it passes into the left ventricle, and is from thence distributed by the arteries all over the body. This opening in the partition is called the *foramen ovale!*

After birth, when the blood begins to pass through the lungs, this passage closes up. By the eighth day it is generally obliberated, often much sooner, though occasionally it has remained open longer without inconvenience. In some cases the foramen ovale does not close at all. The child has then what is called the *blue disease!* The whole body is of a uniform leaden, or blue color, and the whole system is generally languid and sluggish. The blue color is caused by the dark blood of the veins mixing with that of the arteries. These children mostly die early, but some live to be five or six years old, and one I saw twelve, but this is rare. No remedy can be had for this affliction, and I have never known it to cure spontaneously. Some children are so very dark for a few days after birth as to cause great alarm. This is owing to the foramen ovale being very open and closing slowly. No apprehension need be experienced in such cases, as it soon subsides.

The impure blood from the upper part of the fœtal body, which is brought down by the superior vena cava, also enters the right auricle, but does not pass from thence through the foramen, like that from the inferior vena cava. By a peculiar arrangement this blood is made to pass down into the right ventricle, and from thence along the pulmonary artery, the same as in the adult state. Only a very small portion, however, passes into the lungs, the great part being taken along a tube called the *ductus arteriosus* into the great artery called the aorta, where it begins to turn down to the lower part of the body. In consequence of this, the arterial blood going down to the lower part of the body, is mixed with this portion of impure, venous blood, brought by the ductus arteriosus from the superior vena cava ; while that going to the head, and upper part of the body remains pure. And this is the reason why the lower part is always so much smaller than the upper part, previous to birth ; it receives less pure nourishment. The head and chest appear, at an early period, almost as large as the rest of the body.

This circumstance also explains why, in the great majority of cases, the *right* arm is preferred to the *left*, and has more real power. The place where the ductus arteriosus pours the impure blood into the aorta, is almost immediately opposite to where the artery is given off which feeds the left arm. In consequence of which, in most cases, a small portion of this impure blood becomes mixed with the arterial blood, and the left arm is, therefore, in the same situation as the lower limbs, and like them is comparatively imperfectly developed. The right arm is not liable to any such deprivation. In some cases the insertion of the ductus arteriosus is lower down, so that no such mixture occurs. Both arms are then equal, and this accounts for the fact that in some persons there is no difference. In some cases, no doubt, early habit may overcome this natural inferiority, and even give the preference to the left arm; but such instances are rare.

The ductus arteriosus closes up about the same time as the foramen ovale.

The two veins which convey the impure blood back to the mother, to be purified, originate from the iliac artery, pass up the sides of the bladder towards the navel, enter the sheath of the cord, and so reach the placenta. They are obliterated about the third or fourth day after birth, and assume the form of a cord.

The real source of *all* the blood in the body of the child is a mystery; it would certainly appear most likely for the whole of it to be derived from the mother, but there are many circumstances which make it probable that the child may form some itself, by digesting the fluid it is supposed to absorb. This view is supported by the fact that there is found in its bowels at birth, and even before a greenish substance like excrement, called *Meconium*. This has every appearance of being the product of digestion, though some suppose it to be derived from the liver It occasionally contains hair, and other anomalous substances.

CHAPTER XI

EXTRA-UTERINE CONCEPTION, AND UNNATURAL OR MONSTROUS GROWTHS.

IT sometimes happens that a Fœtus is formed *outside* of the Womb, either on the Ovary, in the Tube, or in some part of the Abdomen, as among the intestines, for instance. These are called *Extra Uterine Conceptions,* and their origin has long been a mystery. It was long thought that such cases proved the old doctrine of Conception, which supposed that the Semen was conveyed to the Ovary and impregnated the egg there, otherwise, said its advocates, how could the Fœtus ever be found outside the Womb if Conception takes place inside ? In my first work on *The Origin of Life,* this old Theory was laid down *as a Theory,* because nothing better was known, but since then the new discoveries have enabled us to explain these occurrences more rationally.

The true cause of an extra Uterine conception is this : Any sudden and violent emotion, as a *fright,* for instance, will sometimes reverse the action of the Fallopian Tubes, so that they will convey anything *from* the Womb towards the Ovaries, or contrary to their usual course, so that if an egg should have passed down near to the Womb, but not have quite left the Tube, it might be taken back again during this reverse action. Now, according to our previous explanation, it will be seen that the egg may be impregnated, in some cases, while in the uterine end of the Tube, because the Semen occasionally penetrates so far, and it is therefore possible that an egg so impregnated may be conveyed to the other end of the Tube, or even outside of the Womb, by this reverse action. It is not necessary for the development of the egg that it should be in the womb, but, on the contrary, it will develop in any part, if it can attach itself to some blood-vessel, though it will never form into a perfect human being except inside the womb. In these cases, therefore, when the egg after its impregnation is taken to the other end of the Tube, or to the outside, it is possible for it to grow in this way, though imperfectly, and thus form an extra Uterine Conception.

I have two beautiful models representing actual cases of this kind.—It may even be taken, by the motion of the body, after it becomes loose, to various parts of the pelvic, or abdominal cavities, where it will attach itself and develop in the same manner. In other cases it has been known to imbed itself in the walls of the womb, and develop there. Several instances of Extra Uterine Conception have come under my notice, and I have bestowed considerable attention upon them. Sometimes the development will be indefinite, having no resemblance to a human being; while at others it will be tolerably perfect, and attain a large size, as large in some instances as a fœtus of five months. It is always however, a montrosity, imperfect in some particular. The placenta and cord are found, as in the Inter-Uterine Conception, as also the amnion and chorion, but only occasionally a membrane analogous to the decidua, this being properly a product of the Uterus alone. The expulsion of these products cannot, of course, be effected in the ordinary

way, they have either to be removed by an operation, which is rarely resorted to, or else left to
nature, in which case they may terminate in various
ways. Some authors say they will occasionally be
absorbed, and so dissappear. More generally, however, labor pains come on at the ordinary time,
decay commences, an abscess is formed, and the
remains of the fœtus work through the opening. If
she does not immediately succumb, the wound may
then heal and the woman perfectly recover her
nealth. Cases of this kind have often been met
with. I remember one in which all the parts did
not come away under six months; the head was
nearly perfect. Sometimes the pains will return
every nine months, for a long time, before decay
commences. In other cases, instead of decaying,
the fœtus, with its appendages, will become callous,
and form into a hard tumor, which may remain
during the individual's life, without causing serious
results. I saw a lady very recently who had
carried one of these tumors for nine years! And I
assisted at the dissection of another in whom it had
existed for thirteen years. It was as large as the
head, and fixed on the right side of the abdomen,
apparently just underneath the skin. These accidents, though serious, are not necessarily always
fatal. Females have keen known to suffer from
them several times in succession, though sometimes
the next conception will be perfectly natural. Very
generally, however, the first case is followed by
barrenness.

§ FORMATION OF ONE CHILD WITHIN ANOTHER.

Fœtal development will sometimes occur under

more extraordinary circumstances even than those already mentioned. One foetus may be contained within another. A case of this kind occurred at Verneuil, in France, in the year 1804. A child named Bissien, who differed in no external particular from other children, but always complained of something being the matter in his left side. A small tumor appeared there early, but the development of his body and mind went on as usual, and nothing particular was noticed till he was thirteen ▮▮▮▮ of age. The tumor then suddenly increased ▮▮▮ he began to pass from his body a quantity ▮▮▮▮d matter mixed with long hair, fever set in ▮▮▮▮ died when about fourteen. Upon making a ▮▮▮▮tem examination, there was found, between ▮▮▮▮stines and spine, the remains of a foetus. ▮▮▮, nails, hair, and bones, were not like those ▮▮▮▮ infant, but evidently indicated that the in-▮▮▮▮tus was as old as the one it whom it was ▮▮▮▮ Such cases are extremely rare, and I believe this was the first that was properly observed or explained. Singular as it may appear, it can be readily explained, if the description we have given of the process, and organs of generation be borne in mind.

In all such cases there have been two eggs impregnated, as in a case of twins, but only one has developed into a child while in the womb and the other has become enclosed within its body. The egg thus enclosed may retain its vitality, but not develop for an indefinite period, perhaps not till many years after that child has been born, and very likely there are many cases in which it never does. There is nothing more extraordinary in its development, however, when it does take place under such circumstances, than there is in an Extra Uterine Conception in the mother's body, because the conditions are the same. The most wonderful circumstances is that the egg should remain so long dormant and still be able to grow after such a lapse of time, but this way we cannot explain.

I have met with several cases of included fœtuses in dissecting animals, and a Physiological friend informed me that he once found one in a man of thirty, which was so perfect that he could perceive it to be of the male sex. This man was, therefore, really pregnant with *his own Twin Brother*.

As a proof of our explanation of the causes of Extra Uterine Fœtuses it may be stated that, in every such case when its history could be traced, a fright or other accident had been experienced about the period of conception. It is a singular fact also that the most of such cases have been *from illicit intercourse*, in which females of course are often liable to the fear of discovery and exposure, and which, from its character, is always liable to be disturbed.

The most convincing proof, however, that extra uterine conception is owing to fright, or disturbing violence, has been obtained by experiment upon Animals. It has been found that a blow upon the head, if it be given about the time of conception, will nearly always cause an extra uterine development. It is dangerous, therefore, for association ever to be practised when any disturbance may be experienced immediately after. If conception has already taken place such violence or fright may materially affect the development of the new being, by suspending the vital power for a time. Thus a celebrated Physiologist gave a female dog a violent

blow on the head, at the time of conception, so that
she was partially paralysed for some days, and
when she brought forth her young, all of them,
except one, either had *no hind legs*, or were deformed, or puny and weak. In another similar
experiment four deformed young ones were born
and three others were formed extra uterine. The
four eggs had therefore evidently reached the
womb at the time of Impregnation, while the other
three were at the uterine end of the tube, which
having its action reversed took them to the
outside.

§ FALSE CONCEPTIONS.

A VARIETY of abnormal productions are found in
the uterus, called moles and false conceptions,
which are in no way connected with impregnation,
such as tumors, polypi, &c. The mole of generation is an abnormal development of the impregnated
ovum. It has various forms, but most frequently
resembles a mere shapeless mass of flesh, enclosed
in an envelop full of fluid. On carefully dissecting this substance we can usually discover some
traces of the fœtal structure ; at other times we
find nothing but the bag of fluid. Sometimes the
production will remain attached to the mother by a
kind of cord and placenta, and develop into a shapeless monstrosity ; at others it will be entirely dis-
connected. These growths probably originate
from a blighted ovum, which retains sufficient life
merely to develop, but not to organize. I have
known them to attain a large size, and some females
to have many of them in succession. What causes
moles we do not know, nor can we always distin-

guish one from a natural pregnancy. Occasionally they assume the most fantastic shapes, and resemble the most incongruous objects. It is this circumstance, no doubt, which gave rise to the statements we sometimes hear, and read of, in old works, of women bringing forth *animals, plants, &c. !* I have seen some moles, myself, which could be easily mistaken for such things, by persons who did not attentively examine them, and whose imaginations were a little lively. A kind of imperfect Animalcule, called the *Hydatid,* is also found in the uterus. It merely resembles a bag of jelly, and floats in a fluid. Its size varies from that of a pea to a chestnut. Sometimes only one is found, at others a number. When removed from the fluid in which they live and put in warm water they will often move, which shows them to be alive. Similar beings are formed in the liver and kidneys. Their origin is unknown.

§ DEFORMITIES AND MONSTROSITIES.

Monstrosities. These anomalous productions, called also *lusus naturæ,* are of various kinds. They may either have more parts than natural, or less, or unnatural parts. Sometimes there is a confusion of parts only. Thus we sometimes have a fœtus with two heads, or an additional number of hands or feet. And sometimes we have them with only one leg or arm. Then again we see others with supernumerary parts that resemble no member in particular. And at other times we find some of the parts transposed, particularly the viscera. The causes of these accidents are not well understood. An opinion prevails very generally that they are altogether owing to some personal violence, or strong mental emotion experienced by the mother during pregnancy. Thus fright, sudden joy, or the sight of any disagreeable object are thought to be able to produce them. In many cases this opinion is probably correct, so far as the mere fact is concerned, but some very absurd notions are entertained as to the manner in which these causes operate. I shall, therefore, endeavor to give a scientific explanation.

A deficiency of any part, or an imperfect development of it, is evidently caused by something disturbing the vital process, and depriving that particular part of its power of growth, either permanently or for a time, but what those causes are it is impossible to tell. Sometimes the toes, or the fingers, or some of the limbs become imperfect in this way, and sometimes the heart, or some other internal organ, and children have even been born with no heads.

The disturbing cause may either operate from the first, and then there is no trace of the part, or it may operate at a later period, and then the part is merely smaller and more imperfect than the others. Thus sometimes we see one arm or one leg only half as large as its fellow, and sometimes the whole body is dwarfish and the head large. At other times the roof of the mouth is imperfect, or an eye, or the ear, so as to cause congenital deafness and blindness, and sometimes the upper lip is imperfect causing *hare-lip*.

There is no foundation, however, for the notion that these deficiencies are always caused by frights or fancies, or that the mother can produce them by injuring herself in the same part, or by placing her hands on it merely, as many suppose. In many such cases there is no doubt, if the truth could have been known that the deficiency existed before the fright was experienced, but people are apt to suppose that it must have been caused by the fright merely because it followed after it.

Sometimes when there are two Ova impregnated, instead of both forming perfectly, as in twins, or one being included within the other, as in the case of the boy Bissien, they will become so intermixed as to be grafted, as it were, one upon the other, or grow together. The parts where they touch, then, do not form and these only develop certain portions of the different fœtuses connected together. In this way are produced those monstrosities that we see with two heads, two bodies, or many arms, or legs. If there should be more than two Ova join together, of course, the confusion of parts would be greater, and the monster still more unnatural.

Two perfect twins are also liable to grow together, if they touch, and so become connected, in any part. Thus some have been found joined at the back, others at the stomach, and some by the side, like the *Siamese Twins*, between whom there is a ligament.

Most of these monstrosities are probably caused by some disturbing agency at the time of conception, or during pregnancy ; but monsters may also result from imperfect eggs, as before explained, and also from imperfect or deformed Animalcules.

They may originate with the male, therefore, as well as with the female, and I have known a man who had three deformed children by one wife, and two by another, owing to imperfect Animalcules, as I proved by observing them.

It is certain, however, that cases occur sometimes that may well excuse the common belief, especially as people generally are not in the habit of properly connecting cause and effect. Thus a pregnant mother has seen a man who has lost his arm, and her child when born has been similarly deficient. No doubt, however, other pregnant women might have been worse affected by the sight, and yet have had perfect children, and probably she would have had the one-arm child just the same if the man had not been seen by her. It is more likely that her child's arm was not formed at the time of her fright, from some other cause, for if it were, we must suppose that the fright *destroyed it*, and then comes the question, how was it disposed of, and in what way was it carried off?

In Fleming's Zoology a remarkable instance is given of a Cat, who was much terrified while with young, by having her tail severely trodden upon, and who brought forth, at the usual time, five kittens, only one of which was perfect, all the others having *their tails destorted* in a singular manner, and all alike. This, however, was from real bodily injury, affecting the vital power, and not from *Imagination.*

§ REMARKABLE CASE OF A FŒTAL MONSTROSITY.

THE case represented in the following cut is one recorded a short time ago in the London Lancet. It was the mother's thirteenth pregnancy, and her previous children had been quite perfect. She had received no *fright* of any kind, nor had she been subject to any unusual *longings.*

It will be observed that the upper part of the

PLATE XII.

Singular Monstrosity

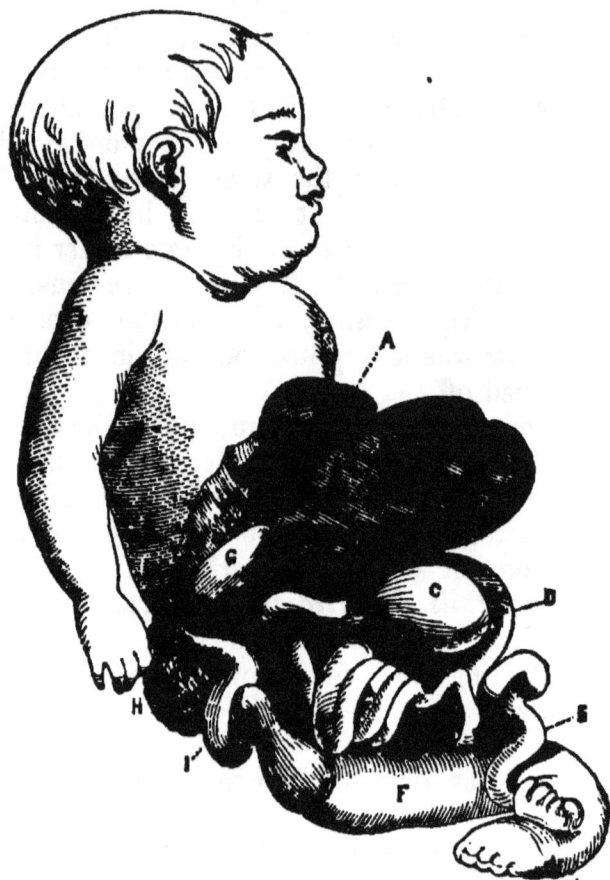

A The Heart.—B. The Liver.—C. The Stomach.—D. The Spleen.—E. Small Intestines.—F. The Large Intestines.—G. H, The Kidney's.—I. The Ureter.

The feet and legs are conjoined, only the toes being separate.

This appears to me more like a case that might arise from an imperfect Seminal Animalcule.

body and the head are quite perfect, but that from
below the chest and the middle of the back, all is
imperfect, displaced and deformed.

About a month previous to her confinement she
had a slight flooding, which, however, increased,
and every day more and more blood was lost, up to
the time of delivery. This, however, could not
have caused the monstrosity entirely, because it is
evident the deformity must have existed before the
eighth month, and was doubtless the result of some
abnormal direction of the nerves and bloodvessels.
The deficient nutrition of the parts, however, owing
to the loss of blood by the flooding, may have made
the case much worse.

In all cases of *deficiency* of any part, there is
always an absence of the nerves and blood-vessels
of that part, and in all cases of wrong position, or
deformity, the blood-vessels and nerves are wrongly
directed, or turned from their usual course. In the
same way, if we tie a ligament round the bark of a
Tree, so as to compress the sap-vessels, the Tree
will bulge out at that part, or be *deformed*, and if
we cut through the sap-vessels entirely, the parts
above will die, or be *deficient*.

CHAPTER XII.

TWINS AND SUPERFŒTATION.

TWINS that are both born at the same time, and of the same age, have evidently originated from two eggs impregnated at the same time, and Triplets from three, and so on. It is a question, however, whether it is possible for one impregnation to occur after another, while the female is yet pregnant. This is called Superfœtation, and its possibility is by some denied, though there is every reason to believe in its possibility within certain limits. Dr. Ryan remarks :

" Physiologists are at issue upon the question of superfœtation, that it is possible for a pregnant woman to conceive a second time. According to Aristole, a female was delivered of twelve infants, and another of twins, one of which resembled her husband, the other her lover. Some writers maintain that superfœtation is possible during the first two months of pregnancy ; the majority hold it possible in a few days after conception, before the uterine tubes are closed by the decidua. This is the received opinion, though cases are on record which justified Zacchias and other jurists, to conclude, that superfœtation might occur until the sixtieth day, or even later. Nothing is more common than to see a full grown infant born, and another of the second, third, fourth, fifth, or sixth month expelled immediately after. I need not cite authorities upon this point, as obstetric works abound with examples. But a few examples may be given. Dr. Mason published an account of a woman who was delivered of a full grown infant, and in three calendar months afterwards of another, apparently at the full time. A woman was delivered at Strasburgh, the 30th of April, 1748, at ten o'clock in the morning, in a month afterwards M. Leriche discovered a second fœtus, and on the 16th September, at five o'clock in the morning, the woman was delivered of a healthy full-grown infant. Degranges, of Lyons, attests a case ; the woman was delivered at the full time, the 20th of January, 1780 ; in three weeks afterwards she felt the motions of an infant, and her husband had no intercourse with her for twenty-four days after delivery. On the 6th or July (five months and sixteen days subsequent to delivery) she brought forward a second daughter, perfect and healthy. On the 19th January, 1781, she presented herself and both infants before the notaries at Lyons, to authenticate the fact. Buffon related a case of a woman in South Carolina, who brought forth a white and black infant ; on inquiry, it was discovered that a negro had entered her apartment after the departure of her husband, and threatened to murder her, unless she complied with his wishes. Dr. Mosely relates a similar case. A negress of Guadaloupe brought forth a black and mulatto, having had intercourse with a white and black man the same night. Another negress produced a white, black, and a piebald infant. A domestic of Count Montgomery's produced a white and black child at one birth. Gardien relates a similar case on the authority of M. Valentin. A mare has produced a foal and a mule, she having been impregnated by a horse, and five days afterwards by an ass.

"Another argument, which I have never seen, occurs to me from analogy, which deserves mention, namely, that each dog will produce a distinct puppy ; this no one can deny, for the offspring will resemble the different males that fecundate the bitch in succession. If a number of healthy, vigorous men were to have intercourse in suc ssion, immediately after the first conception, I thi x it probable and possible that similar superfœtation would happen. I am proud to say that Dr. Elliotson is an advocate of superfœtation ; he explains Buffon's case this way. Magendi is of the same opinion. Medical men must bear in mind that women have had three, four, and five children at one birth. Various cases of infants of different sizes, being expelled in succession, are recorded in our own periodicals.

"One of the Pennsylvania newspapers, in 1827, recorded the case of an Irish lady, who in eighteen months had at three births twelve living children, all born prematurely. She and her husband were healthy fresh-looking people, and only two years married. This case is not recorded, as yet, in any of the American Medical Journals ; but if it prove to be authentic, it will be the most extraordinary case of fecundity recorded in any country. Cases of twins, triplets, quadruple, and quintuple births are of very rare occurrence ; but of these more particularly hereafter. Dr. Golding, of this city, delivered a woman of six infants during the year 1829."

It is, perhaps, possible that eggs may be formed

sometimes during pregnancy, and possibly also the Animalcules may make their way between the Deciduous Membrane and the walls of the Womb to impregnate them, and thus Superfœtation may occur. I think it likely, however, that some of the cases mentioned may have been caused by there being *a double Uterus*, and each one having become the seat of impregnation, independent of the other, and at a different time. Some of the cases of resemblance may also have originated in the way explained in the article on The Permanent Influence of the Male over the Female Organs.

It is a vulgar error to suppose that twins will not breed, or that one of them will be sure to be barren, observation having shown that there is no foundation whatever for such a notion

CHAPTER XIII.

DURATION OF PREGNANCY, AND PERIOD WHEN THE CHILD CAN LIVE.

These are two questions of great interest, and about which there has always been much dispute. In my work on Midwifery all the positive information known is given in full, and I shall therefore quote what is there stated.

The duration of pregnancy, or the precise term of Utero-Gestation, is not fixed. It appears, from accurate observation, that there is no absolute period determined by natural laws, and therefore there is none laid down by human enactments. An approximation can be made, by taking the average of a number of cases, and the period of limitation may also be determined in the same way. The most usual period is about nine months, or from thirty-five to forty weeks, some females going beyond the thirty-six weeks, and others not so long. First children are frequently born under the nine months, and more so than those that come after ; this is a fact not generally known, and ignorance of it has often given rise to unjust suspicions. It is quite possible for a female to be delivered, with the child at full period, in a little over eight months after marriage, without there being any just grounds whatever for suspecting unfaithfulness.

Dr. R. Lee, in his Lectures on the Theory and Practice of Midwifery, gives the best summary that we have in the language, of our information on this subject ; I will therefore quote from his work making such comments and additions as I may think advisable.

" The Roman law fixed the period of gestation at ten lunar months. The civil code of Prussia ordains that a child born 302 days after the death of the husband shall be considered legitimate. By the law of France, the legitimacy of a child cannot be called in question who is born 300 days after the death or departure of the husband. The laws of England declare that the usual period of human utero-gestation is nine calendar months, or forty weeks ; farther than this they do not fix a definite period : the law is not exact as to a few days. Nine calendar months contain only 275 days, and only 273 or 272 if February be included. To fix bastardy on a child in Scotland, absence must continue till within six months of the birth, and a child born after the tenth month is accounted illegitimate.

" The difficulty of determining the precise time when impregnation takes place in the human subject, renders it almost impossible, in any case, to calculate with absolute certainty the duration of pregnancy. We are, however, in possession of a sufficient number of observations to establish the fact that the ordinary period is about forty weeks or 280 days ; but it is certain that it does occasionally exceed or fall short of this period by several days. As we never can be certain of the precise day between the periods of menstruation, when conception occurs—whether it takes place immediately after the last period, or before the expected period, or midway between these—it is obvious that all copulations founded upon the cessation of the catamenia must be extremely uncertain. The error of the calculation will be still greater if the catamenia should have appeared, or a discharge like the catamenia should have occurred once or twice after conception. Impregnation most frequently takes place soon after menstruation, but in others it does not happen till a few days before the expected period ; so that two women may have menstruated at the same time, and one may have reached the full period three weeks before the other ; and to this extent, or nearly so, an opinion founded on this disappearance of the catamenia may be erroneous.

"Calculations of the duration of pregnancy, founded upon what has been observed to occur after casual intercourse, or perhaps a single act, in individuals who can have no motive to tell us what is false, are likely to be much more correct ; and the conclusion to be drawn from these is, that labor usually, but not invariably, comes on about 280 days after conception, a mature child being sometimes born before the expiration of forty weeks, and at other times not until the forty weeks have been exceeded by several days. A case came under my observation very lately, in which I had no doubt the pregnancy existed 287 days : the labor did not take place till 287 days had elapsed from the departure of the husband of this lady for the East Indies. Some women are always delivered before the end of the forty weeks, according to the usual calculation, and their children are mature.

"In the evidence given on the Gardner Peerage cause, the period of utero-gestation was limited, but not strictly, by some of the witnesses, to forty weeks, or 280 days ; by others it was extended to

311 days.   Dr. Merriman, whose opinion is always
entitled to much respect, think the greatest number of women complete gestation in the 40th week,
and next to that in the 41st.   Of 114 pregnancies,
calculated by him from the last day of menstruation, and in which the children appeared to be
mature, 3 deliveries took place at the end of the
37th week ; 13 in the 38th ; 14 in the 39th ; 33 in
the 40th ; 22 in the 41st.; 15 in the 42d ; 10 in the
43d ; and 4 in the 44th week.

" How long before the expiration of the 40 weeks
a child may be born with the power of supporting
life has not been determined.   Where I have induced premature labor for distortion of the pelvis
before the end of the seventh calendar month from
the last menstruation, I have never seen a child
reared.   The lady of the clergyman in Fife, whose
case has lately given rise to so much discussion,
was delivered 175 days after marriage, and the
child lived five months.   To what extent gestation
may be protracted in some cases beyond the 280
days it is very difficult to determine, and the opinions
of the most eminent writers differ upon the subject.
I should suspect some great error in the calculation where the period of gestation exceeded 300
days.   But the experiments made on the lower
animals prove that there exists in them a great
variation between the shortest and the longest
gestation ; and it is difficult to comprehend why
there should not be a difference in this respect in
the human species."

In a trial which took place in this country, in the
county of Lancaster, Pa., as reported in the *Medical
Examiner* for June, 1846 it was decided that

Gestation may be prolonged to *three hundred and thirteen days!* The female swore that conception must have taken place on the twenty-third of March, 1845, and the child was not born till the thirtieth of January, 1846, or over *eleven months.* The judge directed the jury to return a verdict in her favor, and I suppose this case establishes a precedent for America.

In a recent number of the *Medical Gazette,* I find a case reported, wherein the period was said to be prolonged still farther. A man left his wife in New South Wales, he coming to England, and *twelve months* after he left she was delivered of a child, which she claimed to be legitimate. He denied this, however, and the judge in the Consistory Court decided, without hesitation, in his favor. Taking the medium between these two cases, therefore, it appears to be decided that the *extreme imits* is somewhere between *eleven* and *twelve* months! It must be recollected, however, that both were perfectly arbitrary, and that, for anything known positively on the subject, both may be either right or wrong.

Except when labor is brought on prematurely by violence, it always commences at what would have been one of the monthly periods ; or in other words, after a certain number of *full months,* and never at any time between! If, therefore, a female passes over the *ninth* month, she will probably go to the *tenth.* This has been proved by extensive observation, and is only another proof of the regular method in which nature conducts all her operations. The same law is also observed in abortions, which generally take place at one of the months, unless brought on suddenly by violence.

Dr. Ryan remarks that "Hippocrates, Aristotle, Galen, Pliny, Avicenna, Mauriceau, Riolan, La Motte, Hoffman, Stchenk, Haller, Bertins, Lieutaud, Petit, Levret, Louis, Astruc, &c., maintained that pregnancy usually terminates at the end of the ninth calendar month, but might be protracted to the tenth, eleventh, twelfth, and some of them said to the fifteenth.

"It is also decided by a preponderating majority of the profession, in all countries, that the term of utero-gestation is not uniform ; in other words, not invariably limited to nine months. This position is strongly attested by the analogy afforded by the inferior animals ; for it appears by the extensive observations of M. Teissier, on the gestation of heifers, mares, sheep, swine, and rabbits, that all these animals exceed their usual period of delivery. (Trans. de l' Acad. des Sc., Paris, 1817.)—Further evidence is afforded by the vegetable kingdom, in which we observe in the same field, on the same tree, shrub, &c., different parts of vegetables arrive at maturity with more or less celerity. Petit informs us that many faculties of medicine, forty-seven celebrated authors, and twenty-three physicians and surgeons, concluded pregnancy might be protracted to the eleventh or twelfth month. He cites a case on the authority of Schlegel, in which pregnancy was protracted to the thirteenth nonth ; the child was admitted to be legitimate, au ccount of the probity and virtue of the mother, which induced her shopman to marry her, and she bore two children by him, each at thirteen months. Tracy, a navel physician, relates a case at the fourteenth month. Dulignac, a French surgeon, positively asserts that his own wife quickened at four

months and a half, and on two occasions she went
on to the thirteenth month and a half, and on the
third to the eleventh month. Desormeaux relates
a case of a woman who was maniacal, who had
three children, and whose physician, after all means
had failed, recommended pregnancy. Her husband
had intercourse with her once in three months, of
which he kept an exact account. She was closely
watched by her domestics, and she was extremely
religious and moral ; she was delivered at nine
months and a half. (Velpeau.)—The last author
attests a case which went to three hundred and ten
days, and Orfila two of ten months and a half. I
have repeatedly known women mistake expected
delivery, four, five, and six weeks."

§ PERIOD WHEN THE CHILD CAN LIVE.

THE precise period when the child can live, if
brought into the world, is not determined, any more
than the time it may remain in the Womb. Some
children may be able to live a considerable time
before the full period of Gestation, and others may
not till some time after, there being a great difference in regard to their development.

One may be as fully developed at six, as another
at seven months. The common opinion is that the
child cannot live if born before *seven months*. This,
however, is incorrect. Many instances have been
known of births at six months, and even earlier, in
which the child lived, and became strong and
healthy. Van Swieten mentions the case of one
Fortunio Liceti, who was born before the sixth
month. He was not larger than the hand, but grew
to the average size, and lived to be seventy-one

years old.   Dr. Gunning Bedford mentions a similar
case, in   his translation of Chailly's Midwifery.
There are even cases mentioned of children living
at five months, but it must be borne in mind that it
is seldom possible to determine the exact period.
As a general rule, however, the child does not live
till after the seventh month, though there undoubtedly have been cases where it has lived before the
end of the sixth month. The law adopts the medium
period, and declares the child capable of living at
the end of the sixth month, and not before.   There is
no reason whatever for supposing that it is less
likely to live at eight months than at seven, or that
it will not live at all at eight months, as some do.

CHAPTER XIV.

SIGNS OF PREGNANCY;

FROM THE

MATRON'S MANUAL

OF PREGNANCY.

PLATE XIII.

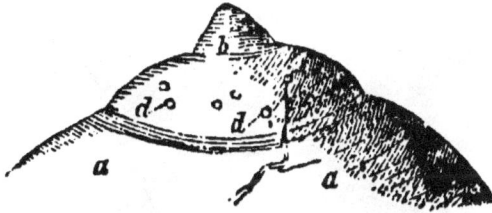

View of the Breast about the Fourth Month.—*a. a.* The Breast.—*b.* The Nipple.—*c.* The Areola, or part which becomes brown; it is elevated above the rest of the Breast as may be seen.—*d. d.* The little Tubercles.

PLATE XIV.

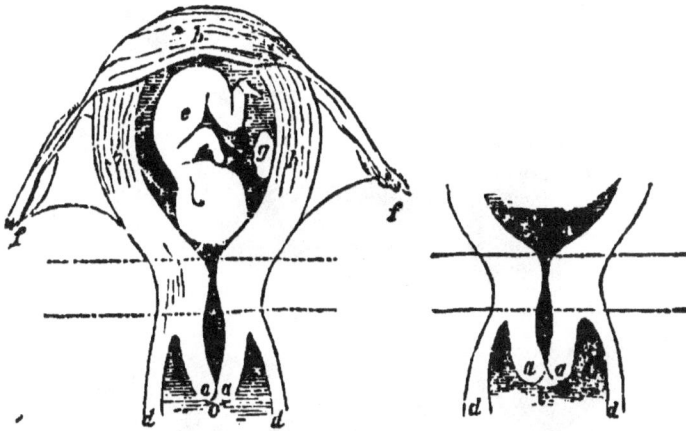

| Primipara, or the first Pregnancy. | Woman who has borne children before. |

a. a. The neck of the Womb.—*b. b. b.* The body of the Womb.—*c.* the Os Tincæ, or mouth of the Womb.—*d. d.* The cut edges of the Vagina.—*e* The Fœtus.—*f. f.* The Fallopian Tubes, Ovaries and Round Ligaments.—*g.* The Placenta.

Most of the changes produced can be readily distinguished by the finger, after seeing this representation, and making a proper comparison between it and the natural state in a former Plate.

PLATE XV.

Womb at about the third, seventh and ninth months.

FIG. 1

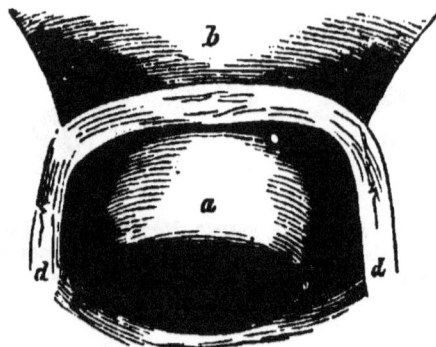

FIG. 2.

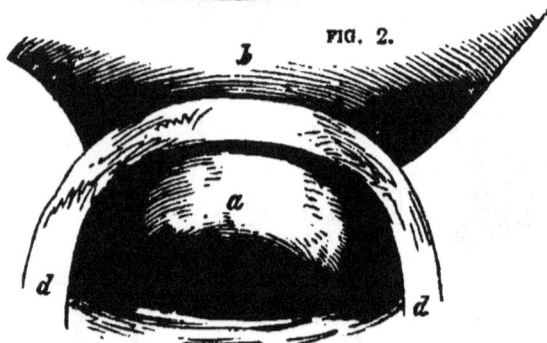

FIG. 3.

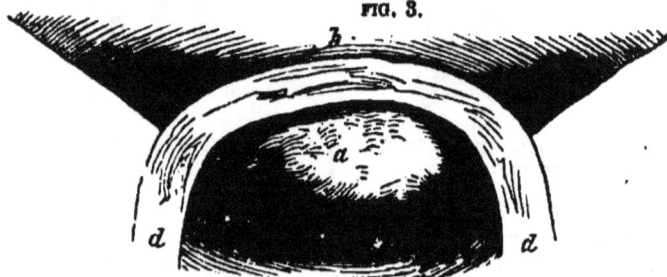

Figure 1, form and size of the body, neck and mouth of the Womb at about the third month.—*Figure* 2, at about the seventh month. *Figure* 3, at the ninth month.
The references are the same in all. *a.* The Neck of the Womb.— *b. b.* The Body of the Womb.—*c.* The Os Tincæ, or Mouth of the Womb.—*d. d.* The cut edges of the Vagina.

PLATE XVI.

The mode of performing the Ballottment

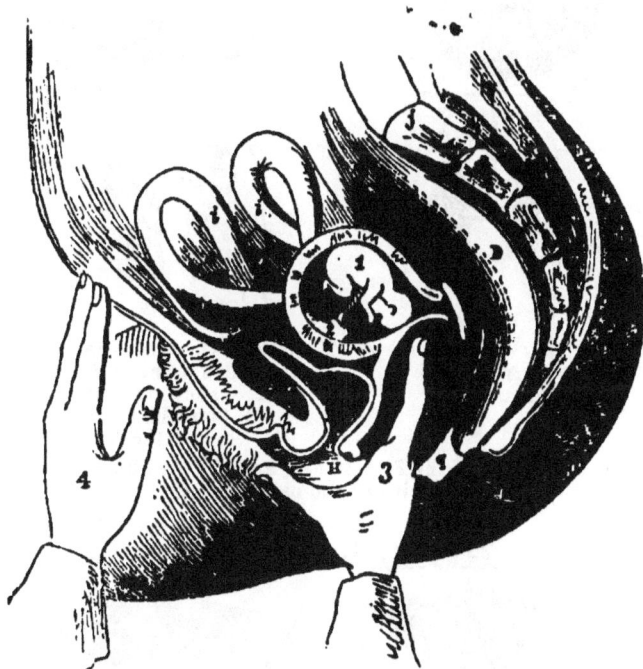

EXPLANATION.

This Plate represents the mode of performing the Ballotment, to detect pregnancy. The outline of the figure is the same as in a former Plate, and most of the organs are lettered the same.

The index finger of the right hand is passed into the Vagina till it touches the body of the Womb, the neck being thrown back owing to the tilting of the Fundus forward. The left hand is pressed firmly upon the Abdomen, just over the pubic bone.

1. Is the Fœtus.—2, The Placenta, connected with the Fœtus by the cord.—3, Is the Index finger of the right hand, within the Vagina —4, Is the left hand.

The development of the Womb, and the change in its position, are very well represented in the Plate, and so are the alterations in some of the other organs. The manner in which the Bladder, A, is pressed out of its usual shape and size, may be seen by comparing this with a former Plate. The shortening of the Vagina, and the expansion of its upper part, are also equally obvious, and the manner in which the mouth of the Womb is thrown back against the Rectum.

PLATE XVII.

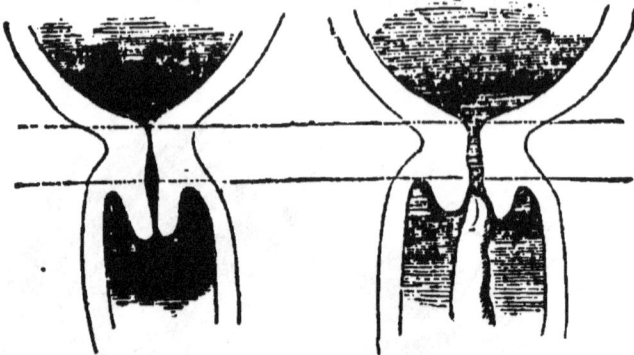

Neck of the Womb in a first Preguancy, very slightly opened.

Neck of the Womb in a female who has borne children before. showing how it admits of the introduction of the finger.

This is at the end of the Ffth Month, and the drawings are about one third of the natural size.

PLATE XVIII.

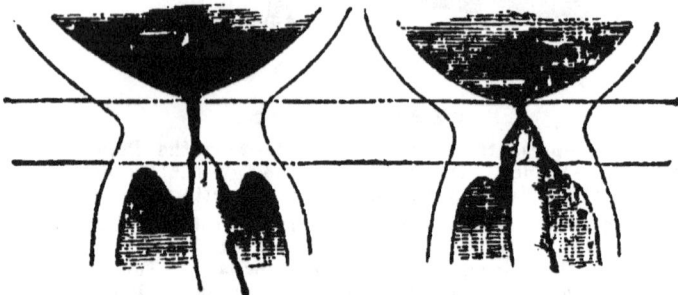

First child.

Woman who has borne children

The neck of the Womb in a first pregnancy, and in a female who has borne children before, at the end of the seventh month.

The part below the lower line here, shows that part of the neck which is contained in the Vagina. It will easily be seen how much shorter this part is, and how much more open the passage is, in the female who has borne children, than in the first pregnancy.

PLATE XIX.

The Fœtus in its most usual position

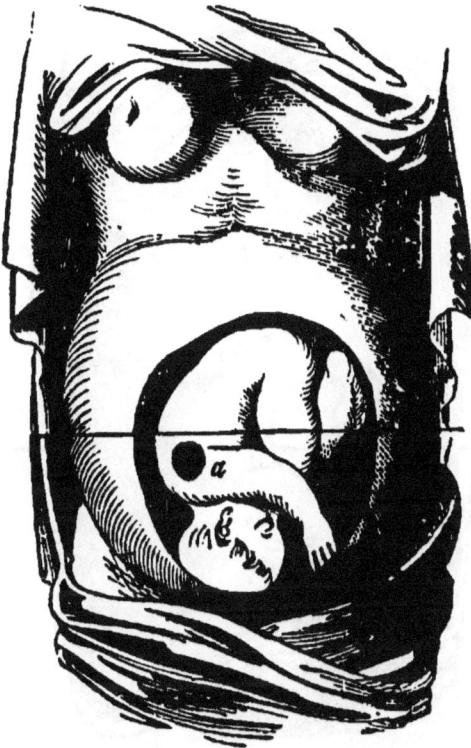

EXPLANATION.

This Plate represents the Fœtus in the most usual position, the head downwards, and the back of it presenting to the *right side*.

The black spot *a*, shows the situation of the heart; usually immediately under that part where the sound is heard the strongest —It is below the same.

PLATE XX.

The Fœtus in the next most frequent position.

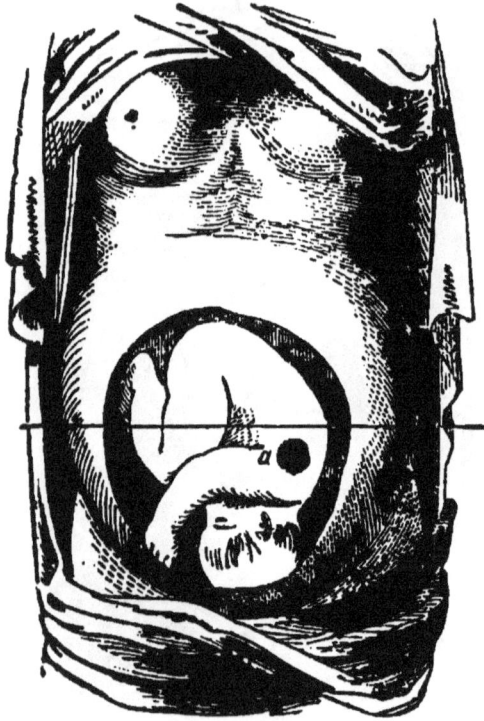

EXPLANATION.

This Plate represents the Fœtus in the next most frequent position, the head downwards, and the back of it presenting to the *left side*.

The black spot 5, 6, was the situation of the heart, as in the previous Plate. It is now below the line, as before, but on the opposite side

PLATE XXI.

The Fœtus in a presentation of the Pelvis, or breech

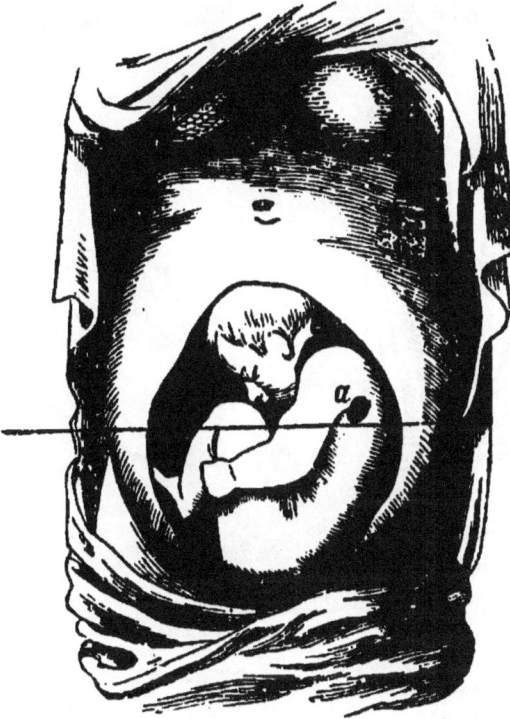

EXPLANATION

This Plate shows the Position of the Fœtus in a presentation of the Pelvis, or breech, which happens, comparatively, but seldom

The black spot a, denotes the situation of the heart, which is here *above* the line, instead of below.

In this case, as in the others, the heart may be on either side of the body, according as the child faces, but always above the line

PLATE XXII.

The position of Twins, as most usually observed

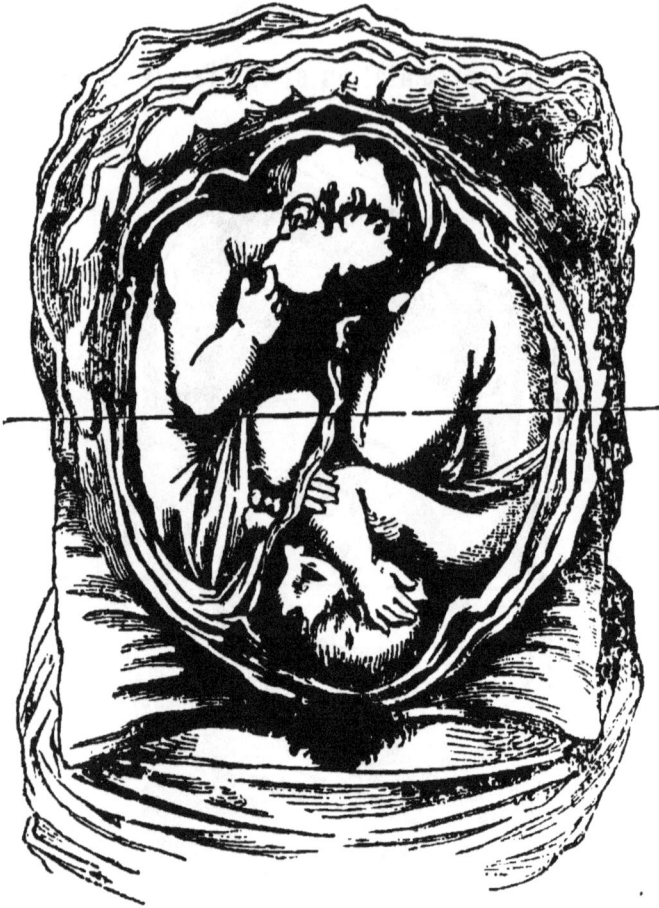

EXPLANATION.

A represents the position of Twins, as most usually observed, one having a head presentation, and the other a breech.

The black spot *a*, on both, denotes the position of the heart, which in one case is above the line, and in the other below.

The head however may be on the right side instead of the left, and so reverse the position of the two hearts, but this is seldom so.

When there are more than two, the confusion and uncertainty becomes still greater.

End of the ninth month.—There is but little difference between this and the previous period. The mouth of the Uterus is more open, and in those who have had children, the finger will pass directly into the womb, and feel the child, but in primipara there is still a small portion of the neck left.

PLATE XXIII.

FIG. 1.　　　　　・　　　　　FIG. 2.

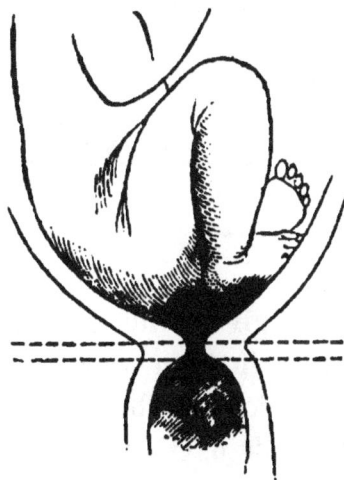

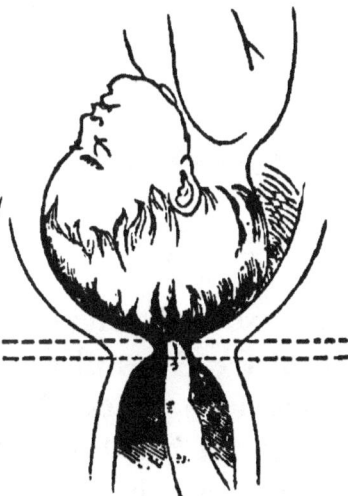

| The neck of the Womb, at near the end of nine months in a Primipara | The neck of the Womb, at near the end of nine months in a woman who has previously borne children. |

Ballotment is now more obscure than before, as the Fœtus is very heavy, and quite low down, and pretty firmly fixed. Auscultation is distinct enough, but not more so than at the previous period. The swelling of the lips, and of the veins of the legs, may increase, and so may the difficulty with the urine ; but the breathing generally becomes easier owing to the Womb having descended a little, and so pressing the diaphragm less.

THE MARRIAGE GUIDE

PART II.

MISCELLANEOUS SUBJECTS

INTERESTING AND IMPORTANT

TO MARRIED PERSONS.

HAVING in the previous Part given a full description of the Generative Organs in both sexes, and explained the process of conception and the nourishment of the new being, we shall next proceed to treat upon certain miscellaneous topics, all of them interesting and important to married people, and many of which have never been popularly explained before

CHAPTER I.

CAUSE OF THE DIFFERENCE IN SEX.

This has always been a fruitful subject of discussion both among Physiologists and popularly, but until recently nothing certain has been known about it. At first sight it may seem very desirable that the cause, or causes, which determine the sex should be known, and that people should have it in their power to decide upon the sex of their children, but probably it is better, at least at present, that it should not be so, for though it might conduce to individual gratification, it is questionable if it would be of social advantage. Nevertheless, I am of opinion that these matters will eventually be perfectly understood, and that the sex of every child will be known previous to its birth. Our knowledge at the present time, it is true, is not perfect on this point, but still much more is known than what is usually supposed, and as such information may occasionally be really valuable, besides being of great interest, I shall lay it before my readers.

All the old ideas on this subject are utterly unfounded, and generally as absurd as they are erroneous. Such for instance as supposing that if the parties lie on the *right* side, during the act of association, the offspring will be *male*, and if on the *left* side, *female*. Or imagining, as others do, that males are more apt to follow from connection in the early part of the day, and females when it is practised in the evening. Neither is there any foundation for supposing that it depends upon which sex the parents most strongly desire, as many know well from experience.

The idea about the *position*, during the act, determining the sex, originated from an unfounded theory of the Physiologists themselves, namely, that the right ovary produced males, and the left females. So generally was this opinion received, and so far did it influence even practical men, that about the year 1827, a Physiologist named *Millot*, published a Book on " *The art of producing the sex at will*," in which he gave directions for producing which ever might be desired. He even gave the names o' several mothers who were said to have succeeded in their wishes by following his directions, but of course did not enumerate those who were disappointed, though experience has fully demonstrated that they were undoubtedly as numerous as the other. In short, the theory, though captivating, is founded on an untruth, and cannot therefore be practically true.

In several instances it has been demonstrated, most conclusively, that each ovary can produce *both* sexes. Thus instances nave been known where one has been destroyed by disease, or where it has been naturally deficient, and yet the female has borne both boys and girls. In one case not only was the Ovary and Fallopian Tube absent entirely on one side, but even the corresponding half of the womb itself was imperfect, and yet she had borne eleven children of both sexes.

Another supposition entertained is, that the parent who has most energy and power *at the time of conception* determines the sex. But, setting aside the difficulty of proving such a fact, it is shown in another article, that the sex is probably not determined till some time after conception. Still, conjointly with other causes, this may have a certain amount of influence.

The fact appears to be that the sex is determined by the joint action of several distinct causes, the principal of which at least *are known*, so that the great majority of children *can be made of whichever sex is desired*, providing certain suggestions are attended to. And I may remark here, that this assertion is not based upon Theory alone, but upon certain observations, and also upon a long series of experiments with animals. The peculiar nature of my practice has of course brought many persons to me for information on this very topic, and I have therefore been able to verify the correctness of my conclusions. *In every case*, unless certain inappropriate conditions existed before marriage which could not be corrected, *I would guarantee either the one sex or the other*, providing my advice was strictly attended to!

To understand how this can be done, I must first state what has been ascertained respecting the influence of relative age. It has been found, by actual observation of some thousands of cases, that the *oldest* parent most frequently imparts the sex, unless the age be so great as to verge upon decrepitude. Thus for instance, when the fathers are younger than the mothers there will be born about *ninety* boys to *one hundred* girls, and very nearly the same when they are of equal age. When, however, the fathers are from one to six years older than the mothers, there will be born *one hundred and three* boys to one hundred girls; and when the fathers are from nine to eighteen years the oldest, the number of boys will be *one hundred and forty* to one hundred girls; but if they be more than eighteen years older, the number of boys will be *two hundred* to the hundred girls.

In the same way, just in proportion as the mothers are the oldest, the number of girls will predominate; till when they are from eighteen to twenty years older than the man there will be *twice as many* girls as boys. It may of course happen, that this rule may not hold good in many single families that may be noticed, but it will always do so when the average is taken of a large number, and the chances of course in the same ratio in every instance. Thus in every case when the father is over eighteen years older than the mother, it is *two chances to one* that the child will be a boy, and in three hundred such births there would be just two hundred male to one hundred females; while, if the mother be so much the elder, the chances and results will be just the same the other way.

The relative age, therefore, has a most potent influence over the sexual formation, but still there are evidently other agencies also, because it does not operate in every individual case, and we must therefore endeavor to discover what those other agencies are. My own impression is, that in the exceptional cases, where the *elder* parent does *not* impart the sex, it is owing to the younger parent being much the more *vigorous*. This view I have had many opportunities of verifying, in confidential communications, and I have almost invariably found it correct. This also shows why it is, that the greater age is no advantage beyond a certain period. Thus for instance, if the father be over *fifty*, while the mother is under *thirty-five*, the rule will change, and the number of girls will predominate. We also find that the greater number of *first* children are boys, especially if born soon after marriage, owing to the father being naturally most powerful then. In illegitimate children on the contrary there are most *girls*, probably because in many of these cases the female is more vigorous than ordinary.—In those countries where polygamy predominates, or where the men have several wives, there are many more girls born than boys, owing no doubt to the male power being weakened by excess, and expended among so many, which causes the female power to preponderate. For this reason polygamy must always continue itself, because the number of females will constantly be greater than the number of males; and if there were no foreign admixture to take place, a nation would probably become extinct, in time, under such an institution.

It is stated, in the article on the influence of connection after conception, that the more frequently it takes place, the more the child will resemble the father, in many particulars, but not necessarily in *sex*. If, however, the mother have as great sexual power, and experiences little or no enjoyment at those times, the father is likely to impart *sex also* as well as general resemblance. This, however, refers only to the first three weeks, during which time the sex is fixed.

In proof of this, I have found, in most instances when female children only were produced, that the mother was of a cold temperment, at least relatively to the father; and on correcting this by appropriate treatment, the sex of their next child was changed. On this point I am very confident, from my observation in a large number of cases. There are many females who are capable of proper excitement at other times, but *not* after conception, owing to some change in the action of the organs, and if connection still continues in such cases, the offspring is nearly sure to be a boy, because the father then predominates. On the contrary, there are other females who never experience excitement till they *have* conceived, and then it is often so great as to preponderate, and very likely to cause a girl to be produced. This accounts for those instances in which children are produced of the same sex as the parents who are the least vigorous; they being, in fact, the most so at a particular and critical period, the   usually otherwise. This explains further, why it is that female children most frequently result from conception in the *first five days* after the period, and male children from conception afterwards. It is in the first days that the female system is most vigorous in its action.

The production of either sex, therefore, is, to a very

great extent, within our power, providing we can fulfil the principal of the above indications. If, for instance, a boy is desired, the father should be older than the mother—say at least five years—and Conception should not be allowed to take place during the first five days after the monthly period. The relative warmth of temperament should also be regulated, so that the female do not preponderate, especially at the time of Conception, and during the first two or three weeks afterwards. If a girl be desired, of course the opposite conditions should exist. And in every case where the age is not appropriate, the other particulars must be the more scrupulously attended to. The means by which the warmth of the temperament may be increased, in either sex, is a portion of the medical art, and is explained in another place. Suffice it to say here, that it can nearly always be accomplished, even in those females who have been always perfectly indifferent. There are, of course, other hints and suggestions that apply to individuals specially but in nearly every case, success will attend the observance of these rules alone.

Many intelligent breeders of animals are practically acquainted with these principles, and will undertake to breed almost any proportion of either sex, by properly mating the parents as to age, vigor, and frequency of association, besides causing the offspring to resemble which they please, and to partake of any general characteristics.

Taken in conjunction with what is stated in another article, respecting the influence of the male in connection after conception, and also with what is stated as to the power of the mother's imagination over her offspring, it will be seen that these facts are of the greatest value, and it will one day be accounted of the utmost importance for every one to be acquainted with them.

From what was stated in the article on Fœtal Development. it would seem, however, that the sex is determined almost the first thing, immediately that the organization of the new being commences. It was then shown that the primary *cellules* of the Vitellus are always *an even number*, and that they form either into *Ovaries or Testicles*, and, of course, determine the sex at once, long before the heart, the stomach, or any other organs are begun. What is it that determines them to form sometimes into one and sometimes into the other, of course we do not know, but it is possible that the relative age and vigor, as already ex-

plained, may do so. At all events those facts are *practically* true, whether they explain this primary truth or
not.

There is good reason for supposing that sex is sometimes
a matter of development, or that the two are originally the
same, and capable of being converted one into the other.
The organs in each correspond to those of the other in a
remarkable degree, as will be seen by comparing them.
The Ovaries are identical in function with the Testes, the
Fallopian Tubes answer to the Vasa Deferentia, the Seminal Vesicles to the Womb, and the Ejaculatory Canal with
the Vagina. The External Lips of the female are similar
to the Scrotum of the male, and the Clitoris is similar to
the Penis, so that we have in each one a corresponding organ to every one found in the other. The Urethra, or
urinary passage, is not connected with the generative apparatus so closely in the female as it is in the male, but it
is not essentially so in either. The Semen can be perfectly
formed, or even emitted without it, as we see in some cases
of deformity; and in some females the Urethra has even
been known to pass down the *Clitoris* the same as it does
down the male Penis.

It is possible, therefore, that these parts may be pri-
marily the same in all cases, and that certain causes may
determine which particular form they shall afterwards assume. In their earlier stages also it may be that one can
be changed into the other, since they differ so little, and in
this way we may account for the influence of the male
after conception.

From what is observed in some animals, and also in the
vegetable world, this conversion of one sex into the other
is actually demonstrated. Thus it is well known that Bees,
when deprived of their Queen, will *make another*. And
this they do by taking one of the larvæ, or grubs, such as
produce, under ordinary circumstances, a common worker,
or Drone, and treating it in a peculiar manner, feeding it
upon different food, and carefully tending it in a different
way to what they ever tend the others. The result is, that
the grub, which would have been an ordinary bee, under
the usual conditions, is by this treatment formed into a
Queen, or perfect female. In this case, then, sex is evidently a result of development, effected chiefly by a peculiar
kind of nutrition. Botanists also know that plants frequently change their sex in a remarkable degree, under peculiar

cultivation, some becoming nearly altogether Staminate, or male, and others nearly altogether Pistillate, or female, though, in their natural condition, they remain uniformly one or the other, or a proper mixture of both.

A still further confirmation of the identity of these organs in the early stages, is afforded by some cases of accidental hermaphrodism. Thus, in many Crustaceous Animals, as Crabs for instance, it is not at all unusual to find a perfect Ovary on one side, and a perfect Testicle on the other. I have observed the same pecularities in Fishes also, and in one case at least it was found in a human being. Birds scarcely ever have the Ovary developed but upon *one side*, the other being merely rudimentary, and sometimes even formed something like a Testicle.

Many circumstances make it probable that the first stage of development of the Primary Cellules is always into *Ovaries*, and if they develop no further, of course the being remains female, and all the other parts correspond. If, however, any additional impulse be given, they develop further, and become *Testicles*, the other parts changing also, and thus forming a male. The male sex is, therefore, the farthest and most perfect development, which may possibly be effected, in many cases at least, by greater vigor, or more frequent approach of the male parent. In the early stages of Fœtal life, the Testes are within the body, nearly in the same situation as the Ovaries naturally occupy, and at a very early period of their growth they are also very similar to them in appearance. In the article on *Doubtful Sex*, many cases are given, in which the organs of one sex resemble those of the other, which still further illustrates this view.

Let the cause or causes of sex be what they may, however, it is certain that we can *practically* produce either Male or Female, as we choose, *in most cases*, by attending a certain precautions, as already shown.

CHAPTER II.

ON CONNECTION AFTER CONCEPTION, AND ITS CONSEQUENCES.

SOME persons suppose that when Conception has occurred no further association should take place between man and wife until after delivery. One reason assigned for such forbearance is, that sexual connection should not be indulged, except for the purpose of procreation. This notion is, however, manifestly absurd, and impossible to be acted upon. There are but few females who can tell when Conception has taken place, till it is considerably advanced, and they must, therefore, either wait a long time after each act, to see if such be the case, or be continually breaking the rule. But, independently of this, there is no doubt whatever, that connection is both proper and beneficial after Conception as well as before, providing it be not repugnant or hurtful to the female, and is not carried to excess. In no case, however, should it be indulged, if it causes her suffering, or is disagreeable to her, for then it will have a most injurious effect upon the *Nervous System*, and may also lead to *miscarriage*. The same evil results may also follow from excessive indulgence, even when not hurtful or disagreeable, and this must, therefore, be avoided.

So far, however, from sexual indulgence being improper in all cases after conception, it is often *required*, and various evils may follow from its denial. When the temperament is warm, and the sexual instinct unusually strong, as it often is during pregnancy, indulgence is imperatively needed, and if it cannot be had, the most injurious consequences may take place. I have known instances of this kind to result in a peculiar nervous frenzy, or partial derangement, and in miscarriage. In short, the indications and obvious requirements of Nature should be the guide in this case, as in all others, and not the dreams and theories of speculating physiologists.

Besides these reasons, there are also others, connected

with the child, which show the important influence of this after-union, in many ways. It is a question often asked, whether the new being is in any way affected by connection after impregnation? and a notion prevails, extensively, that in some way or other it is so. This notion, like many others, has probably originated merely from observation, without any knowledge of its scientific accuracy, but, recently, its truth has been *demonstrated* by experiment, as well as by observation. Several intelligent breeders of Birds and other animals, had long remarked, that the male could influence the offspring *after* conception, as well as before, and they acted upon this knowledge practically, in the production and preservation of particular varieties. Dr. Delfraysse, of Cahors, in France, was the first, however, who recorded any special observations of this kind. He found that the first connection merely *gave life*, or impregnated the egg, and that the after-connections imparted to the young the *colors* of the male, and that the more this after-connection was repeated, the more closely would the offspring resemble the father. In what way this effect is produced it is difficult, in the present state of our knowledge, to even surmise; but, notwithstanding this, the *fact* is one of great importance. It has been suggested that the resemblance to the male, observed in such cases resulted from an effect upon the *imagination* of the female, through the medium of the *sight*, the colors being as it were, impressed upon her mental vision. This, however, is not *always* the case at least, even if it be so occasionally, for a friend of mine, at my request, tried the experiment upon a Hen that had been *blind* during the whole of her laying period, and in her case, the chickens produced from her eggs invariably resembled the male in color, just in proportion to the frequency with which association took place. And in another instance, two Heifers, when put to the male, were both blindfolded, one having but one connection, and the other several. Each brought forth a calf— that from the mother who had but one connection, resembling both parents, *but mostly the mother*, while that from the other, with whom there had been several connections resembled the male parent in almost every particular of color, marking, and general appearance, though she had been carefully blindfolded each time. It is not through the imagination alone, therefore, that the paternal influence is exerted, though it may probably be so in some cases, as, for instance, in that of the Mare and the Quagga, recorded by Sir Everard Home. The Quagga is a species of Ass striped like the Zebra, and one of these, a male, impregnated an English Mare, in the Park of the Earl of Morton, in Scotland. There was but one connection, and the offspring was a Hybrid, or Mule, marked like the father. This Hybrid remained with the mare about four months, and probably she might also have seen it again about ten months afterwards. After this, during the next five years, she had four foals *by an Arabian Horse*, and strange to say, though she had not seen the Quagga during this time, they were nevertheless all marked more or less like him. Now if this singular resemblance was effected through the imagination of the mother, as Sir Everard supposes, the most wonderful circumstance is, that the effect should endure so long, even after the Quagga was removed. It rather makes it probable, even in this case, in my opinion, that some permanent influence was exerted upon the *Female Ovary*, as in some other cases that I shall allude to further on, when speaking of the permanent influence of the male upon the offspring of the female. I am not disposed, however, to deny the influence of the imagination altogether in all cases.

In the human being it is of course more difficult to make corresponding observations, but still it is not impossible. My own professional ministrations have been so confidential, and so numerous, that I have enjoyed opportunities of testing this interesting question more fully perhaps than any one else, and I am fully satisfied that the same rule holds good in regard to human beings as with the animals already referred to. In our own species, however, it is not in respect to the *color of the skin* that the influence of the male in after connection is made manifest, so much as in the color of the *hair* and *eyes*, and in the *expression* of the features, though the peculiar tint of the father's skin, as to being light or dark is often so imparted. Certain propensities, habits, and modes of thought are also given in the same way. I have made many observations of cases in which all the necessary particulars were fully known to me, and invariably I have found that the child resembled the Father in proportion to the frequency with which association was practised after conception.—The mere bodily resemblance seems to be most readily imparted, especially the color and expression of the eyes, and the color of the

hair. The mental qualities, and disposition, are more apt
to vary, unless the connection is very frequent, and then in
the majority of cases they will be like those of the Father.
I have known married persons act upon these principles,
in order to produce certain characters in their offspring,
and with great success.   In all such cases it has been found
that the more frequently connection takes place after conception, the more decidedly the child will resemble the Father, especially in the particulars above mentioned, whilv
if such after connection takes place but seldom, or not at
all, it will on the contrary resemble the mother, in the
same way.—This fact may often be of great service to mar
ried persons, as it gives them a certain power over their
offspring, and enables them to ensure or prevent the transmission of the character of either one at will, if it be desirable to do so.   .
    This influence it should be remarked does not, however,
extend to the *sex* of the child, which appears to depend
upon other causes, and until these causes are fully understood, the above facts lose half their value, because it might
be advisable to impart the character of one of the parents
to a male child but not to a female, or the reverse, and as
long as the sex is a matter of chance, so far as we are concerned, this cannot be done.   The causes of the difference of
sex, therefore, should be attended to likewise, and they will
be found discussed in another part of our work.—When all
these matters are fully understood, I have no doubt but that
any form of body, any disposition, and any given character of mind, as well as either sex, may be given to every
child *before its birth !*—Such a statement may seem strange
to those who have not considered these matters scientific
ally, but to those who have it will be nothing new or sur
prising.   I have known breeders of Birds and other ani
mals, for instance, who would undertake to produce, in a
given number of young, either ninety per cent of males or
females, just as might be desired, and alike in color to a
hair or a Feather, besides being all endowed alike with
certain prominent traits of character.   And when the pro
creation of the human being is as carefully attended to as
that of these inferior beings, the results will be equally
certain, the Organic and Physiological laws being the same
in both, in regard to this function—I leave every person
of common sense to answer the question for himself, whe
ther it is not more important to understand these laws in

relation to the human being than in relation to the inferior animals alone?—It seems clear to my mind that it is only by attending to such laws that the human race can be truly and permanently improved in body and mind, and made to attain its fullest perfection of development. By Education after birth, he can only partially modify and regulate the development of the bodily and mental powers with which the individual is born, and very often their natural force successfully resists the most powerful influences we can bring to bear upon them, and this is the reason why education frequently fails either in preventing evil or in leading to good. By acting upon those laws, however, which govern the child's Organization, mentally and bodily, *before* its birth, every power and quality may be made to have precisely that degree of development which may be most desirable, so that education will *always* produce the results we wish from it, and disease and vice be for ever removed. At present, however, it is scarcely allowable to talk of improving *human beings* by such means, though it is thought quite right, and even praiseworthy, to do so respecting Dogs, Horses, and Cows; as if they were of the most consequence.

My readers will bear in mind that the Law I have now been explaining, when fully stated is this,. That *frequent* connection after conception causes the offspring to resemble the Father, and that *no* connection afterwards, or but *very little*, causes it to resemble the mother. This is undoubtedly true in the great majority of cases, and the degree of resemblance will usually be proportionate to the frequency in the one case, and to the unfrequency in the other. If, therefore, no connection took place after conception, as some would be philosophers contend should be the case, all children would in time resemble their mothers only, and there would be a uniform and unbroken transmission of certain fixed characters, without any variation, which of course would be a great evil, even if it did not in time extinguish the race. This is another proof of the error of such a doctrine.—On the other hand, if the after connection was always frequent, children would as constantly resemble their Fathers, which is equally undesirable. To produce a mixture of the characters of both, therefore, when it is best to do so, the after association should occur, if other considerations do not forbid it, to a moderate extent, according to the peculiar habits, temperaments, and relative vigor and age of both parties. This will, however be better understood by referring to what is stated in another part of this book, on the proper frequency of sexual association.

An interesting question arises, further, when a female conceives by one man whether connection afterwards with another man would cause the child to resemble him, the second partner! Of course, such a question is not easy of solution in regard to human beings, but from observations made upon animals, it seems certain that the second partner *can* really impart his likeness to the child that was begotten by the first! So that the second partner could actually exert more influence, or impart more resemblance, than the Father himself, who only gives *life*, but not form and character!

In one instance I knew a widow who secretly married in about three months after the death of her husband, and while, as it appeared afterwards, she was pregnant by him. The child, however, resembled her *second husband*, though there was almost a certainty that no previous infidelity had been practised, because the individual was at a distance when the conception must have occurred.

It has even been conjectured, by some philosophers, if a female have association, at any time, with a man who exerts a strong influence upon her, that any children she may have afterwards, by any one, will be liable to resemble him, even for many years afterwards

§ PERMANENT INFLUENCE OF THE MALE UPON THE FEMALE ORGANS.

IT is commonly supposed that the influence of the male in the process of conception, is solely confined to the immediate result of that one conception, or in other words to that one child, but there is good reason for supposing that he can influence other children, born afterwards, though they may be by other Fathers. This singular fact is explained by supposing that, in the act of sexual union, the male not only impregnates the Egg, but also exerts a more or less permanent influence upon the Female Organs, owing to which they have a tendency afterwards to bring forth new beings upon the same plan, or resembling each other This was probably the case with the mare impregnated by the Quagga, above referred to, and it explains why the

Foals produced afterwards, though begotten by a horse still resembled the other animal.

Instances of a precisely similar character are sometimes seen in human beings. Thus a female married a second time will have children resembling the first husband, and sometimes even in a third marriage, as I have witnessed myself—Such remarkable resemblances can be explained only by supposing a permanent influence to be exerted by the male ; and probably that influence is likely to be exerted most powerfully by the first partner. The true explanation of these remarkable facts should be generally known, to prevent improper and unjust suspicions, which I have known to be entertained in such cases, and which, in the absence of proper information might well be excused.

Many persons would suppose immediately that these resemblances were simply the result of imagination, but I do not think so, at least not always. In a former article, when speaking of the influence of the male after conception, I gave some facts to show that such results were occasionally seen in cases where the imagination *could not be exercised*, and many of those facts apply to the present question. I have known instances of this influence, both in the lower animals and in human beings in which the influence of the first partner was visible for a long time afterwards, and in which I was assured the imagination had no share.

Breeders of animals are aware of many such facts, and have frequently stated them to me. Thus for instance, when a mare has a mule foal by an ass, it will frequently happen, if she have a foal afterwards by a horse, that it will to a certain extent resemble the ass. This resemblance is most frequently traced in the form of the mouth and lips, and in the greater length of the ears.—A friend of mine, at my request, tried some experiments, on several animals, for the express purpose of testing this curious question, and the result was a striking confirmation of the truth of the explanation I have given. Many of these experiments were so managed that the imagination could not possibly operate, and yet the influence of the first partner was distinctly perceptible during several conceptions afterwards. We can only come to the conclusion therefore that the male does often exert a permanent influence on the female organs, and especially by the first acts of association. In all probability this permanent effect is most likely to be seen when the male is relatively the most vigorot or where the association has been very frequent, but i may be manifested even after a single act, as was shown in some of the experiments made by my friend. Among other singular cases bearing on this subject I may also mention the following, which was told me by an old physician in Scotland, who knew all the parties concerned. A young female was forcibly violated by a person whom she did not know, and under such circumstances that she could not see him; it was known, however, by her friends who he was, but from a wish to avoid exposure, the occurrence was kept secret, though unfortunately she became pregnant in consequence. The child strongly resembled its guilty parent, and what was still more singular, she married, and had two other children *which also resembled him*, though by her husband, the young man having left the country in consequence of his offence.—Every one will see how naturally unjust suspicions might be entertained in many such cases, if they were not explained.

In the procreation of animals such facts may be of the greatest importance. *Life* may be given for instance by the male that has the most constitutional stamina or vigor, and yet particular qualities may also be obtained from others, in which he may be deficient.

CHAPTER III

DOUBTFUL OR DOUBLE SEX.

It is generally supposed that individuals are occasionally born that are both male and female, and it is certain that sometimes it is very difficult to decide upon the sex, through the form of the genitals being so unusual. In the lower animals, perfect Hermaphrodites are not at all unusual, especially in those that are low down in the scale of creation. Indeed, Hermaphrodism becomes more frequent in proportion as we descend, till, in some of the very lowest species, there are none but Hermaphrodites, each individual being both male and female, impregnating itself, and bringing forth its own young without the concurrence of any other individual. In none of the so-called Hermaphrodites in the human being, however, is this ever the case. They cannot perform the functions of both sexes, though uninformed persons suppose they can, not even when the resemblance to both is most perfect. All such cases are either of one sex, with some deformity which also makes them resemble the other, or else they are mere monstrosities, and, properly speaking, of no sex at all.

The greater number of so-called hermaphrodites are truly females, in whom the *Clitoris* has assumed an unusual development, so as to resemble the male Penis. In some instances this development has been so large, and the power of erection in the part so complete, that it could be used like the male organ, with another female, and thus an imperfect connection could be held, but it, of course could not lead to conception, owing to their being no secretion of semen. In other cases the Womb has been extended from the Vagina, and while in that situation has been used for a similar purpose, and supposed, by ignorant persons, to be truly a male organ. A proper investigation, however, soon reveals the truth in all such instances.

In men we sometimes find the Scrotum cleft, and an opening through it into the bladder, which has been taken for a Vagina. In such formations it is occasionally possible for one of the same sex to have connection. by this unnatural passage, but, of course, without any result, there being neither Womb nor Ovaries, and, of course, no Ova.

Cases of sexual monstrosity are found of infinite variety, all of which it is neither necessary nor useful to describe.

Many of these deformed females who are called hermaphrodites, also resemble the male in other respects, such as the form of the Pelvis and shoulders, the shortness of the hair, and tone of voice, and also occasionally in having an imperfect beard. This has still further led to wrong conclusions, and has tended to confirm the popular misapprehension. M. Béclard, describes a curious case of this kind, and I have met with several such myself. In one instance that I saw, a young person of sixteen, who had always been considered and treated as a boy, was found, upon full examination, to be really a girl. The Vagina was completely closed by a membrane across its external mouth, and the Clitoris was at the same time much enlarged, so that there seemed to be something like a male organ, but no indication of the usual female passage. This led to the mistake, which probably would never have been rectified but for her falling sick, and complaining of peculiar pains in the abdomen, the character of which induced an examination, which led to the discovery. It was with the greatest difficulty that I could convince the parents that they had mistaken the sex of their child, whom they insisted in considering a boy. I felt certain, however, that the pains complained of arose from *Menstruation*, and that the usual flow would be seen if the Vagina was not closed. I, therefore, made a thorough examination of the membrane, and determined to puncture it, so as to open the passage, which I ascertained existed beyond. A small incision was accordingly made, through which a probe readily passed to the usual depth of the Vagina, without any difficulty This was kept open, and gradually enlarged till the finge could be introduced, when the *Womb* was distinctly felt at the top, and in a short time after the Menstrual flow oc curred, and continued regularly. The only deformity now existing was the enlarged Clitoris, and this, at the earnest request of the parents, was amputated, till it was no larger than usual. She was now perfectly female, and, in a short time, little or no difference could be seen between her and most other young women of the same age. If this nad not been done, she would always have been considered an imperfect male, or an hermaphrodite, and would have led a life of misery in consequence. I have since heard that she afterwards married and became a mother. It is worthy of remark, that previous to the operation, her general appearance was certainly more that of a boy than a girl, the hair being quite short, the voice rough, and the Pelvis quite narrow. Very soon after the operation, however, and especially after Menstruation had begun, the appearance changed rapidly, so that in a short time she differed but little from other young persons of her sex. The hair grew long, the voice softened in its tone, and the Pelvis rapidly attained its full dimensions.

In the year 1818, an hermaphrodite was exhibited in London, but, on examination by a medical class, she turned out to be a female with an enlarged Clitoris.

A celebrated Prussian physician, Rudolphi, gave a description before the Academy of Sciences, in Berlin, in the year 1825, of the most perfect case of admixture of the sexes perhaps ever seen. It was a child that died soon after its birth, and which was found to possess a Testicle on one side and an Ovary on the other, besides a Uterus, Vagina, and Penis. In this case the two sexes were undoubtedly united, but had it lived, no doubt both sets of organs would have been inactive, or one set would have disappeared and left the other. No single instance has ever been known, in the human species, in which both sets of organs performed their functions in the same individual. Uninformed people judge from mere external appearances, and these are often deceptive.

A curious instance occurred a short time ago, in one of the Eastern States, in which an individual, who had always passed as a man, voted at an election, which was decided by that one vote, but the losing party objected to it, on the ground that the voter was a *woman*. It being a case of doubtful sex, what decision was come to I never ascertained, but the question was a curious one, and must, of course, be decided by medical examination.

In many of these cases, the inclination of the individual is sufficient to decide the question, as they nearly always desire to associate with those of the opposite sex.

Perhaps the most complete case of hermaphrodism, among the higher order of animals, was observed by Dr. Harlan, on an *Ourang-Outang*. It had Ovaries, Fallopian Tubes,

Uterus, and Vagina—being the complete female apparatus, and also two Testicles, with the Epididymi and Vasa Deferentia, and also a perfect Penis, being the complete male apparatus.

Among neat Cattle there are often found instances of a curious admixture of the sexes, in what is called the *Fre Martin*. They occur in this way. When a cow has twin calves, one male, and the other apparently female, the male will grow up into a perfect bull, but the other is often of no sex at all, or rather of both. There is, to a certain extent, a development of both sets of organs, but each imperfect, and sometimes they will both admit the male and also attempt to associate with the female, but, of course, neither act is productive.

§ SINGULAR CASE OF FEMALE HERMAPHRODISM.

The case represented by the following cuts, is that of a female who died in the Fever Hospital, Leeds, England. Her previous history was unknown, and as no one claimed the body, it was sent to the dissecting-room, when the curious conformation of the Genital Organs was first noticed.

It will be seen that the Clitoris is so developed as to resemble a real Penis, and that it also has a perfect passage or Urethra, down it, communicating with the bladder, and down which, in all probability, the urine could flow. In every other respect the organs are in nowise different from those of other females, but the Clitoris could, in all probability, erect and perform the part of a Penis.

Fig. 1, shows the appearance when the Clitoris was lifted up towards the abdomen, and Fig. 2 when it was hanging down, in its most usual position. In its collapsed condition it measured about two inches and a half in length, or about half the average size of the male Penis, and, when erect, must have measured *four or five inches* in length. Its diameter was probably about an inch and a quarter, and its structure evidently indicated that it was capable of perfect congestion and erection. Every other organ was normal, except the Ovaries, which were *very large,* and, in appearance, much resembled the male *Testicles !* They were undoubtedly female in their action, however, for she had, in all probability, been pregnant, and the *Corpora Lutea* were readily distinguishable.

PLATE XXIV.

View of the Organs when the Clitoris was raised up towards the Abdomen

FIG. 1.

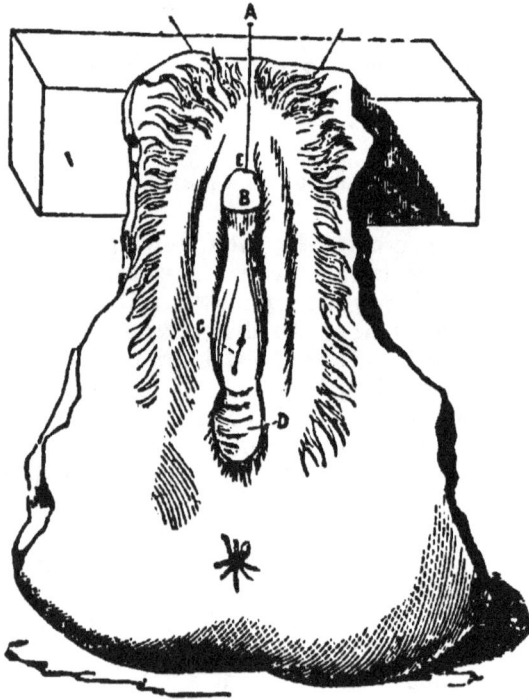

EXPLANATION.

A. A Probe passed down the passage in the Clitoris.—B. The *Glans of the Clitoris*, or Penis.—C. The Probe passing out of the lower end of the passage down the Clitoris, close by the Meatus Urinarius, or mouth of the passage into the bladder, which was the same as in other females.—D. The folds, or rugæ, in the entrance of the Vagina.—E. The commencement of the passage down the Clitoris at the top of the Glans.

PLATE XXV.

View of the Organs with the Clitoris hanging down in its natural position, when not Erect

FIG. 2.

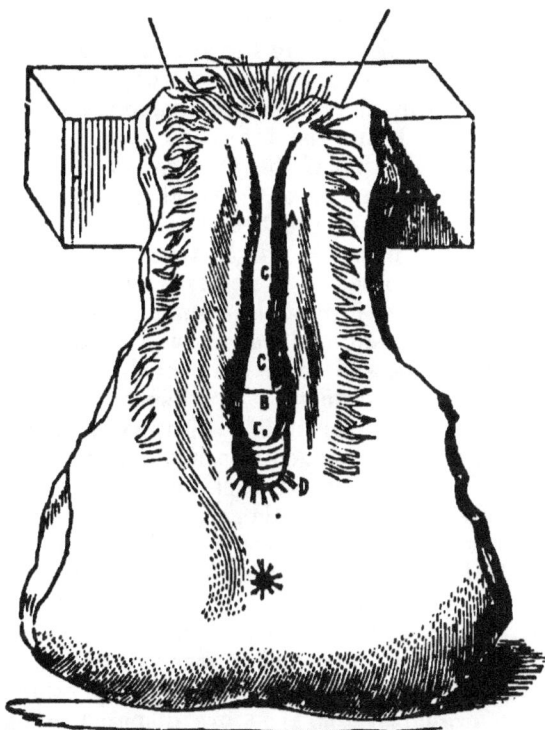

A, A. The Large Lips.—B. The Glans of the Clitoris.—C, C. The body of the Clitoris, or Penis.—D. The Vagina.—E. The opening in the Glans.

It is probable that the Urine actually passed down the passage in the Clitoris when that hung down, but that it passed out of the natural opening, (at C. Fig. 1.) when the Clitoris was held up. There seems little doubt of this organ having been fully capable of the usual functions of the Penis, with another female.

CHAPTER IV.

INFLUENCE OF THE IMAGINATION OVER THE GENERATIVE
FUNCTIONS, AT EVERY PERIOD.

As a general rule, there can be no doubt that the sexual instinct is first awakened by the Generative Organs, but after it has been once called into action, it may be afterwards awakened by the imagination alone, which also exerts a peculiar and marked influence over its manifestations. It is certain that if the Generative Organs do not exist, there will never be any sexual desire, which is a proof that the action of the brain is merely reflex, or secondary, and not primary. It is true that some Infants have been known to excite themselves even before the organs were perfectly formed, but such anomalies are evidently owing to a peculiar local sensibility, constituting a disease of the parts, and in no way invalidate the obvious principle we have laid down. In all such cases the unnatural and precocious sensibility disappears immediately when the organs are restored to a healthy condition.

Sexual desire, therefore, at first, originates from a positive *want*, arising from organic action, the same as hunger arises from want of food. Very soon, however, this want awakens the Imagination, which often acts so forcibly as to increase the desire a thousand fold. This is especially the case in cities, where there are so many causes to call forth the instincts prematurely, and to keep its gratification almost constantly denied. Some peculiar temperaments also, and certain organizations, are more disposed to a preponderance of this desire than others.

That acute observer, J. J. Rousseau, has well exhibited the effects of the Imagination upon the sexual instincts, particularly in his *Émile*. Buffon had remarked, before him, that young persons were more precocious in cities than in the country, simply because they were fed on more stimulating food, and were warmer housed and clothed. Rousseau remarked, however, that this explanation is not the true one, but that it is owing more to difference in manners and habits, and this is undoubtedly correct In those places where the people live a quiet, simple life, with nothing to excite the imagination, sexual manifestations are not seen till late in life, and then not strongly ; but where the manners are free, and social observances lax, it is the reverse, though their nourishment may be poor and scant. It is undoubted that food and clothing exert a great influence, and in some cases more than in others, but the imagination often exerts a greater, particularly over the first manifestations, as is well shown in the article on Menstruation.

It is probable that there are many causes inherent in the present constitution of society, which, in spite of all we can do, have an invariable tendency to inflame the imagination on these subjects, and to direct attention to them at an early period. The very concealments which are now necessary, even becomes provocatives, and, perhaps, have more to do with these evils than we suppose. Rousseau remarks that children have a peculiar sagacity in seeing through all these concealments, and in detecting every artifice that is made use of to blind them. The mysterious language that they hear, and the half-hidden acts of tenderness that they see, he remarks, are only so many *stimulants to their curiosity*, and, in all probability, they learn more from these attempted precautions, than from any other lessons

Even DRESS, necessary though it be, and conducive to true modesty, as it undoubtedly is calculated to be, has yet had its share in these teachings. The half-concealment— half-disclosure which it leads to, and sometimes even the *exaggeration* which it causes, excites curiosity, and gives the imagination a boundless and mysterious field to roam in. Such evils are perhaps unavoidable in the present state of society, but the conviction arises irresistibly, to all who consider the subject fairly, that in a more enlightened age they will be corrected.

Between the two sexes there is a wide difference as to the manner in which the Imagination acts, owing to the difference in their characters and organization. In the young woman there are two powerful sentiments which oppose each other, and which by their antagonism originate those caprices and eccentricities which are so captivating at the same time that they are so tantalizing. In the first place she naturally desires to *please*, and all her arts and actious, towards the other sex, have this object in view. It is essential to her happiness, to her very existence even, that she should endeavor to be liked, or loved, and no misery is so great to her as the consciousness that her endeavors are in vain. That being that has not this desire of pleasing is not a *woman*, in character, though she may be a female in Organization.—In the second place there is an innate sentiment in woman of *modesty* or *shame*, which controls her desire to please, and prevents her from exhibiting that desire in the way she would wish to do. These two sentiments are, therefore, continually struggling for the mastery, and their alternate and intermixed manifestations produce that bewildering but universally adored mystery the *female character.* Sometimes one of these sentiments preponderates and sometimes the other, and sometimes they properly control each other, and this gives us a key to all the apparent vagaries which this peculiar character presents. When shame preponderates we have prudery, when the desire of pleasing preponderates we have forwardness or coquetry, and when both are properly active we have that affable, engaging demeanor, corrected by true modesty, which makes woman truly entitled to the name of *Angel*, and commands reverence even when it does not awaken *Love.*

So intimately are these two sentiments connected with the female character that we see them exhibited at the earliest age, even little girls being Prudes, Coquets, and true women, equally with those of more mature years.

With man this is totally different. He desires more to *be pleased* than to please others, and has but little of that sentiment which would lead him to conceal his feelings. He, therefore, makes the first advances, and presses his suit, while woman coyly resists, and pretends indifference, even when her ardor is really equal to his own. Upon two such different characters it is obvious the Imagination must exert a very different influence, and with a different degree of force. From peculiarities in her organization, explained in the article on menstruation, the Female is most under its dominion, and it is in reference to her, therefore, that its power over the Generative Functions is most marked, though it is manifest enough in both.

Many cases in which the Imagination is supposed to have exerted a peculiar power, especially in pregnancy, have really been produced more by the Imagination of other people, but still there are authentic cases sufficient upon record, some of which are instructing as well as interesting.

The celebrated Descartes had for his first love a young Lady who squinted, and never after could he admire any one who saw straight. His Imagination associated all her charms with that peculiar obliquity of vision, and could not see them if that was absent.

Raymond Lully, the great Philosopher and Chemist, was violently enamored of a beautiful Spanish Lady named Elenora, who returned his affection, and even encouraged his advances to a certain extent, but whenever he pressed her to grant him the last favor, invariably refused, though evidently not offended at his importunity. He discovered eventually that her objection to a closer intimacy arose from her having a *Cancer* in the Breast, which she wished to keep secret, and thus there was a perpetual struggle between her lover and her shame. This discovery instantly cooled all his ardor, but did not extinguish his love. His Imagination instantly pictured to him how delightful it would be to effect her cure, and then claim his happiness as a reward, thus ensuring both her love and her gratitude. All his talents and time were henceforth devoted, almost without intermission, to this special object, and no doubt his mind constantly revelled in the delightful anticipation of success. Unfortunately, however, he did not succeed, the disease was proof against his science, and probably more powerful than his love.

I once knew an instance myself where a young man's desire was quenched instantly, and permanently, on his marriage, by the discovery that his wife was marked across the bosom by a large *Nævi*, which looked like a burn. Her bust was faultless in *form*, and his Imagination had no doubt often pictured it as being equally beauteous and perfect in every other respect; when this blemish was so unexpectedly discovered, therefore, all his feelings underwent a complete revulsion, and disgust took the place of admiration.

Many similar instances might be given, and perhaps more cases of mutual unhappiness after marriage arises from such discoveries than is usually supposed. Especially may this be the case where young females are induced, or forced, to marry old men or those who have been debauchees, as is too often the case. A melancholy instance of this kind occurred but a short time ago, not far from New York, which resulted in the suicide of the unfortunate victim, her horror and disgust when the actual condition of her husband was known completely overpowering her reason. Many often under such circumstances drag out a miserable life in constant despair and grief, while their friends, and the public generally, offer congratulations upon the excellent alliance they have formed.—In very many cases the Imagination, working under the veil of ignorance, forms such perfect pictures of the object loved, both bodily and mentally, that humanity as it actually exists can never come up to them, and the consequence is that the reality is sure to disappoint. The ardent Imaginations of females make them peculiarly liable to this romantic dreaming, and they are, therefore, more frequently the victims of this disappointment, which they feel acutely, and may even never forget.

How far the Imagination may influence the Sexual Functions it is of course difficult to tell, though it is undeniable that it does so to a great extent. In my work on *The Male System*. This has been well exemplified by cases, a few of which, with the remarks thereon, I shall quote.

§ INFLUENCE OF THE MIND OVER THE GENERATIVE ORGANS.

It is a fact not generally known that the mind can **exert** an influence over the Generative Organs of a most decided character. Not only can desire be engendered or annihilated by mental impressions, in despite of all other conditions, but the actual growth, or development of the organs themselves can be retarded or accelerated by the same means. I have known men who never felt sexual desire, and whose organs were very imperfectly developed until a late period, and then quite suddenly the long-suppressed feelings were experienced, and the parts began to grow, simply from the stimulus of seeing some person of the opposite sex who was adapted to make the proper impression upon their minds. Such instances are, indeed, by no means rare, as every person of experience must know, and they prove that, in many cases at least, a certain impression must be made upon the *mind* before the mere animal feeling can be experienced, or the physical development take place; or, in other words, they prove that with some persons tnere are only certain *individuals* of the opposite sex who can call forth those feelings in them, and that if they never meet with these individuals it is probable that such feelings will never be experienced, or at least only to a slight extent.

A knowledge of this fact will often explain to us many of those distressing cases of indifference and dislike to be met with between parties, and will also be a valuable guide in giving advice, particularly in those instances where there is only apparent impotence without any real deficiency.

There seems to be good reason to suppose that the sexual instinct is materially dependent upon a particular part of the brain, though we cannot tell what part it is, nor whether it is a mere development of it that is needed or some peculiarity of structure or organization. It is not at all uncommon to find men perfectly organized, in every respect, with vigorous minds, and with every other faculty in full play, but yet almost wholly destitute of desire for sexual enjoyment. In some of these cases it is true the Generative Organs are small, or evidently inactive, but in others they are of full average development, healthy and active. In such cases we can only account for the singular indifference exhibited by supposing that the part of the Brain which regulates the reproductive instinct has not had sufficient power, or else that the *proper object* has not yet been presented to the senses, as before explained.

Besides this particular influence the Generative Organs can also be much affected by the general action of the Brain and nervous system, the same as all the other organs. Thus if a man exhaust most of his nervous energy in thinking or in muscular energy, the other functions including the generative, must be proportionally weakened. I have met with many instances of this among men of business, many of whom would become quite impotent when more than usually absorbed in their pursuits, and regain their powers in a short time after their care and anxiety were lessened. The following case of this kind I select from my note-book as being more than usually instructive. The patient, a young man of twenty-eight, had been married three years, and had one child; he was very fond of his wife, and she in return reciprocated his affection. He had never been addicted to excesses or abuses of any kind, and until about six months before I saw him was in the full enjoyment of his generative powers. About that time, however, he experienced a sudden and severe loss in his business, which had previously been very prosperous, and the care, anxiety, and incessant exertion he underwent, in endeavoring to extricate himself from his embarrassments, brought on various physical and mental troubles that he had never before experienced. Among the rest he found himself perfectly *impotent*, having completely lost both power and will. This distressed him very much, both for the loss itself and also from apprehension that it was the beginning of general decay. In this dilemma he came to consult me, and was exceedingly anxious to know my opinion as to the prospect of his ultimate recovery. After a careful examination, I felt convinced that there was no actual loss of power, but merely a temporary absence of the requisite nervous stimulus, owing to the excessive mental labor and anxiety he had undergone; I therefore inquired as to his future prospects, and was gratified to learn that he was not quite relieved of his difficulties and was beginning to regain his usual health and spirits. On learning this, I unhesitatingly assured him that in a short time his generative powers would return, and more especially if he could abandon all care and thought about them. I gave him a slight stimulus, and some general directions as to diet, external treatment and exercise, and arranged to see him twice a week. In one month afterwards he was as well as ever, though he had been for nearly seven months as impotent as if the organs had been totally destroyed.—I have also frequently had business-men remark to me that they were liable to experience more or less deprivation of sexual power, and to feel much less desire, at those periods of the year when trade was most active, and their minds in consequence more absorbed. An author also told me that when writing any very particular part of a book, or when anxiously expecting the criticisms of the press after its issue, he was always for a time perfectly impotent. In the lives of several severe students we have further corroboration of this fact, many of them having been remarkable for their coldness and incapacity, particularly those engaged in absorbing abstract studies, like the mathematics. Sir Isaac Newton is said to have never known sexual ardor, though in every respect a perfectly formed man, and it is probable that this was in a great measure, if not entirely, owing to his incessant and all absorbing studies. In short there is no question but that intense mental occupation lessens sexual ardor in most persons, and that it may sometimes even extinguish it altogether. This is a fact of considerable importance both medical and moral, and one that should be more fully considered than it has hitherto been. There is no doubt that a great part of the licentiousness which exists, particularly in youth, is in a great measure brought about, or at least made much worse, by mental and body *idleness.* If the mind is not occupied by some proper and congenial study, that will pleasingly engage it at every leisure moment, a habit will soon be formed of indulging lascivious thoughts during such vacant periods, and if at the same time a due proportion of the vital energy is not absorbed in physical exertion, the sexual organs will soon become so constantly and intensely excited that such thoughts will become paramount over all others. I once pointed out the philosophy of this to a gentleman who came to consult me both for himself and for his son, aged seventeen. The father was nearly impotent from intense occupation in business, and the son was nearly dead from constant licentiousness and intemperance. I found on inquiry that the young man had been brought up as a *gentleman,* and was not even expected to employ himself with anything useful; in consequence of which, from mere idleness, he resorted to licentiousness and drinking as a regular occupation, till he was scarcely capable of anything else. *Moral suasion* was utterly useless to effect a change, and habit was too strong for the fear of consequences to break through, so that it seemed as if nothing could be done but abandon him to his fate. His father bitterly deplored the condition of his son, and earnestly entreated me to give him any information I thought likely to be of service in preventing similar misfortunes to his younger brother.

On explaining to him how the sexual power and propensity is influenced by a proper exercise of the rest of the system, the philosophy of his own and his son's condition was immediately apparent. "Yes," exclaimed he, "I have exhausted myself by over-exertion, and at the same time, I have left my son a prey to his licentious desires merely from idleness. I now see plainly enough that had part of my burden been laid on his shoulders it might have saved *both,* but from mistaken kindness, and false pride, I condemned *him* to a life of inactivity, and consequent depravity, and myself to a drudgery that has left me a mere ruin of what I was." Now this is a case instructive to all, and there are many others in society precisely similar.

Certain feelings are also very influential over the generative functions, but only temporarily, or with particular persons. Thus some men have found themselves suddenly impotent, with certain females, merely from disgust at something that was unexpectedly displeasing in them, and others have experienced the same difficulty from the fear of discovery or infection. Some men will experience a total loss of power on finding their companions too cold, or too ardent, or meeting with some unusual difficulty, but perhaps the most frequent cause is *Timidity*, or self-distrust. I have known several men, every way competent, who were so possessed with the idea of their own incapacity, that they invariably became impotent whenever they attempted an approach to the other sex. This timidity is sometimes exhibited in the most striking manner, the patient being intensely agitated, and so nervous that his whole frame trembles, and his bodily powers sink so much that often fainting ensues. This peculiarity appears to be constitutional, and is often seen in those who are by no means *nervous*, in the ordinary acceptation of the term, and who are collected enough in regard to other matters. The only remedy for such an infirmity is constant association with *one object*, in marriage, by which means a proper familiarity is induced, and in time the individual loses his distrust and becomes convinced of his perfect capability, In most of these cases there is a real *excess* of power, rather than a deficiency, and the very intensity of the feeling tends to prevent its gratification, by completely absorbing all the vital energies. I have frequently been consulted by persons so circumstanced as to the propriety of marriage, they fearing that the failing could not be recovered from, and it has been with the greatest difficulty that I could persuade them to the contrary. In every instance, however, I have found marriage to effect a cure, though it might not be immediate. Some have worn off their distrust very soon, others have experienced it for months, but eventually have been surprised that they ever did so at all. It is the fear of failure that causes it, with these people, and when that fear is once found to be groundless the cure is complete. In some few of these

cases a little medical assistance is available, but is (f a
nature not necessary to point out here. I once saw a man
who had been married for three years without being able
to associate with his partner, and solely from this cause.
In all probability he *never* would have done so, had it not
been for the advice he received, and yet there was no real
deficiency of any kind.   The celebrated John Hunter
gives us a similar instance, which he met with in his practice.   The patent was perfectly incompetent, solely from
the fear of failure, which so operated upon him as to always
make him fail.   Mr. Hunter was persuaded there was no
other difficulty, and that it was merely necessary to break
this spell, he therefore required of him, as one essential
requisite of the treatment, that he should remain with his
companion, but on no account whatever make any attempt
for six nights, let his desire be ever so strong.   The result
was, that before the period fixed had gone by his desires
were so strong he found it difficult to obey the injunction,
and feared he should have too much power instead of too
little.   In fact the cure was complete, without any further treatment.   The only thing required in such cases is
a judicious and honest physician, who will first ascertain
that there is no real deficiency, and then explain to the
patient the real nature of his case and the means by
which it may be relieved.   If this be done in a proper
and sympathizing manner a cure may always be effected,
but by a wrong course of procedure the evil may be confirmed.

A too great intensity of the sexual feeling itself will
sometimes cause impotency, by overpowering the patient
before the act can be properly consummated.   I have
known instances of men who always became so intensely
excited that they fell into a kind of dreamy stupor, and
had involuntary emissions while in that state.   This, however, can always be remedied by proper treatment.

Several instances have come to my knowledge of men
being impotent, at their marriage, from their first discov-
ering some disagreeable fact respecting their partners.
In one instance the lady had a small abscess on the arm,
which she had hitherto concealed, and doubtless thought
it a matter of little or no consequence, as her health was
good, and her appearance remarkably pleasing.   Her partner, however, thought differently, and such was the effect
upon his mind that he could never afterwards experience

the slightest desire towards her. In some cases such simple discoveries as false hair, or false teeth, have had a similar effect. It is not so much that the circumstance is excessively disagreeable in itself as that it is *unexpected*, and its discovery destroys the dream of comparative perfection hitherto indulged. With uncultivated and unimaginative people such causes might operate but slightly, or not at all, because they form no such ideal image, but with men of refinement it is different. There is no doubt but that a good deal of the dissatisfaction, and loss of power, which many men experience after marriage is, owing to this circumstance. They are ignorant of the real physical and moral nature of the being they take to their bosoms, and have formed a picture of her in the imagination very different from the reality, so that when the truth is known, their feelings undergo a complete revulsion. This ignorance sometimes extends to the most ordinary functional phenomena of the female system, and the first knowledge even of that has, to my own knowledge, produced a very disagreeable and lasting effect. In short, it is in this as in everything else, ignorance and concealment produce evils that only knowledge and mutual confidence can prevent or remove.

It is still a question, however, whether the Imagination of the mother can affect the child *before birth*, and if so in what way, and to what extent? The popular belief in its influence this way is well known to be very strong and probably it has some foundation though there is no question but this belief is carried too far. The well known case in the Bible, in which Jacob caused his father-in-law's animals to bring forth striped young, by placing peeled wands before the mothers, shows that this notion was entertained long ago, and the wonderful *marks* attributed to *longings* which we see every day shows that it still exists. (Genesis, chap. xxx.)

Hippocrates, who wrote some thousands of years ago, ... that a celebrated Queen was accused of Adultery, because she was delivered of a *black* child, herself and husband being white. The great Physician, however, remarked that at the foot of her bed there hung the picture of a *Negro*, and he at once cleared her from the difficulty, by asserting that this picture had influenced the child through the medium of her imagination, it being constantly before her. A contrary case is recorded, by the

Historian Heliodorus, of an Ethiopian Queen, who brought
forth a *white* child in consequence of looking, at the moment of conception, upon a picture of Andromedus.—At
the present day such explanation of how these cases came
about would not be received, any more than that of the
Irishwoman, who attributed the production of a young
wooly-headed, thick-lipped African, whom she brought
forth, to the fact of her having *eaten some black Potatoes.*

These are not mentioned here as authentic cases it will
be borne in mind, but merely to show the bent of the pop
ular belief.

In many old works which people are still in the habit of
reading, merely from the *name,* such as "*Aristotle*" for
instance, pictures are given of children resembling *animals,* which are there represented to have come either from
the mother seeing such, or from having actually associated with them. All these, however, are gross exaggera-
tions, and many of them even mere fabrications. In none
of these works is there anything approaching to *science,*
but on the contrary the merest rubbish and trash, utterly
worthless for any purpose whatever.

Among more probable cases may be mentioned that of a
lady who had a child covered with hair, and with hands
fashioned much like the paws of a bear, and which she
attributed to having often seen a picture of John the Bap-
tist, clothed in a bear's skin. Malebrande also tells us
of another infant which was born with all its bones broken
and its joints dislocated, in consequence of the mother
having seen an unfortunate criminal broken alive on the
wheel. In short such instances are numerous, and they
show how firmly this belief is grafted on the popular mind,
whether it be true or false.

It is quite common to observe, on the skin of new-born
infants, certain brown, yellow, red, blue, or black marks,
which are generally supposed to have been produced by
the mother having *longed* for something while pregnant.
These marks vary much in their form, size, and appearance, and are usually of so indefinite a character that a
little stretch of the imagination may easily make them
resemble anything. It is scarcely necessary to remark,
that there are but few females, if any, who do not *long* for
something during their pregnancy, and if this cause could
produce such marks but few children would be without
them, whereas they are, on the contrary, rather scarce.

The fact is that when one of these marks is discovered upon an infant the mother begins to think of something she very much wished for, and then she easily sees that the mark is like it, but it is very seldom the case t..at any one else perceives the resemblance, unless it has previously been suggested to them.   I have known one of these *Nævi Materni*, as they are called, taken for half-a-dozen different things by as many different people.

The real cause of the mothers' marks is a disease of the skin which produces an alteration in its texture.   In general they are of little consequence, and remain station ary as long as the individual lives.   It is seldom that success attends any attempts to remove them, and as a general rule they are better left alone, the effects of an operation being more likely to disfigure and injure than the mark itself.   There is one kind, however, which differs from all the others, and which requires attention.   This kind presents the appearance of little red warts, with flattened tops, connected with the skin by small necks, and full of blood-vessels.   These are called *Fungus Hæmatodes*, and they are caused by obstructions in the little vessels under the skin, which makes the blood accumulate in minute tumors, or *aneurisms.*   These may continue to grow, or even ulcerate, and lead to serious consequences; it is therefore best to remove them.   This is done either by tying a silken string round them, to gradually strangle them off, or to use a sharp knife.   In many cases, however, they may be destroyed by simply washing them in alum water, or a solution of sulphate of copper, or in keeping a silver coin pressed flat upon them for some time.

The fear that many people have of causing these marks is quite amusing, and has sometimes been acted upon for particular purposes.   Thus I saw sometime ago, in a medical work, an account of a lady in England who induced her husband to buy a carriage and horses, which she longed for, by assuring him that if he did not do so the child with which she was pregnant would be *marked with them!*

In no case does the mother ever announce *before the birth* what kind of a mark the child will be born with, and yet if she knew about the longing that caused it she ought to be able to do so.   It is always *after the mark is seen* that its resemblance is sought for, and then of course *something* can be thought of that may at least be *supposed* to be like it.

In one of the French Medical Journals, some years ago, M. Girard gave a very curious and instructive instance of the fallacy of this popular belief. In the course of his practice he became acquinted with three pregnant females, all of whom had been so strongly impressed by some object presented to the mind that the children were expected to be marked, but neither of them were so. On the other hand three others, who had experienced neither frights nor longings of any kind, had their children terribly deformed with Nævi. And this is in fact daily seen, numbers being born *with* marks though the mothers did not long at all, and others being free from them though they did long, and intensely too. In fact, if their longings could do what some people suppose them capable of there would be few children without marks, for nearly all females experience these imperious desires. Another circumstance, too, should be borne in mind,—if the imagination can exert such a power over the child as to cause deformity, it can also equally cause *beauty*, or give any particular *feature*, or *sex*, so that every mother must be supposed to have the power, by her imagination, to make her child be just what she pleases. Experience, however, shows that this power does not exist, and no mother who longs for a son can be certain of bearing one by so doing, nor can she by her imagination give a Grecian nose or auburn hair. If this *could* be done we should have none but *Venuses* an) *Apollos* born, but unfortunately for the gratification of fond mothers it cannot be, and this fact alone proves the imagination is not so powerful as some suppose it to be.

It should be remarked, however, that the Generative act is certainly the most exalted that the animal organization can perform, and requires the greatest expenditure of vitality. The union of the two sexes is accompanied by an excitement more intense than is ever experienced at any other time,—in fact it results in a positive *convulsion*, and often of partial derangement of mind, as if the two parents while giving life to the new being almost, for the instant surrendered their own lives. This is the case at least when the conditions are perfect on both sides, but though this excitement must of course be always experienced by the male, yet the female may be perfectly passive. In such cases it may be questioned whether the act is really so perfect as when both are in the normal condition, and whether this remarkable salivation and expenditure of vitality is not really necessary in both, to properly impress the new being, and make it active and vigorous. It is possible, as before explained, that conception may occur without any emotion whatever being experienced by the female, but there is very good reason for supposing that the child ren resulting from such conceptions are imperfect, by being deficient in mental and bodily vigor. In fact, experiments of artificial impregnation, upon animals, have proved this, and have shown that the vivid and overpowering emotion of sexual excitement should be experienced by *both* parents, in order to give that impulse to the new organization which is necessary to its most perfect development.

This accords with the popular notion respecting *illegitimate* children, who are generally believed, and with sufficient reason, too, to be on the average more talented and handsome than others. It is supposed that the intense warmth of temperament which, in most of these cases, leads to the breach of morality and social propriety, is advantageous to the new being, because it is conceived with more energy and power. The imagination of the parents is also more acted upon by the very circumstances of their association. The necessity for deceiving others, and of practising secrecy in their meetings, together with the charm of mutual confidence, and perhaps the indulgence being a *forbidden* one, all conspire to produce an excitement greater than the ordinary circumstances usually give rise to.

It is certain also that children who are conceived during sickness, or when old age has vitiated the parents' energy, are never so vigorous and healthy as others.

After Fecundation, the new being remains for nine months connected with the mother, and its development within her body, is as much a natural function of her organization as is Digestion or the Circulation of the Blood. Now both these functions, in common with all others, are well known to be affected by moral causes to a great extent, which alone would make it probable that Gestation is also. Thus Grief, Joy, or sudden Fright, will often prevent Digestion entirely, and so derange the action of the Heart that the circulation will completely cease, as in Fainting. There is every reason to presume, therefore, that these emotions can also influence Fœtal development, and modify the new being both in body and mind. Indeed many cases have been known which directly prove this and no doubt the moral temperament and bodily condition of many human beings is thus in a great measure determined before their birth.

In connection with this subject, it is most important to bear in mind that the child must be formed entirely *from the mother's blood.* Excepting the male Animalcule, which forms no portion of the general organization, there is not an atom of its material that can come from any other source. The condition of the mother's blood, therefore, is of great consequence to its future well-being, for if that be imperfect, or diseased, the body formed from it must be so likewise. Now it is well known, that the state and even the composition of the blood is very much affected by the state of the mind, and by the emotions experienced. In despondency and grief the blood is imperfectly formed, being thin and watery, and it circulates sluggishly through the Heart. On the contrary, joy makes the circulation brisk and nutrition perfect, so that the blood is rich and pure, while anger makes it boil through the veins, and changes its very composition. In Fever it is well known the blood is so altered that when drawn from the body it speedily putrifies, and it is almost the same during a violent fit of rage, as I have seen when bleeding for a fit of Apoplexy brought on by that cause.

It is not bodily disease only, therefore, that can change the quality of the blood, but also the state of the mind and feelings, which must be capable, therefore, of affecting the child through the medium of the blood.

Now when we reflect how sensitive females usually are during Gestation, and how many causes then annoy and disturb them, it is readily perceived that their offspring must of necessity be much under their moral influence, or in other words be affected through the imagination. This influence, however, is exerted in a general way, and not for the protection of merely local effects, like *marks.*

It is deeply suggestive, also, to the reflective mind, to contemplate the fact that when a female is pregnant with a female child there are *three Generations* nourished by the same blood at the same time! There is the mother herself,—the child in her womb,—and within its body the rudiments of the *Ovaries* from which, if it ever become a mother, its children will be formed! Who does not see from this how literally true it is that the physical sins at least, of the parents, are visited both upon the children

and the children's children! There are conditions of the
blood which no doubt can in this way affect both the child
that is forming and also its future children, through the
rudimentary ovæ, and those conditions may originate from
the Imagination. A violent fit of anger in a mother, therefore, or of any other powerful emotion, may cause suffer
ing and disease both to her child and her grandchild.

Another fact may also be mentioned, to prove that the
child can be influenced by moral emotions. It is well
known that many diseases of the Womb, and also miscar
riage, are often caused by fright, anger, and grief, and it
is scarcely possible to believe that the child in the Womb
is not influenced by the same causes. During times of
great public excitement and danger, as in revolutions and
civil wars, it has been observed that miscarriages are more
frequent, and that more of the children born then are idi-
otic, or become insane, than is usually the case.

It is true that there has not yet been discovered any ner
vous communication between the mother and child, but
this by no means proves, that the emotions of the mother
cannot influence her offspring. The blood itself is regard
ed by many physiologists as being truly *living*, and this
certainly is connected in both. But whether it be living
or not, it is certainly the material from which both are
formed, and there is no question as to the emotions of the
mother affecting it.

In works on Medical Jurisprudence many trials are recorded in which the power of the mother's imagination
has been called in question, but it has never been legally
admitted. About forty years ago, a Mulatto female, in
New York, became the mother of an illegitimate child, the
father of which she asserted was a Negro, named Whistelo,
who was accordingly arrested and brought to trial, as he
denied the fact. The child was not at all like that of a
Negro in any particular, being whiter, and with straigh
hair, but Dr. S. Mitchell contended it might have been in
fluenced by the mother's imagination, and that conse
quently Whistelo might have been the father. The court,
however, thought otherwise, and it was unanimously and
very properly decided that the father must have been a
White man, or a Mulatto, and consequently Whistelo was
acquitted.

Many of these resemblances which are supposed to originate with the imagination of the mother may really

arise from other causes, as shown by the case of the Quag
ga. given in the article on The Permanent Influence of the
Male upon the Female.   In fact, that article should be referred to in connection with the present one.

It is a familiar fact to medical men, that many diseases
are transmitted from the mother to the child while it is yet
in the Womb, and also that many drugs can influence it
under the same circumstances, but this must of course,
take place through the medium of the blood.

The Ague, Small-Pox, and the Venereal Disease, are
frequently given to a child before its birth, and possibly
also many diseases of a more chronic nature.

To show how crude the popular notions on this subjec'
are, and how little they are founded upon correct information, it is only requisite to state that many people believe
it is the child itself that *longs*, while in the Womb, and
they think the *mark* can be taken away by giving the child
the object it wanted immediately it is born.   Thus I have
known an infant of two days old given a piece of *beef-steak*
to take away the supposed image of one on its cheek.

Some suppose the marks are only given at quickening,
others at six months, some at three and others again at
any time.

CHAPTER V.

DEFICIENCY AND TOTAL LOSS OF THE GENERATIVE POWER.

THIS is a subject that has never yet been fully treated upon in a popular way, though it is unquestionably one of the most important and interesting. In my work on the *Male System,* I remarked, that "This is a part of our subject of the very first importance, and yet beset with such numerous and peculiar difficulties, that precise knowledge about it is extremely difficult to obtain. In regard to many things of the greatest moment, connected with man's virile powers, but little or nothing is known, even by medical men, who are, generally speaking, taught nothing about them, in their earlier studies, and have but few opportunities of learning afterwards. Dr. Curling remarks, when speaking of the Testes, 'Their functions are so involved in those of other parts, are influenced by such peculiar causes, and are so dependent on and modified by particular events and circumstances, that the investigation of them, when disordered, necessarily becomes of a complex and difficult character. The product, too, of these glands, is one, the qualities of which it is almost impossible to appreciate, and which during life is never afforded in a pure and unmixed state; and further, taking into account the repugnance felt to such inquiries, it is scarcely surprising that the subject has been but imperfectly investigated, and rarely treated of by the pathologist and practitioner. Indeed, the little information we possess respecting it is chiefly to be found under the head Impotency, in works on medical jurisprudence, in which it is cursorily considered, principally in relation to points of medico-legal interest, and scarcely at all in relation to practice.'"

This is strictly true, and it will, I dare say, surprise many persons, to learn that physicians, generally speaking, know little or nothing about such matters. Such, however, is the case, as is well known to those who have occasion to apply them, either for advice or information. I have

found it absolutely necessary to set out in my investigations, on many important points, as if *nothing* were known,
and hunt out the requisite information by the tedious but
sure process of actual experiment and extended observation.   Very many of the statements made in this work will
probably surprise those who see them for the first time,
wing to their novelty, and to their variance with old notions.   None of these statements have been made, however,
without good and sufficient evidence having been obtained
of their correctness, while the old notions with which they
conflict, are merely suppositions and assumptions, utterly
destitute of any foundation whatever.   This is especially
the case in regard to the functional and sympathetic causes
of *Impotence*, and also its medical and moral *treatment,*
which may be truly said to be, nearly invariably, of the
most *quackish* character, even when practised by the most
eminent medical men.   The notions of non-professional persons, respecting such things, are frequently as correct as
those of their medical advisers, and their own empirical
treatment is often the most successful.   It is but very recently, that the true action of many powerful agents on
the Generative Organs has been ascertained, and I assert,
without hesitation, that many practitioners, some even of
considerable celebrity, are as truly ignorant in regard to
it as the patients they undertake to treat.

In pursuing my own investigations into these important
and interesting subjects, I have left no means of acquir-
ing information untouched.   Besides studying and experi-
menting, as far as was proper, in thousands of cases that
came under my notice professionally, I have fully experimented upon hundreds of animals, to the utmost extent
that humanity would allow.   By these means I have ascertained many important facts, and studied the action of
many powerful medical agents, which could not with pro
priety and safety have been tried upon human beings first.

Functional or sympathetic disability of the Reproductive Organs appears in two forms, *Impotence and Sterility,*
which are frequently, but erroneously, confounded together.   Sterility means a total absence of the Reproductive principle, and must always be accompanied by impotence or inability to associate with the other sex, except
temporarily in certain peculiar cases; but a man may be
impotent without being sterile.   Absolute sterility is generally incurable, because it arises from destruction or dis-

organization of the Testes, and it is, therefore, only in the way of preventing the evil, by removing its causes, that we can do any good, but impotence can very frequently be *cured*, as well as prevented. Besides impotence is the more frequent affection, and is often merely the forerunner or first stage of sterility, and it becomes, therefore, the most important subject to consider.

The various kinds of deformity, deficiency, and acute disease that cause destruction of the generative power, have already been fully treated upon, (in my work on the Male System, and we have now only to explain those mysterious sympathetic and functional agencies, which, though they are often more powerful, are yet so different in their operation, and hitherto so little studied, that but little is generally known respecting either their nature or mode of action.

In the female though there are many causes of sterility, there is but one cause of positive impotence, and that is, deformity or absence of the Vagina. If this canal exists, and is of sufficient size, she can always receive the embraces of the other sex, though they may be fruitless.

With man, however, this is different; not only may he be sterile from various causes, but also impotent. Desire may be strong, and the semen abundant and perfect, but still he may be unable to convey it within the Female Organs. There may be no power of erection, or the passage of the Urethra may open in the wrong place, or it may be obstructed by stricture; in all which cases the man is impotent, though not necessarily sterile, for if his semen could be placed, even artificially, in the Female Organs, it would impregnate.

All these defects are capable, in most instances, of being remedied, as I have shown in my work on the *Male Organs*. The Penis can not only be made to erect, but to grow when too small, and sometimes can even be *made*, when it is nearly totally absent. Its proper sensibility can also be created or restored, and the Urethral passage can be either restored to its proper dimensions, or made to open in the right place, so that in every respect it can be made capable of performing its peculiar functions.

In like manner the Vagina can be either enlarged or opened in the female, and the only cause of impotence in her, can, therefore, be removed, as shown in my **book on** *The Diseases of Woman*.

With sterility, however, it is not always so easy to deal, depending, as it often does, upon peculiar organic deficiencies, or resulting from mysterious sympathies, it frequently baffles all our endeavors to understand or relieve it. As far as advice can be given, however, I shall treat upon it fully, and I believe that the cases to which the present article will apply, amount to a very large preponderance of the whole.

The Ancient Greek and Roman females used to hang a wood or metal image of the Male Organs round their necks when they desired children, as a charm, firmly believing that it had power to make them fruitful.

In the long-buried cities of Herculaneum and Pompeii, many of these images are dug up, some of them being most elaborately and beautifully carved. · They are generally about an inch long, though some are of the natural size. A friend of mine, a short time ago, presented me with several of them. In Cochin China—as I have been assured by a medical man, long resident there—it is the custom, when a female remains long barren, for the priest to give her a wooden model of the Male Organ, which has been blessed by him, and which she uses herself. This is supposed to remove the sterility, and is implicitly relied upon.

Even in our own times and country, charms are often practised for the same purpose, and medical means are employed, almost as ridiculous, and quite as useless. In some parts of the world, the waters of certain springs are supposed to make women conceive, and many resort to them for that purpose. A famous well of this kind once existed at one of the monasteries in England, and it certainly did seem to well deserve its celebrity. It was found, after a time, however, to lose its powers to a great degree, and, singularly enough, it failed just in proportion as the worthy *Abbot* of the monastery grew old. This, however, was accounted for, by supposing that with increasing age he had less strength to *pray*, and his prayers, in connection with those of his fair patient, were always needed to effect the sure.

Perhaps the most frequent cause of impotence and sterility in the male, however, is *Spermattorrhœa,* or excessive seminal loss. This may arise from many different causes, but principally from excesses and from masturbation. It may occur in two ways, either *visibly,* as in those who lose *t in sleep, or during the motion of the bowels, and it may also take place in an *unseen* form, which is the worst of all.

There is, in fact, scarcely anything more important for a man to know than the causes, effects, and treatment of this terrible affliction, and there are *few indeed* who do not practically experience more or less of its consequences.

It is undoubtedly, the most frequent of all the causes of impotence and sterility, and also of premature decay of the system generally. Every man, young or old, ought to read the article on *Spermattorrhœa* in my book, on the Male Organs. If the knowledge there given was universally possessed in time, it is incalculable how much suffering, disease, and untimely death would be prevented.

It should also be borne in mind, as explained in a former article, that the male is often sterile from *imperfection of the Semen*. Sometimes there are no Animalcules at all, and at other times they are dead, in either of which cases he is sterile, or incapable of impregnating. If the imperfection is not of long standing, however, he may not be impotent, but may still be able to practise association; though, eventually, even that power will be lost, for the organs soon lose all sensibility if they are not stimulated by perfect Semen.

In some men the Animalcules disappear, or die, for a short time only, from disease, or from taking drugs, and afterwards re-appear. In others again, I have found that they only appear at *a particular time of the year*, so that these individuals can impregnate then, but at all other times are impotent.

The power of the Testicles, however, and also their size, is capable of being much increased by proper medical treatment, even in the worst of cases, as shown in my work on *the Male Organs*.

The worst cases of sterility in the male are those connected with a *wasting of the Testes*, which may take place from numerous causes, some of them apparently trivial, to which all men are more less liable. To guard against such evils, however, is easy, with proper information, such as is contained in my work on the Male Organs.

There are also certain mysterious causes of sterility, the nature of which we cannot understand. Thus some females will conceive by one man and not by another, and some men will impregnate one female but not another, which shows that there is a certain *adaptation* needed between the two, though we cannot tell in what particular that adaptation consists.

There are often cases, in both sexes, where there is neither sexual desire nor capability till some particular object is found, as shown in a former article on the Influ- ence of the Mind over the Generative powers, and also in the Articles on the Power of the Imagination, and on the Brain, all of which should be referred to in connection with this subject.

§ IMPOTENCE AND STERILITY IN THE FEMALE.

The principal causes of these disabilities in the female have been explained in the previous articles, particularly in those upon the *Ovaries* and *Menstruation*. The non- formation of the egg, its not passing down the Tube in time, and the non-retention of it in the Womb, are among the most frequent causes, though medical men generally know nothing about them. Many married couples are also childless because they do not associate *at the proper time*, as explained in the article on Conception.

At the present time there are but few causes of barren- ness in Females but what can be removed, except those de- pending upon imperfect or deformed development, and even many of these are capable of being remedied. The Vagina, or mouth of the Womb can be opened or enlarged, *The Fallopian Tubes can be opened*, and the Ovaries can be stimulated to act in cases where they have been dor- mant for years.—All which operations come constantly within the scope of my practice, and with very few ex- ceptions they are uniformly successful.

The operations of opening the mouth of the womb and the Fallopian Tubes are quite new, especially the last, and they are both very often needed. In nearly all cases when a female has painful menstruation, attended by a dis- charge of membranes or clots, it is owing to a constric- tion of the mouth of the womb, which also prevents con ception. The operation for opening it therefore relieves both the suffering and the sterility.—Opening the Tubes is a difficult operation, but perfectly safe, and by any one well practised in it may always be successfully performed.

The treatment most frequently required in females is that for stimulating the Ovaries to form the eggs, and strengthening the womb to retain them sufficiently long, a weakness or irritability of one or the other of these Organs being the most frequent cause of female sterility known.—A want of sexual feeling is also a cause of barrenness sometimes, indirectly, and the production of it leads at once to conception. In nearly all cases, however, this peculiar sensibility can be produced, to any extent that may be required, and by means comparatively simple, and perfectly harmless. Diseases of the Womb and Vagina also often lead to sterility, especially Leucorrhœa, or *the Whites*, the discharge from which *kills the Animalcules*, and thus prevents conception.—I have known many females barren from this cause who conceived very readily, by simply using an injection of warm water before connection, to cleanse away the acrid discharge.

Moral causes do not operate so strongly and uniformly with the female as with the male, because she is in a great measure passive, and may even be made to conceive in spite of herself.

Many unsuspected causes of sterility will be given in our next chapter.

CHAPTER VI.

INFLUENCE OF DRUGS OVER THE SEXUAL POWERS.

IN no work upon the Generative system ever published except my Treatise on *the Male Organs*, has this subject been fully and practically treated, and from no other source therefore can information upon it be obtained. I have there described, as will be seen below, the effects of all drugs that act in a decided manner on the Generative system, and so completely, that but little remains to be added, to adapt that explanation to our present purpose.

Cantharides, or Spanish Flies. This article is popularly supposed to have an undoubted stimulating effect upon the sexual powers, and many persons will be surprised to learn how little foundation there is for such a belief. In fact, upon most persons, Cantharides have but little or no effect at all in that way; except they are given in such quantity as to be poisonous, and then they only act by causing severe inflammation, not only on the genitals but also in all the neighboring parts. It is quite common for even a small dose to create great irritation of the bladder, with complete inability to discharge the urine, and this may take place without any unusual sexual excitement at all, though most usually, the generative organs are stimulated more or less. —It is a great mistake, therefore, to suppose that Cantharides have a constant and specific action on the sexual organs, for they merely create an intense irritation, which affects these organs along with others, in the same way that many other irritant poisons do.—All the popular notions on this subject are utterly unfounded, and quite opposed to the truth.

It is very seldom that Cantharides are of any service whatever in the treatment of Impotence or Spermattorrhœa, though a combination of these with other articles is useful in certain cases. They form the main ingredient in all the quack stimulants for the generative organs and the use of them in this way unfortunately causes great mischief. Numbers of young men are permanently ruined, from

Spermattorrhœa, through taking these preparations of Can tharides, and I have known many married persons render ed hopelessly sterile from using them as stimulants. I had one distressing case of a young man, who was persuaded by a thoughtless friend to take some Spanish Flies as an experiment, to see if they would not increase his desires and powers. The quantity he took was only a moderate dose, but the effects were most alarming. He completely lost all power of discharging the urine, though the Blad der was full almost to bursting, and experienced such ago nizing pain in the prostate and urethra that he was nearly delirous. Priapism took place, but so far from being at tended by increased pleasure that it added to his sufferings, and yet he could not prevent it. Fortunately, he had timely assistance, and the immediate danger was obviated, but immediately after, he began to be troubled with involun tary emissions in the night, and eventually when urina ting, so that he became completely impotent, and so weak he could scarcely stand. I cauterized him, and used every other means the case would allow, but in spite of all, the trouble continued to some extent, and probably always will. He had been suffering, however, over four years when I saw him.

I also had a case of a young person of the other sex who was seriously injured by Cantharides, given as a trick, and who had involuntary discharge of urine ever after wards.

Camphor.—The action of Camphor upon the genital organs is sedative rather than stimulant, and when taken improperly or in excess, it may almost entirely destroy the sexual feeling, at least for a time. It is, therefore, given in cases of priapism, and in excessive excitement, whether from sexual or physical causes. If Cantharides or any other irritating poison be taken, Camphor is usually a val uable palliative, and it is sometimes of great service in certain forms of Spermattorrhœa. If taken in too large doses, however, or for too long a time, it will cause invol untary emissions.

Nitrate of Potash or Saltpetre.—It is commonly sup posed that this substance acts as a direct sedative to the sexual organs, and that if taken in any considerable quan tity, it will destroy all feeling, but this notion is a very erroneous one. Like all other diuretics, Nitre stimulates

• Genital Organs and if taken in too large doses it will

even produce inflammation, like Cantharides. Instances have been known where a discharge from the urethra has followed its use, like that of Gonorrhœa, and afterwards involuntary emissions have been experienced.

Ergot of Rye, or Secale Cornutum. This substance, as is well known, is used to expedite delivery in females, which it does by increasing the action of the womb. Its use, however, is dangerous, except in proper hands. From recent observations, it appears to stimulate the male organs also, and the men of those parts where it grows among the rye are noted for their ardent desires, while the females frequently miscarry. The Ergot cannot be given alone, either with safety or advantage, but its combination with other articles, forms a valuable remedy, both for impotence and spermattorrhœa. It is one of the ingredients of a stimulating and invigorating medicine which I use extensively in my practice.

Coffee and Tea.—Both these articles, but especially coffee, act as direct stimulants to the generative organs and if taken in excess, may produce all the effects of the most powerful drugs. I have known coffee cause priapism, lascivious dreams, and involuntary emissions, and nearly always its continued use will counteract any treatment that can be followed for relief.

Phosphorus.—This article is similar in its action to Cantharides, but much more energetic, and consequently it is much more dangerous in wrong hands, but when properly administered, it is frequently of great service. It is one of the ingredients of the invigorating medicine which I formerly spoke of, with which I have often produced the most unexpected restorations to power and health. Phosphorus should, however, never be experimented with by those not familiar with its action, for in some cases it will lead to the most disastrous consequences, and its evil effects are not easily recovered from.

These remarks were intended to apply more especially to the male, but they are equally applicable to the female also. In fact, to females they may often be of more importance than to males, because the female system is more easily affected by many of these Drugs, and they act upon them with more intensity. I have known little girls affected in a most deplorable manner by having such drugs given to them, and I am confident that the practice is productive of more mischief than is generally suspected.

Some Females are even affected in a very curious man ner by mere *scents*, or *odors*, such as are used in the *Toi- lette*, as shown by some singular cases in my *Diseases of Women.*

Phosphorus is certainly a most powerful stimulant to the Generative Organs, and also a most dangerous one.— Instances have occurred of men being made perfectly deli- rious with *Satyriasis*, from merely taking an ordinary medicinal dose of it, and women from the same cause, have become so furiously excited as to forget every considera- tion of prudence and decorum. In one instance a Physi- cian found his patient utterly unable to subdue the ardor that consumed him by any means whatever, until complete exhaustion ensued and he died. In less than thirty hours this man had cohabited *sixty-five* times, without erection having subsided or the flow of semen ceased.—Similar ef- fects are also observed upon animals, showing that the power of this Drug is specific. A Chemist having thrown out some of his refuse preparations, in which was some Phosphorus they were partly drunken by a Drake, who immediately afterwards commenced cohabiting with his female companions in the most furious manner, and con- tinued to do so till he fell down dead.

When incautiously used however, this Drug is exceed- ingly dangerous, and many cases of severe suffering have resulted from its unwarranted employment. Not only will it cause delirium, but it will also create the most burning and destructive inflammation of the Stomach and Intes- tines, which nothing can subdue. So perfectly does it pervade the very substance of the body that, in many cases of death from its use, the corpse has been perfectly *luminous*, and the phosphorus has been distinctly smelt in the blood. A physician, who dissected a body of this kind found that even his hands, and the instruments he had used, were luminous, and smelt quite strongly of it.

Even workmen who employ Phosphorus, as Match Makers for instance, unless they are very careful, are apt to suffer seriously in consequence of breathing its fumes. In some cases the Bones have even decayed, and ulcers have formed of the most malignant character.—Children have been poisoned by eating the phosphorized ends of matches it is well known, and I have known people made quite sick by only breathing the fumes when striking a friction match.

Ether and other similar articles, have occasionally

a singular effect upon the generative instinct, and awakes it when nothing else will. In many cases where Ether has been taken to produce insensibility, during surgical operations, the patient has been, in imagination, enjoying the pleasures of amative indulgence during the whole period. This has even been the case with Females while in Labor, and insensible from Ether, several having con fessed, that so far from suffering, they actually experi enced the *warmest* feelings, and imagined they were enjoy ing the embrace of their husbands.—In some of these cases females have experienced these feelings under such circumstances *for the first time,* and never after did so while awake.—A short time ago, I knew an instance of a young married lady who took Chloroform to have a tooth extracted, and instead of putting her to sleep it created a singular amative excitement, which in her half uncon scious state she could not control. Her advances to the Dentist were obvious enough, but fortunately he was a man of honor, and took no advantage. In a short time the excitement wore off, but she had a distinct recollec tion of her situation, and was most deeply mortified and hurt when she thought of it. At other times she was rather indifferent to such pleasures, especially after the above occurence. In some peculiar cases I use these agents in my practice, but only under certain circum stances.

Aromatics and Spices.—These have in general a stimu lating effect on the generative organs, the same as on other parts, but their power varies very much in different per sons, and under different circumstances. There are vari ous spice mixtures and combinations in popular use for this purpose, but they should not be indiscriminately used. Sometimes they are highly injurious, like all other stimu lants, and even when they do cause an increase of power .or feeling it is only temporary, and often followed by directly opposite effects.

In short, none of these articles operate specifically, in a benefical manner, on the generative organs, though cer tain combinations of them may do so under particular circumstances, like the medicine I have referred to as being used in my own practice.

There is one drug brought from the East Indies, the *Cannabis Indica,* which is the most regular in its action, and produces the most constant beneficial effects of any thing yet tried. It appears to act as a special nervous stimulant, exciting that part of the brain which influences the sexual organs, so that they feel directly an increase of power. It also causes great mental activity, disposes to cheerfulness, and induces a feeling of warmth and comfort over the whole system. Those who have taken it in a proper manner, are delighted with its effects, and never complain of any after-depression or re-action in any way. If given improperly, however, or in too heavy a dose, it first causes excitement of the wildest character, with an uncontrollable disposition to bodily activity, and afterwards a complete mental and physical prostration. In short, it is most powerful, either for good or for evil, according as it is used, and is the only means we possess, in numerous cases, of restoring sexual power and desire. In the East Indies it is commonly used, like Opium in China, for the purpose of producing pleasurable excitement, and also for removing impotence.

A plant producing this drug grows in the United States, and with due care a similar preparation may be made from it to that received from the East Indies. I have experimented with both, and when prepared by himself I have found the native product fully equal to the foreign. The Botanic physicians use the plant for various other purposes, but none of them seem to be aware of its possessing the properties I have described. Indeed the way in which they prepare and administer it, prevent those properties from being exhibited.

Medicines that excite the sexual organs are called *Aphrodisiacs*, and in various parts of the world they are in great demand, though but seldom administered, so as to be of any real service. As I have already remarked, some of these medicines, when properly used, have undoubted aphrodisiac powers, but they are by no means applicable in all cases. They may frequently fail of producing any good effect whatever, and sometimes may even cause irretrievable mischief. The successful admiration of them, therefore requires a perfect knowledge of their properties, and an extensive observation of their effects under all circumstances. It is for this reason I have not given any recipes for these drugs, for no one can tell when they should or should not be used, unless they know something about them, and the effects of taking them improperly may be so serious that mere experiment with them is highly

In a particular class of cases I have long been using a combination of the Cannabis, with other articles, which I find to possess the most extraordinary powers, the preparation of which I have been repeatedly importuned to disclose, both by patients and medical men. At present, however, I do not feel called upon to make this disclosure, because I know the great mischief which would result from using such a preparation improperly, and I know also how few persons there are familiar enough with its powers and properties to use it rightly. My own experience has made me acquainted with signs by which I can tell, *in every case* whether it is proper to be used or not, and I will answer for its never producing evil effects when I advise it. So wonderful and unexpected have been the effects of this preparation, in numerous instances, that if I chose to be unscrupulous, and sell it indiscriminately, I have no doubt but it would be used more extensively than any other medicine has ever been, for any purpose whatever. I do not think it proper to give it, however, in any case, till I know whether it be appropriate or not, and this I can always tell on receiving either a verbal or written description of the history, progress, and symptoms of the disease. I do not hesitate to say, that I have seen more restorations to sexual power, and more cures of *Sterility*, in both sexes, from the use of this preparation than from any other means, and I do not hesitate to pronounce it, in certain cases, *an infallible remedy*.

Medicines that *decrease* the sexual powers are called *Anaphrodisiacs*, and I believe they have all been mentioned.

Every young man should also read attentively the remarks upon the influence of *Tobacco* and *Alcohol*, in my work on the Male Organs. The real power of these drugs is but little known, and the mischief they do to the sexual organs is unsuspected. Married persons should also be acquainted with many of the facts I give, as they will show that in many instances the most temperate use of these articles is hurtful, and that they often cause Impotence and Sterility, as well as Insanity.

Odors and Scents.—It will scarcely seem possible, to those who have not considered this subject philosophically, that a mere *scent* can have any effect at all over the generative powers, but such is undoubtedly the fact. The different parts of the Nervous system are so mysteriously

and sympathetically connected that any impression, however slight, made on one nervous fibre may react upon
others in a remote part of the organization, and thus exciting the olfactory nerve by any peculiar odor may react
upon and excite the sexual organs, as powerfully as if they
were directly irritated.

Some persons are much affected by *odors*, which operate
either as stimulants or as sedatives to the nervous system,
and sometimes produce peculiar effects. That there are
odors that speedily excite the sexual instinct is beyond
question, some naturally and others artificially, though
different people experience their effects in very different
degrees. There are also others that exert an opposite
influence, though seldom in so decided a manner. Very
sensitive people, particularly those in whom the sexual
instinct is naturally strong, may be as much excited by a
mere scent as by a medicine conveyed into the stomach, as
I have frequently seen. *Hysteria* is often excited in this
way in females, as I have shown in my work on the Diseases of Women, and various forms of nervous excitement
frequently supervene in the other sex from the same
cause.

It may be stated, as a general rule, that all powerful
odors *may* produce effects of this kind, and they are, therefore, better avoided, particularly the habitual use of them.
There are some particular scents that exhibit this power
more constantly, and to a greater degree than others, and
several of these are articles of common use in the *toilette.*
An enumeration of these would embrace many of the
choicest *perfumes* used, but it is scarcely possible to par-
ticularize among so many, nor is it necessary, as the
whole are better avoided. The very *origin* and *natural*
use of some of these indicates clearly enough the purpose
Nature intended them to fulfill, in the animals from which
they are taken, and I cannot but think that few *females*
at least would use them, if they really knew what they
were. *Musk*, especially, is an article of this kind, the
aphrodisiac effects of which I have sometimes seen exhibited in the most unequivocal manner.

The readers of classic poetry will call to mind the story
of the *Indian Prince*, who exhibited such marvellous
powers merely from smelling the flowers of the *Nymphæ
odorata*, and also several other instances in which the
aphrodisiac power of different odors is distinctly alluded

to, showing that the general truth was known centuries ago. Some of these accounts are of course much exaggerated, but most of them are founded upon actual truths, as I have in some cases proved, and I believe the statement about the *Nympha* is one that is entitled to consideration.

In Turkey, an Odoriferous *Pastile* is in common use in the Harems, and is reputed to have great stimulating power. It is compounded principally of Musk, Civet, Ambergris, Cinnamon, and a variety of Vegetable Oils. One of these is constantly worn in the dress, and sometimes it is powdered and rubbed over the person.

Some of these scents, as Musk for instance, are probably the *sexual odors* of the animals from which they are taken, and are intended to attract the other sex. This may possibly account for their peculiar power, and make it less singular. Dimerbrock relates an instance of a man who rubbed Musk upon his genitals, before cohabiting, and who became so swollen and excited in consequence, and his partner likewise, that they could not separate till a variety of refrigerant means had been resorted to. And in another instance it was observed, that one of these scents excited an insane person, though he gave no such indications without it.

Experiments have shown undoubtedly, that the peculiar odor of the Genital Organs, of either sex, will excite the other sex, though the individuals may neither be visible nor known to be near.

CHAPTER VII.

ON THE PREVENTION OF CONCEPTION.

THIS is a subject which many persons may think not necessary to be treated upon, but there are peculiar reasons why it ought not to be passed over in silence. It has been, of late years, so much talked of, and so many unscientific works have been published, pretending to give information about it, that every one is familiar with the idea. To say that there *are* means of preventing conception, is only stating what every person has already heard, or believes, and is, therefore, nothing new. Even if such information was likely to be productive of great evil, as some imagine, it is now impossible to prevent its dissemination, and it is, therefore, useless to avoid the topic. I think, however, that the danger apprehended from it is altogether fallacious, and the fear arises from a wrong view of the case, as shown in the article on Conception, to which I refer my readers for the arguments.

Many of the practices resorted to for preventing conception, are altogether ineffective for the purpose, and some are decidedly hurtful, but this not being known, people resort to them, and are both deceived and injured. It is, therefore, the duty of every physician to show the inutility and danger of such practices, and not to shun the subject.

Independently of this, however, there are many great and good men who think that *harmless* means of preventing conception may be practised with propriety, or even become *advisable* in peculiar circumstances, and that there may be nothing either immoral or improper in their use. It is well known for instance, that there are many severe diseases to which females are subject, that never can be removed while they conceive, but which, if uncured, are sure to become fatal, and probably also descend to their children. Some females also have deformed Pelvises, and can never bring forth live children, while others are *certain to die* if the child remains in the Womb till it is a certain size. Besides these cases, however, how many

there are that remain in constant ill-health and suffering
from continued child-bearing, without the possibility of
relief or escape. In our country, fortunately, there are
but few persons that cannot find means to maintain a family, though it be large, but still, with many it may be a
severe struggle to do so, and a constant increase may condemn the parents to poverty and difficulty, and the children themselves to neglect.

Now it cannot be denied that people are situated under
all these different circumstances, and that the continual
increase of their families entails all these evils both upon
them and their children, but whether this affords a sufficient reason for limiting the number, must be left for
every person's own decision. I am acquainted with many
moral and religious people who think that the practice,
under such circumstances, is perfectly justifiable and pro
per, and some even consider it a duty. Others, however,
think the contrary, and hold that every evil or inconvenience ought to be undergone, whether poverty, sickness,
or even death, rather than avoid it by such means. For
my own part, I would neither give advice nor offer an
opinion on the subject, as I consider that all persons should
decide for themselves, and that their decision concerns
themselves alone. My duty is simply to show the injury
of those practices now in use, and also to show, where it is
absolutely needed, that safe and efficacious means can be
employed.

It is not generally known, that it is the regular custom
in medical practice, when a female has a deformed Pelvis,
or is otherwise incapable of being delivered at the full
term, to *produce Abortion* at any early stage. This, however, is the invariable custom, and in practical works upon
midwifery, the means are explained. (See, for instance,
Chailly's Midwifery, translated in my *Matron's Manual.*)
This is done because it is thought better to sacrifice the
Fœtus only, at any early stage, than to let *both* die, as they
assuredly would, if the gestation were allowed to proceed.
Now it may well be a question in such cases, whether it
would not be better to teach how to prevent the conception
altogether, and I leave it for others to decide which is the
most objectionable, *prevention* or *Abortion?* I am confident also, that much of the horrible practice of procuring
Abortion, now so prevalent among married people, is
caused by the want of simple and reliable means of pre-

vention. No matter what may be said, there are thousands who are so circumstanced, that they will endeavor, at all hazards, to avoid increasing their families, and it is simply a question whether it is not better to teach them prevention, than to leave them only the other alternative.

There are few persons except medical men, who have any idea of the extent to which the revolting practice of Abortion is now carried, nor of the awful consequences that frequently follow from it. Every female who undergoes any of the disgusting operations practised for this purpose, does so *at the risk of her life*, and to the almost certain destruction of her health if she survives. I have had many of these miserable victims come to me afterwards for advice, and more wretched objects cannot be conceived. Some of them have been almost torn and cut to pieces, and others so injured, that their lives hung as it were by a thread. Those that take drugs for this purpose are also equally exposed to risk, and suffer in their health to an equal extent, so that their lives become a positive burthen to them. In short, this is one of the most terrible evils of the present time, and every one must earnestly desire to see it abolished, or some lesser evil take its place. Every female may be told with truth—and, indeed, every one ought to know—that there are *no safe means of procuring Abortion*. It is true that some few may undergo the ordeal in safety, but none can depend upon doing so, and the chances are ten to one that death, or the evils above referred to, will follow!

A general knowledge of this fact would, no doubt, do much to prevent the practice, but, still it would not do away with it altogether, unless some reliable means of prevention were known. Strange as it may seem, many of the worst sufferers have assured me that they would undergo the same risk again, rather than have more children, and some have even said that they would *die* first. In such cases, therefore, there is simply a choice between the two practices of abortion and prevention, and I am confident there are thousands who feel in this way.

A gentleman called upon me a short time ago, who was suffering from a terrible scrofulous affection, which had appeared since his marriage, and by which his first child was afflicted in an awful manner. He assured me that both himself and his wife would rather suffer death a thousand times than be the authors of such another miserable being, and that they thought it would be a most grievous sin for them ever to be parents again. In another case, the mother had periodic attacks of insanity after she had borne two children, one of whom had already shown symptoms of the same terrible affliction, and they, with good reason, feared that if they had others, the same calamity might befall them. Now, in such cases, I leave those who condemn prevention altogether to decide what should be done. For my own part, as I remarked before, I leave all to decide for themselves, according to their conscientious notions, and I think that no one person's decision, let it be what it may, should in any way affect another person. In a word, I think it is every one's own affair.

Besides such instances as the above, I often meet with others equally distressing, and such as are common enough. An industrious, hard-working mechanic, called upon me once and stated his case, in the hope I could give him advice. He had four children, the eldest only eight years old, and after every confinement since the first, in consequence of an injury then, his wife was from three to six months completely bed-ridden, and unable to attend in any way to her household duties. His employment was often restricted, and his means so limited, that hired help was out of their power, and there, said he, "My wife had to lie, day after day, and week after week, and see every thing go to ruin in the house, with the children dirty and ragged, without being able to rise and help herself." Now this may be considered an extreme case, but there are thousands of others that approximate to it, and people, so situated, naturally ask of their medical adviser, "What shall we do?" If these men give them no reply, as is generally the case, and no other means are offered to them, the dreadful practice of Abortion is too often resorted to.

I know some people will say that it is possible for such persons to avoid having a family without using *preventive* means. And so it is; but the deprivation required *will not* be undergone by the great mass, and cannot be undergone by others without the most immoral consequences. It is sheer absurdity to suppose that the promptings of Nature can be totally unheeded, except in peculiar individual cases, and illicit intercourse and vicious habits of self-indulgence would certainly follow a total deprivation of the marital right in most instances.

Many medical men and philanthropists have perceived

these difficulties, and have pressed a consideration of them, but few have chosen to give actual advice. I think it is best to leave it altogether an open question as to the propriety of prevention, or in what cases it is allowable, but still to put all who choose in possession of the proper means. They can then decide for themselves as to employ ing or rejecting them, and the hurtful means now resorted to for the purpose—to say nothing of the *criminal* ones at a later period—will naturally fall into disuse.

The most obvious means of prevention are those alluded to in the Bible, as having been practised by *Onan*, and which have doubtless been in use for thousands of years. If the seminal fluid be not placed within the Vagina, of course there can be no conception, and all that is required, therefore, is to cease association before the emission oc· curs. But, independently of the uncertainty of this being done, at least in many cases, it is not *advisable*. There is good reason to believe that, in every act of association, the presence of the male principle within the female organs is always required, even when there is no conception. It is, in all probability, more or less *absorbed* in every case, and even when it does not impregnate, it prevents irritation and exhaustion. In fact, without it, the act is merely a species of Masturbation—unsatisfactory and injurious. It is also extremely hurtful to the male, and in a way not at all suspected. When emission occurs without the female organs, it is always more incomplete and slower than when it occurs within, owing to the absence of the customary warmth and pressure, and of that peculiar influence which the organs of one sex exert upon the other. A portion of the semen, therefore, remains undischarged at the time, and escapes slowly afterwards, thus giving rise to a weakness and irritation of the Urethra and Seminal Ducts, which, in time, becomes permanent, and lays the foundation for *involuntary* losses and final impotence.

I have known many married men much injured in thi way, without being able to even conjecture what had hurt them. And I am confident that much female exhaustion and nervous irritation result in the same way.

The *partial* adoption of this plan is not liable to the above objections to quite an equal extent, but still it is so, more or less, and it is, perhaps, still more difficult to practise. But, independent of these considerations, it cannot be relied upon, for conception may follow if the seminal

fluid be placed in *any part* of the Vagina, as before ex
plained, or perhaps even in the External Lips. It is true
it is not so likely to occur under such circumstances, but
still it may do so.   In some men the Penis is imperfect, the
opening of the Urethra being *under*, and some distance
down, instead of being at the end, so that they can never
eject the semen to the top of the Vagina but only into its
lower part.   Still these men may be fathers, though not so
frequently as others, unless with certain females.   Dr.
Dunglison, in his *Human Physiology*, remarks of this im
perfection, that " we cannot, therefore, regard it as an ab
solute cause of impotence, but the inference is just, that
if the semen be not projected far up into the Vagina, and
in the direction of the Os Uteri, impregnation is *not likely*
to be accomplished ; a fact, which it might be of moment
to bear in mind, *where the rapid succession of children is
an evil of magnitude.*"

This plan, therefore, diminishes the *liability*, but does
not totally *prevent*.

The next most general plan is the use of *Interjections* after
association, either for the purpose of removing the Semen,
or of destroying its power.   For the purpose of removing
it, however, they cannot always be relied upon, for sufficient will often be retained in the folds of the Vagina, to
cause conception, notwithstanding the injection.   For the
same reason, no certain dependence can be placed upon in
troducing any object into the Vagina before association, as
a Sponge for instance, which, on being withdrawn, may
bring the semen with it.   In many cases this succeeds, but
often it will not, because a small portion of semen is sure
to be left on the walls notwithstanding, and that many impregnate.   There is another objection also to this, which
should forbid its general use—the object introduced, of
course, comes immediately before the mouth of the Womb,
and then prevents the contact of that part with the male
organ.   Now this contact is often necessary for the production of a proper state of excitement, as formerly explained,
and when it does not occur, there is simply an injurious irritation to the female, without any gratification.   I have
known it also cause irritation of the Meatus in the male.

The use of injections to destroy *the power* of the semen
would seem to be the most reliable means, and, when of the
proper kind, they are so, but the unscientific use of them
has led to serious evils.   The way in which they operate

when effective, is by *killing the Seminal Animalcules*, and any injection that will not do this, will not prevent conception. There are many substances that will apparently kill them, but which only leave them paralyzed, so that they afterwards recover, and there are other substances that will destroy them, but only when used so strong as to injure the female organs. The solutions of various Salts, for instance, act in this way, such as Alum, Sulphate of Zinc, Chloride of Zinc and Sulphate of Iron, none of which, according to my experiments, will always kill the Animalcules, unless used stronger than is allowable with safety to the female. Very many I have met with seriously injured by the constant use of powerful injections of this kind, some having inflammation of the Womb and Vagina, some excoriations, and others hemorrhage. Besides which, they in a short time destroy the sensibility of the parts entirely, and lead to total indifference and sterility. The only articles proper to be used in this way, are such as destroy the Animalcules without acting on the female organs, and there are but few that do so. I know of only one article that acts in this way with certainty, and it is both scarce and difficult to obtain, so that it is not likely to come into general use. It is a vegetable substance, which destroys the Animalcules almost instantaneously, but has no effect whatever on the female organs. I wish it, however, to be distinctly understood, that I do not desire, by this statement, to *advertise* the article, as I have neither the desire nor the intention of making a trade of it in any way. It may be of importance to medical men, and to those whose *lives* are in actual peril, to know that such an article has been discovered, and that is the only reason I mention it.

The employment of injections is objectionable, however, on other grounds. It is not advisable, as before stated, to remove the Semen from the Vagina, nor to prevent its being deposited there, because it is better for it to be absorbed, even when there is no impregnation. In all cases also it is necessary for them to be used *immediately* after emission, and the too early separation, together with the anxiety and revulsion of feeling attending upon the *preventive* act are both agitating and injurious, to say nothing of inconvenience. Some females, also, absorb the Semen so quickly that the injection can scarcely be used in time, and with some men the emission is so slow that the first part may impregnate before the whole has been expelled. To be in any degree certain, therefore, when using injections, it is necessary for the act to be to a certain extent incomplete, and this often causes a weakness in the male and nervous irritation in the female.

The employment of a *covering* to the male, in the form of a thin skin tube, called the *Condom*, is of course effi cacious as a preventive, but is liable to many of the above objections. The emission is never quite perfect when it is used, and the mutual contact of the male and female organs with each other being prevented, as well as the contact of the Semen with the Vagina, there is not a com plete gratification, and to the female great nervous irri tation often follows.

Among some persons a plan has been adopted more injurious than any of the above, though not known to be so. It consists in forcibly compressing the Male Organ close to the Scrotum, just previous to emission, so that the Semen cannot escape. Some men think that by such means nothing is lost, and that the connection does not exhaust them, but this only shows their ignorance of their own structure. In all cases where the compression is practised, the emission is as complete as if nothing of the kind had been done, only it takes a different course. By referring to the plate showing the internal Male Organs it will be seen that the Semen passes into the urinary passage, from the Prostate Gland, through certain little openings called the *Ejaculatory Ducts*, close to the Vera Montanum, or little protuberance in the middle of the passage, close to the Bladder. Now the Vera Montanum is so formed, being pointed forwards, that it *directs* the Semen along the passage towards the external opening, which is the course it should pursue, but when compression is prac tised, so as to close the passage, it cannot escape in this direction. Under these circumstances, therefore, it is compelled to flow by the large end of the Montanum and *enter the Bladder*, from whence it is expelled afterwards along with the urine. The consequence of this is that it soon begins to take that course always, whether compres sion be practised or not, and the man becomes sterile in consequence. He is also liable to inflammation of the Urethra, Vera Montanum, and Bladder, and suffers from Spermattorrhœa. till eventually his powers are lost alto gether. It is, in short, a most destructive practice.

M. Parent Duchatelet gives us some curious information respecting this practice in his work on " Prostitution in Paris, which may be read with profit both by the Physiologist and Philosopher.

I may, perhaps, as well remark here, incidentally that some young victims of Masturbation practise the same thing, under the mistaken idea that no evil ensues from their vice if the *emission* does not take place. The folly of this will, however, be apparent from the above explanation.

Those females who think they can escape being impregnated by simply avoiding all excitement, and pleasurable feeling are more deceived than those who rely on any of the other modes, as former explanations have shown.

It is evident, however, that the Prevention of Conception, when association is practised, is not so easy as some have suppposed, and that it is not altogether harmless either.

Those who really *need* information as to the means of *Preventing Conception* may address Dr. HOLLICK, Box, 3606, P. O., New-York City, and he will send the information if the case makes it proper to do so.

CHAPTER VIII.

TOPICS OF SPECIAL INTEREST.

§ INFLUENCE OF FOOD AND DRINK OVER THE SEXUAL
POWERS.

THOSE who think that food and drink exert little or no direct influence over the sexual powers are greatly mistaken. They in fact operate most powerfully, both directly and indirectly, as I have shown in my work on *the Male Organs*.

It is very essential to the preservation of the sexual power that the general health should be good, and that there should be no serious derangements of any of the vital functions. When the general health is impaired and the vital energies are low, the sexual organs are sure to be weakened, and usually more in proportion than any of the others. Owing to their extensive sympathies also they are sure to be affected by the diseases of all the other organs, and not unfrequently this sympathetic injury becomes very serious. The stomach particularly exerts a great influence over the generative organs, both beneficial and injurious. Long-continued dyspepsia is nearly always accompanied by weakened sexual power and desire, and even temporary attacks of indigestion will, for a time, produce similar effects. On the other hand a healthy stomach, with perfect digestion and nutrition, is highly conducive to sexual vigor. We may even go much further, and show that high feeding is nearly sure to over-excite the genital organs, or in other words that gluttony leads to licentiousness. This is a truth too often lost sight of in the education of children, many of whom, though predisposed to sexual ardor, are stimulated with rich food and exciting drinks till their passions become overpoweringly strong.—In short, the stomach exerts a most decided sympathetic influence over the generative organs, and we are thus enabled, by proper attention to the diet and drink, to either increase or weaken their power to a great extent.

Some kinds of food stimulate the sexual organs while other kinds leave the contrary effect upon them. Shell-fish, as before stated, are usually stimulating, owing to the phosphorous they contain, but other fish have seldom such power Flesh-meat is stimulating merely because it is nutritious, but it is a great mistake to suppose that it is of necessity more so than vegetables. There are some vegetables that are often more stimulating than flesh, especially those that are *farinaceous* or contain much starch, as the potato, for instance, which, when of good quality, contains most of the elements the body needs. Most strong tasted or aromatic vegetables have a stimulant effect, such as Celery, Parsnips, Onions, and *Asparagus*, especially, and so have all seasoning herbs, such as Mint, Sage, Pennyroyal, and Thyme. Spices and condiments have a still stronger action, especially the Peppers and Nutmeg.—Mushrooms stimulate some people very much, and Truffles still, more, and even Olives exert a marked influence at times. The flesh of birds I think is not stimulating, except that which is red, such as ducks and geese. I have several times been assured that eating freely of the *Canvass-back duck*, when in season, has been highly beneficial to those who were weakened by excess, probably partly from its own nature and partly from the wild Celery on which it feeds. Of all meats, however, *Turtle* has the greatest reputation for exciting the generative organs, and I think with good reason. It is undoubtedly highly nutritious, and it appears also to contain some *heating* principle, which specially affects those parts.

As a general rule all watery vegetables, such as turnips, cabbage. and squash, have no such effect as those enumerated, and are therefore proper when we wish to keep down excitement. Acid fruits also come under the same category, and indeed fruits generally, except some highly-flavored ones. such as peaches, and pine-apples, which are undoubtedly *aphrodisiac*, except they disagree with the stomach.

Tomatoes are rather stimulating, and so are most kinds of beans, especially the Lima Beans, but peas are not so. Wheaten bread or wheaten flour in any form, is more stimulating than the flour of any other grain, while Indian meal is probably the least so. When we desire an anaphrodisiac effect therefore, Indian bread should be used, with mush, samp or hominy, instead of wheaten bread or potatoes. Rice is unstimulating, but sage, tapioca, and arrowroot are the reverse.

In regard to drinks it may be stated that all alcoholic liquors are highly stimulating when first taken, but they soon lose their power if used too long or intemperately, and then they become injurious. Wine has a more strengthening effect than spirits of any kind, and ale or porter is still better than wine. Those who desire to keep their passions down should not take either wine or malt liquor in any quantity.—Most of the cordials in use are highly exciting, owing to the spices they contain, and so are many of the so-called bitters.—Coffee is almost as stimulating as wine, and should never be used by those who are disposed to involuntary emissions, nor by those whose desires are too strong. Tea is different from coffee in this respect, and is therefore the better drink in such cases. Milk, though highly nutritious, is not stimulating, and it therefore forms an excellent drink for those who are disposed to emissions or exciting dreams; such persons, however, will do better to use cold water only, and they should also avoid all *warm* fluids, no matter how simple, because warm drinks always excite the flow of urine, and of course stimulate the sexual organs also. Those who *cannot* use the cold water only may safely drink soda and mineral waters as much as they choose, or lemonade if it agree with them.

The Turks regard all kinds of *Fish* as being stimulating to the sexual powers, and they resort to them on that account. Some kinds besides shell fish may probably be so, because some of them undoubtedly contain Phosphorus, which is the real cause of their power when they have any.—A French writer, Hecquet, gives us a curious account of an experiment made by one of the Sultans, to test this. He had two Dervishes brought before him, men who mortified the flesh in every way, and who practised the most rigid celibacy. He had them fed upon the most stimulating and nutritious meats, till they became quite stout and strong, and then commanded them to be constantly attended by two of the most beautiful young females in the Harem, who were directed to use all their arts to excite the amorous desires. The Dervishes, however, resisted all these powerful influences and maintained their celibacy inviolate. He then directed them to be fed on *Fish*, and to be waited upon in the same way. This course was found to succeed, the rigid Dervishes forgot their vows, love triumphed, and the influence of this peculiar diet was fully established.

Young meats are not nearly so stimulating as those or mature animals, nor so nutritious —. In roasting meat, especially Beef, when it is properly done, there is a peculiar and delightful odor given from what is called the *bark*, or *brown*, which indicates the presence of a principle termed *Ozmazone*, which is not found in Veal, or lamb. This principle is highly stimulating, and generous, and undoubtedly conducive to generative power.

In well prepared soups we smell the Ozmazone, and then they are of service, but without it they can do but little good.

Good rich Beef, roasted, especially the outside, is perhaps as good an article for strengthening the sexual powers as any that could be eaten, and it may often be used alternately with some of the other articles mentioned with great advantage.

Fat is of little service for this particular purpose, it having a direct tendency, as is well known, to *form fat*, which is not required.

§ PROPER TIME FOR SEXUAL INDULGENCE.

THE importance of this subject is greater than at a first glance it might appear to be, and in giving advice, as a medical man, I often find it necessary to refer to it, as will be seen in my work on *the Male Organs*.

Perhaps, however, the most important suggestions, as regards the preservation of the procreative power, are those relating to its actual use.—It is well known, respecting all the other vital functions, that their healthy performance and preservation depends materially upon their being exercised at proper times, and under proper circumstances, and it is the same with the generative functions. Many persons think, because the genital organs are usually capable of action at any time, and under almost any circumstances, that it is therefore of little consequence what time is chosen, or under what circumstances it may be. This, however, is a great mistake, as any one may soon discover by studying his own experience.

The *time* for sexual indulgence should be so chosen that the temporary excitement and after exhaustion resulting from it, may not interfere with any of the bodily or mental functions, nor distress the system by necessitating too much effort during any needful exertion. Ignorance of this important rule, and consequent neglect of it, very often leads to great inconvenience, and even serious mischief. Sexual indulgence just after eating is nearly certian to be followed by indigestion, even if it does not cause immediate vomiting, owing to the temporary loss of nervous power thereby produced, which arrests the action of the stomach. Just *before* eating also the same evil may follow, from the stomach being made so weak that digestion cannot properly commence, and the food consequently ferments. Many times I have heard men confirm this truth, when explained to them, though they had previously never dreamt that their troubles arose from such a cause and when our previous explanations are borne in mind, respecting the *nervous sympathies* of the sexual organs, the philosophy of it will be evident. The proper time for this indulgence therefore, in reference to taking food, is at a sufficient interval after eating for digestion to be nearly accomplished, and before another meal begins to be needed By observing this rule the action of the stomach is not interfered with, and no indigestion or nausea are likely to follow. It is true, that most men experience a *stronger desire* for indulgence *immediately after* a full meal, particularly when stimulating drinks have been used, but this does not prove that they choose the best time. The desire they then experience is merely a factitious one, produced by the general excitement of the whole system, and the exhaustion afterwards felt is nearly always in proportion. In the same manner a man, while under excitement from alcohol, may feel disposed to great bodily activity and may exhibit astonishing strength, but when the stimulus is withdrawn he feels a corresponding prostration and lassitude. This is the reason also why sexual indulgence should not be sought during such excitement, for the disposition is nearly sure to be stronger than natural, and the over-excitement is followed by proportionate exhaustion. In *Poetry*, I am aware, *Venus* and *Bacchus* are associated together, but Poetry is not always *Physiology*, nor even *common sense*, nor should the licentious furor produced by wine be in any way considered as the promptings of nature.

Upon the same principles it is obviously injudicious to seek indulgence just previous to any mental effort being made, because the vital energy will be too much exhausted to allow of such effort being made with advantage. Nor is it advisable immediately *after* any great mental effort, because it is injurious to have *two* causes of exhaustion in action at the same time.—The same remarks also apply to *muscular exercise*, which should neither immediately follow nor closely precede sexual indulgence, for the reasons above given.—In short, the period chosen should be one when both body and mind can enjoy repose, at least for a short period, both before and after, and when none of the functions are likely to be disturbed.

The time of day is a matter of secondary importance or rather no preferable time can be named, because it must so much depend upon how the individual is circumstanced. That of course will be the best time when the above-mentioned rules can be most fully observed. Some medical writers suggest the evening, because the business of the day is then over and the repose of night is to follow, and this probably is the best period, generally speaking.— Others again recommend the morning, because there is then the greatest vigor, and in case of conception the *offspring* may be benefitted thereby. This, however, I feel assured, is a bad suggestion, for the business of the day will be very apt to oppress a man who starts exhausted, and the various functions of his system will very likely be imperfectly performed. The notion about the offspring being influenced at *the moment of conception*, by the state of the male system, I have already shown the fallacy of, because that moment may not nearly correspond with the period of association.

The celebrated *Buffon* was accustomed to indulge just after his dinner, and possibly in his particular case it might have had no ill effect, but most certainly the practice cannot be generally advised, and there are few persons but what would be injured by it.

Perhaps the best course, when a man is much exhausted by the fatigues of the day, is to take a first sleep, for two or three hours, and then wake up for the purpose, devoting the remainder of the night afterwards to undisturbed repose.

§ EFFECTS OF OVER EXCITEMENT AND ABSTRACTION OF MIND.

Abstraction of Mind, or its complete absorption in some much-liked pursuit, is highly unfavorable to the manifesta-

tion of sexual powers. Many men who were really strong
and vigorous in their sexual systems have been comparatively impotent from mere pre-occupation of mind, as some
of our former articles have shown. Such is the case also
with females, who are very apt, when absorbed in their
domestic duties, and in the anxieties attendant upon a
family, to become completely indifferent to amative enjoy
ment. Indeed it is a common remark that most of them
soon fail in this respect, and seldom maintain the ardor
they experienced at first, and no doubt for the above rea
son Those that remain childless, or who have no care
and anxiety, do not experience this deprivation, but on the
contrary their power of enjoyment increases.

A celebrated Medical Author, relates an instance of a
great Mathematician who married, and who, though every
way capable, was utterly unable to consummate fully the
act of sexual union. Always before it was complete some
of his mathematical *Problems* would come up in his mind,
and so completely abstract him, that Love was momentarily
forgotten, and the excitement went down. His Lady com
plained to the physician above-mentioned, and asked his
advice. He recommended her to partially *intoxicate* her
husband some night. with Champagne, and induce him to
seek her society while experiencing the, to him, novel ex-
hilaration. She did so, and the result was as desired, so
that in a short time she became a mother.—During the
unusual excitement of the time his mathematics were forgotten, and Love had the desired opportunity to triumph.

Several instances have been known where over-excitement has led to *Apoplexy*, and to *Paralysis*. I know a
young man now, who became completely *blind* from excessive excitement when first cohabiting with a female.
And I was told a case of a husband who actually died
while embracing his wife after a long absence. In another
instance, a man became insane from over excitement, on the
occasion of his marriage, and a female who was exceedingly amorous, completely lost the use of her limbs in the
same way. Palpitations of the heart, nervous tremblings,
and partial loss of sight are frequent occurrences at such
times in both sexes, and when excessive are apt to become
permanent.

§ DURATION OF THE SEXUAL POWER.

The duration of the sexual power, like any other, materially depends on the manner in which it is used, and this should therefore be duly considered by those who think the preservation worth striving for. A certain amount of natural indulgence is probably essential, *in most cases*, to perfect health, but when that amount is exceeded of course more or less permanent injury results, as before shown. Every individual should, therefore, endeavor to discover, for his own guidance, the proper limits to his gratification, and if he will attend to what has been previously stated on this point, that limit may be readily ascertained. By doing this a *real gain* will always be made, for the extra duration of the power which this will ensure will more than compensate for any temporary denial.—With those people whose systems are in regular action, and whose health is nearly uniform, the observance of a *regular period* is found to be advantageous, and highly conducive to the preservation of the virile power, as it prevents both excess and gradual decline.

These hints and suggestions, though apparently simple and common-place, are nevertheless of great value, and if duly observed would probably do more towards preventing untimely decay than all the medical treatment ever practised. Decay is caused, in numerous instances, *by a number of small causes* operating together, and if each of those be removed, as it may generally be very readily, the decay is of course prevented. People are too apt to take notice only of the more striking agents of destruction, passing unnoticed these apparently simple ones, as being of small consequence, while in reality they are the most important.

There are few persons of good health, who will attend to the above suggestions, and the advice formerly given, but what may preserve their powers to an indefinite period of their existence, particularly if they practice *cold local bathing* over the parts, and avoid all improper excitement. There is no particular time of life when the powers of the male system decay, but they may be preserved to extreme old age, as many cases have proved.—Old Parr, for instance, was condemned to do Penance *when over a hundred years old*, for an amorous intrigue, and he had several children after that period.

In females, however, the power of generation ceases at the turn of life, but not the power of association, which of course remains the same. It is a remarkable fact also, that the disposition and the capability of enjoyment remain as strong after that period as before in many, which, would seem to prove, that association is quite proper as a means of *indulgence* only, or certainly the desire for it would become extinct.

The explanations already given will show that both power and capability of enjoyment may be either increased and made to endure, or decreased and early extinguished according to the mode of life which the individual pursues. There are, however, many modifying circumstances not generally taken notice of, but which are of considerable importance. Some of these are pointed out in the following extract from a former work.

There is no question but that association between persons properly adapted to each other is less exhaustive, and may be more frequently indulged, than between those who are naturally unfitted to be companions. And it is also certain that the circumstances under which the association occurs may very much determine the effect it will have. It is requisite, for the act to be truly pleasurable and advantageous, that it should be fully approved both by the feelings and the judgment, otherwise it will be more or less regretted, and more or less injury will follow, no matter what amount of mere animal gratification be experienced. This is the reason why mere licentious debauchery is always followed by remorse, and ill health, while legitimate association in marriage, with a loved and respected partner leads to no such evil results. It is a fact equally important to individuals and to society at large, that the institution of marriage is conducive both to health and to happiness, and that the duration of life, in both sexes, *is longer in that state than in any other.* Many men fall into a great error in regard to this subject, and suppose that they can realize *more pleasure* in the unlicensed indulgence of the single state than when married. *This is, however, a fatal mistake*, for they really enjoy less, and are after all dissatisfied with themselves, while the duration of their powers is materially shortened.

Some little time ago, I had a very interesting conversation on this subject with *Swedenborgian*, who remarked that any of the principles laid down in my lectures exactly corresponded with his *spiritual* views on marriage, and that his own experience fully corroborated the truth of what I had stated. He told me that in his youth, he was unfortunately led into a licentious course of life, and experienced in consequence all that *self-accusation* and loss of real pleasure which I described, but that since his marriage, and in consequence of the important truths learned from Swedenborg's writings, he had subjected his passions to the control of reason, and had led, as he expressed it, *a new life.* He assured me that, with the partner of his bosom, association was *never followed by exhaustion* to either, but on the contrary by a feeling of *increased strength and pleasure* to both, and I have no doubt but he spoke the literal truth, for I have been frequently told the same by others. *He* regarded this as a *spiritual* effect, while *I* looked upon it as a simple *physiological* one, but be that as it may the fact is an important one, both as regards health and morals. These subjects, however, will be fully discussed in a work on *the Reproductive Functions and Marriage,* which I have been for a long time preparing, and which will be shortly issued. It has been delayed in order to institute a number of experiments, and an extended series of observations, to clear up all doubtful points and make the explanation complete. (The work referred to is *The Guide.*)

Another important requisite for the healthy action and extended duration of the sexual power, in both, is a near correspondence in *age.* Experience has proved beyond doubt that when there is *great desparity* of age, in marriage, the elder person *is nearly sure to benefit at the expense of the younger,* sometimes even sufficiently to compensate for the loss resulting from great excess. This fact was acted upon medically in former times, and is now even, in some countries, by procuring young females to sleep with old men, so that they may be strengthened thereby, which they nearly always are, though the females suffer a corresponding loss, and not unfrequently waste and die in consequence. Such unnatural practices are therefore properly discountenanced now, both by reason and morality, though we sometimes see a near approach to them in marriage. It is even known that when children sleep with old persons they suffer from it, and sometimes even die, without the causes of their sickness being sus-

pected. In all probability.young men who marry old
females suffer in the same way, and to an equal extent,
providing they are as exclusive in their companionship,
but there are many causes that may make it otherwise in
their case.

What constitutes a great disparity of age must of course
depend upon various circumstances, besides the number of
years. Some persons are younger at *forty*, or even *fifty*.
In respect to health and probable longevity, than others
are at twenty-five or thirty and this must be taken into
account. Generally speaking, however, there should not
be much more than *ten years* difference under any circum
stances, and only half that is better, the man being the
elder.—Besides health, this principle of similarity of age
has an important bearing upon the relative number of the
sexes born, as shown in my *Matron's Manual*, to which I
refer those who wish for more extended information on the
subject.

The explanation af the above-mentioned fact is probably
this,—all living bodies are constantly giving off portions
of their substance, in the form of insensible perspiration,
and these particles thrown off are in the same state, in
regard to age and health or disease, as the body from
which they emanate. The same bodies are also as constantly *absorbing*, both by the lungs and by the skin,
whatever is presented to them in a proper form, which
partly counterbalances the loss. Young healthy persons
are therefore always giving off a stream of fresh wholesome
material from their bodies, and old or diseased persons as
constantly give off a stream of morbid and decaying
matter, which explains why it is that the young suffer and
the old benefit when they live together. The waste of the
old persons is in part made up by absorbing the fresh ex
halation from the young, and they become thereby
rejuvenated, while the waste of the young persons is only
made up by absorbing the decaying exhalation from the
old, and they in consequence speedily decay and become
old likewise. The celebrated Hufeland, in his "*Art of
Prolonging Life*," gives some curious instances of the
practical application of this fact which are highly interest
ing, in a scientific point of view, though morally repre-
hensible. Among others he tells us of an old man who
had the superintendence of a kind of almshouse, in which
were a large number of young girls, in whose society he

passed nearly the whole of his time. He contrived to have a number of them always around him, so that he was constantly in an atmosphere as it were, of youthful exhalation, and by these means he preserved his life to an extreme old age, with all his powers in full vigor. A similar practice, to a certain extent, has even been adopted in London and Paris very recently, as was discovered in the evidence on a Police Trial. It appeared, from the statements made, that a number of poor young married females were hired to attend, at certain establishments, for so many hours in the day, to associate with superannuated old men. And not only did these young females associate in company with the aged patients, but they also supplied them with what ought to be kept for infantile nutriment alone,—in short, they acted as *wet nurses* to them!—The results of the practice were said to be *very satisfactory*, but fortunately there is not sufficient degradation and poverty in this country to make it available here, though I have known it attempted.—With persons of equal age, and similar condition of health, the exhalations are similar, and there is an equal loss and gain on both sides. During sexual excitement the insensible exhalation is much increased, and therefore the effects above-mentioned are more evident where there is association, and this perhaps explains, as my Swedenborgian friend remarked, why it is that in *a proper marriage no exhaustion at all is experienced*, there being merely a reciprocal interchange exactly corresponding in both.

§ PROPER AGE FOR MARRIAGE.

The proper age for marriage cannot always be determined by the number of years the individual has lived, some being fully as much developed at fourteen or fifteen as others are at seventeen or eighteen. The Law, of course, fixes a definite period for each sex, as it is requisite to do, but nature makes many variations. The ancient Greeks fixed the period of marriage very late, from an idea that it would ensue more vigorous offspring. Some of their lawgivers assigned thirty years for the female and from thirty-five to forty for the male, but others decreased this extreme period five or eight years, still leaving it, however, very advanced. The ancient Germans, according to Tacitus never allowed young persons to marry, but compelled the strictest celibacy in the male till five-and twenty, and in the female till twenty-one. This rule we are assured was never infringed, and they believed that the children were more strong, healthy, and long-lived in consequence. At those times perhaps, when none of the artificial excitants of civilization existed, and when all lived, almost from the mother's arms, in the constant practice of laborious muscular exertion, with coarse food and thin clothing, this continence might be practicable, but it certainly is not now.

In other parts of the world, where the habits and social condition of the people are different, we find the opposite extreme, marriages often taking place between mere children, and females of twelve years old becoming mothers. Both extremes are undoubtedly lustful, the too early marriage being, however, undoubtedly the worst, both for parents and children.

A female who delays marriage till after twenty-eight is liable to many uterine derangements, and runs more risk during childbirth than even at a very early age. Perhaps it may be said with propriety, that it is better for a female to marry before she is *twenty-four*, and not till she has turned fifteen at least, or better still sixteen or seventeen. The medium age of eighteen being esteemed the most desirable by experienced Physiologists. Much, however, will depend, as before stated, upon the development of the system, and upon the inclination. Mothers ought to be able to tell whether the development is such, in every respect, as to make marriage allowable or not, and it should be esteemed their duty to ascertain such an important fact.—In the course of my practice I have met with many cases of deplorable suffering, both of body and mind, from neglect in this way.

The proper age for the male is from twenty to twenty five. It is true that he is capable of becoming a father at a much earlier age, but it is not at all advantageous for him to be so, because previous to that time the vital energy is all required to complete the growth of the system, and it cannot be abstracted in the emission of semen without injury. It is an undoubted fact that in most young men, previous to seventeen or eighteen years of age, the Seminal Animalcules are very small, and often imperfect, which shows that though they may impregnate yet it is not probable that perfect offspring will result from them.—There is, however, a difference among males as there is among females, though it is not perhaps so great as a general rule.

§ ADVANTAGE OF TEMPORARY SEPARATION.

It is an undoubted fact that a short absence, or partial separation, occasionally, tends both to increase marital pleasures and to make them endure longer. It also makes conception more likely, as the organs act more energetically after a period of repose, and when stimulated by a short restraint. Many eminent men are said to have been conceived after a separation of this kind, and their genius has been attributed to the greater vigor experienced under such circumstances.—It is said, for instance, that *Sir Isaac Newton's* Father had been absent at sea for a long time previous to his being conceived, and that both his father and mother had strongly desired their meeting after this irksome separation. In many cases I have acted upon this principle, in giving advice, and with happy results, and I have no doubt of its being well worthy of attention practically.

On the same principle, some Authors contend that it is advisable always to leave at least three years between every two births, and they contend it is better both for mother and child. It has even been advanced as an argument why females should know how to prevent conception, because it is thought that a small number of children will be less weakened.

§ PRECAUTION AT THE TIME OF MARRIAGE.

From our previous explanations it will be seen that there may be many little pecularities of organization, and many conditions of the Genital Organs, especially in females, that may make the first association not only difficult and painful, but even seriously hurtful. An imperforate or very strong Hymen, a relatively small Vagina, a partial closure of the Lips, or an irritable condition of the parts generally, may be mentioned among others, and both parties ought, at such a time at least, to know that such impediments occasionally exist. In most of these cases a little care and gentleness may obviate both pain and difficulty, while a want of it may create lasting trouble and dissatisfaction. If young persons, of both sexes, had perused this book, and also my *Diseases of Woman*, these minor difficulties would be easily overcome in every instance, and even more serious impediments would be so well understood, that they would neither alarm nor disgust, as they now too often do. The use of the emollient ointment, mentioned in the article on Enlarging the Vagina, in the Diseases of Woman, is often all that is required, and its general employment, even at such times, is not unworthy of recommendation, nor unnecessary to be spoken of. In all cases however, the existence of impediments of this kind should be known to mothers, or if they are not sufficiently informed, and suspect them, the advice of a medical man should be sought.

It appears to me that no young person should enter into marriage totally ignorant of its duties and liabilities; and common humanity—to say nothing of prudence—imperatively demands that no young female should be condemned for it. I·have known many instances of the terrible consequences resulting from a neglect of this necessary precaution, and, in many cases, when I have been timely applied to, I have been the means of removing impediments and difficulties that otherwise would have led to deplorable results. Owing to my books and lectures, a large class of cases of this kind constantly come under my care, and I therefore, speak on sufficient grounds.

CHAPTER IX.

PHILOSOPHY OF AMATIVE INDULGENCE.

THOSE who suppose that sexual enjoyment is altogether immoral and unworthy of rational beings, and those who regard it as a mere sensual gratification, are both in error. The instinct or desire for it is innate in all beings, and exercises a most powerful influence, both upon individual action, and upon the destinies of nations. That influence may be productive of good or evil, according as those moved by it are ignorant or properly informed, but there is nothing necessarily wrong in the instinct itself, that gives rise to it. The charms of mutual love, the relations of family, and the compact of society, are all dependent upon it, and would never originate without. Dr. Dunglison remarks, in his Human Physiology, that " In Man and the superior animals, in which each sex is possessed by a distinct individual, it is necessary that there should be a union of the sexes, and that the fecundating fluid of the male should be conveyed within the appropriate organs of the female, in order that—from the concourse of the matters furnished by both sexes—a new individual may result. To this union we are incited by an imperious instinct, established within us for the preservation of the species, as the senses of hunger and thirst are placed within us, for the preservation of the individual. This has been termed the *desire* or *instinct of reproduction;* and, for wise purposes, its gratification is attended with the most pleasurable feelings which man or animal can experience."

The true origin of this instinct has been discussed in a former article, and frequent reference to it has been made in connection with various other explanations, so that its influence and uses are tolerably well shown already. It undoubtedly originates from the action of the sexual organs themselves, and its mental manifestations are merely caused by the reflex action of those organs on the brain. In proportion to the activity of the *Testes* in the male, and of the *Ovaries* in the female, is the extent of the sexual power, and in proportion to the number and sensibility of the *nerves* of certain parts is the intensity of sexual feelings and desire. To say that all these are experienced in different degrees, is but stating what is generally known, though few persons know the occasional extent of that difference. While some experience sexual desire so weakly that they can easily overcome it altogether, others feel it so overpoweringly, that every other impulse besides is utterly powerless, and for the sake of one indulgence, all risks are run, and all consequences madly braved. There are people even—females at least—who never even feel the slightest amorous propensities, and there are others in whom they become so imperious as to cause actual mania. It is, therefore, very difficult to be strictly *just*, when judging of the virtues or failings of people in this respect, and the utmost charity should at least influence our *thoughts*, whatever prudence may point out as requisite in our actions. There are, no doubt many immaculate people who owe their virtue chiefly to organic deficiency, which lessens the inclination to indulge, and there are no doubt others that fall, from unusual organic vigor, which, perhaps, few, if any, would have been more successful in withstanding. This is not said, be it remembered, as an excuse for licentiousness, nor to undervalue the power of a well-regulated mind, in controlling these impulses, but merely to state the case as it really exists. That the sexual powers and desires may be either exalted or depressed, by the state both of the mind and body, has already been abundantly shown, and all persons with sufficient knowledge may regulate that state in a great measure themselves. It is the duty, therefore, of those acquainted with such truths to make them generally known, and thereby hasten the time when the mere animal instinct will be controlled, at least sufficiently to prevent evil, by the intellect.

The phenomena attendant upon Copulation, or the actual union of the two sexes, have already been discussed, and also the causes that may be supposed naturally to lead to it. In both sexes, when the union is really desired, and no obstacle interferes, it leads to the highest and most absorbing excitement that animated beings can experience. Both beings are thrown into a species of mental ecstasy and bodily fever, during which all other thoughts and functions are totally suspended, and all the vital forces are concentrated in the Reproductive system. In the female the Uterus and Vagina are engorged with blood the Labia are tumefied and irritable, and the Clitoris becomes congested, erect, and highly sensitive. In the male similar changes are also observed, to fit the organ for its peculiar use. " It is first necessary that, under the excitement of the venereal desire, the organ should attain a necessary state of rigidity, which is termed *erection.* In this state the organ becomes enlarged, and raised towards the abdomen ; its arteries beat forcibly : the nerves become tumid ; the skin more colored, and the heat augmented. It becomes also of a triangular shape, and these changes are indicated by an indescribable feeling of pleasure."—(See Dunglison.)

At this time the adaptation of the male and female organs for each other becomes most manifest, and the *manner* of union is clearly indicated. The Penis being drawn up towards the abdomen, it necessarily has an upward curve, which precisely adapts it, in the usual position, to the curve of the Vagina, and brings the mouth of the Urethra almost directly against the mouth of the Womb. The Cushion of the Mons Veneris prevents injury by external pressure, and the increased flow of Mucus from the Vagina moderates the heat, and lubricates the walls of the passage.

Dr. Dunglison remarks, respecting the male organ, that in. all probability, " The Arteries first respond to the appeal ; the organ is, at the same time, raised by the appropriate muscles; its tissues become distended ; the plexus of veins turgid, and the return of blood impeded. In this way the organ acquires the rigidity necessary for penetrating the parts of the female. The friction which then occurs, keeps up the voluptuous excitement and the state of erection. This excitement is extended to the whole generative system ; the secretion of the Testicles is augmented ; the Sperm arrives in greater quantity in the Vesiculæ Seminales ; the Testicles are drawn up towards the abdominal rings, by the contraction of the Dartos and Cremaster, so that the Vas Deferens is rendered shorter, and, in the opinion of some, the sperm filling the excretory ducts of the Testicle, is in this manner forced mechanically forwards towards the Vesicles. When these have attained a certain degree of distension, they contract suddenly and powerfully, and the sperm is projected through the ejaculatory ducts into the Urethra. At this period the plea-

urable sensation is at its height. When the sperm reac nes
the Urethra, the Canal is thrown into the highest excitement; and the Ischio-Cavernosus' and Bulbo-Cavernosus
Muscles, with the Transversus Perinei and Levator-Ani are
thrown into violent contraction ; the two first holding the
Penis straight, and assisting the others in projecting 'the
sperm along the Urethra. By the agency of these muscles
and of the proper muscular structure in the Urethra, the
fluid is expelled, not continuously, but in jets, as it seems
to be sent into the Urethra by the alternate contractions
of the Vesiculæ Seminales. These muscular contractions
are of a reflex character, being independent of the will
and incapable of being controlled by any exertion of it.
They are induced, as in deglutition, (swallowing) by a special excitant—the food in one case, the sperm in the other.

This highest point of enjoyment is termed the *Orgasm*,
and in some it is so intense, that all consciousness of everything but the intense pleasurable excitement ceases. The
duration of the orgasm is short, it being over immediately
the flow of Semen is ended, which it usually is in a few
seconds. This momentary ecstasy is followed by a state of
dreamy languor and exhaustion, which is often not devoid
of pleasure, though of a different kind, and there is an almost invariable desire for repose. So intense is the orgasm
in some cases, that the individual utters loud cries, and becomes delirious, or, occasionally, insensible. The exhaustion afterwards is also sometimes very great, and the individual will be almost unable to move.

In the female an Orgasm is not always experienced, and
may even know not what it is, though they may be capable
of considerable excitement. When it does occur, it is exhibited in the same way as in the other sex, though often
much more intensely, being accompanied by cries and
convulsive motions of the most energetic character. The
after-exhaustion is usually not so great in them as in the
other sex, and the dreamy languor is more pleasing. It
wil. often endure for hours.

In the male there can, of course, be but one orgasm at
once, because no other can be experienced till a fresh supply of semen has been secreted, which requires more or
less time. Some, however, can have two or three secretions in an hour or two, but it is unusual, and the effort is
always very exhaustive and hurtful. I have known an instance in which a man has forced eight or ten orgasms in a

single night, but, in such a case, I have no doubt there was a peculiar conformation of the organs, owing to which but a small portion of semen was emitted at once, and probably no more altogether than most men emit at once. In general, no repetition of the act is desired under several hours, or, perhaps not for days, and it is certainly improper for it to be sought earlier then.

In the female the orgasm is not caused by any secretion, like that of the semen, and, consequently, the excitement is not necessarily subdued by the first, but several orgasms may follow each other in quick succession. This is sometimes carried to a great extent, each one becoming more vivid than the others, till fainting ensues. In general, however, there is but óne, as with the male, and when there is a proper *adaptation*, the two orgasms correspond, which mutually heightens the pleasure of both, and conduces to conception, though not necessary to it in all cases.

The after state in females is not always the same, but is often one of sadness and weeping, or of violent Hysterics. Some females even say that this is always the case *when they conceive*, and that they thereby know when that event occurs. It has been even said by some that during a vivid Orgasm, resulting in conception, they could see, mentally, the new being they were about to bear, and one female assured me that in this way she had a perfect view of the form and features of her child as it afterwards appeared at birth.—Perhaps we ought rather to believe that the image so strongly impressed on her mind, at such a moment, was given to the child in consequence of that impression.

In most females there is a sudden and increased secretion of mucus from the vagina, at the moment of the Orgasm, which is erroneously thought by the uninformed to be a species of semen, but it has nothing whatever to do with conception.

In most females the Orgasm is very difficult to be produced, and they therefore seldom experience it, and in some even it is never felt. In others, however, it is produced very readily and will even occur during sleep, or from exciting the breasts. Owing to this peculiar Nervous susceptibility sexual excitement will also often follow various moral emotions, and an Orgasm will occasionally supervene without their being any licentious tendency. This peculiar liability is in fact the cause of many female enthu siasms, which are often only the results of this powerful emotion directed by circumstances, and education. When strongly experienced, if conscientious motives are powerful enough to forbid its natural indulgence, it takes some other direction, and imparts that fervor and devotion which is so amiable a part of the female character, and which all admire though few suspect its origin.—This nervous suspectibilty, however, is unfortunate for them in some respects, as it makes them liable to undesirable influences, and often overcomes them in spite of themselves.

It has been asserted, by a very eminent Physician, that it is simply owing to the susceptible state of the sexual system that many females are so readily *impressed*, as it is termed, by *mesmerism*, and similar nervous excitements, and that those who are uninfluenced by such agents are always of cold temperaments. The truth of this, as a general rule, every medical man of experience must have perceived, and in some instances it has been proved by unfortunate and unlooked for occurrences, not at all creditable to the morality of the *operators*, nor recommendatory to the *science*. (?)

A short time ago I induced a Lady, who was formerly much addicted to mesmeric practices, to give me her experience, written down, and a curious revelation it is. She confessed that whenever she was capable of being acted upon, mesmerically, the mesmeric state was always preceeded by one of sexual excitement, often amounting to a perfect Orgasm, and that if this feeling was not experienced she could never be mesmerised. Sometimes the exhalation of the nervous system was so great she could with difficulty control herself, and so many Orgasms would follow each other that she would be completely exhausted, and would faint away. According to her statement, the mesmeric sleep, or ecstasy, was nothing but the dreamy languor following a sexual orgasm, and though it may not be precisely the same in all similar cases yet I am satisfied it is in most. I have seen exhibitions of this kind with young females in which I could plainly perceive, from observation of such phenomena, that sexual excitement, though modified and disguised, was the moving impulse. Several respectable ladies have also assured me that they were fully aware of this, from their own partial experience, when being mesmerized for the pretended cure of disease, and they both refused to submit to such influences again or to allow their daughters to do so. In short, I am satisfied that such influences are often dangerous to morals, and also destructive to health.

Similar results to the above often follow intense devotional excitement, when carried so far as to overpower the reason,—such for instance as the wild fanaticism of a camp-meeting, or protracted revival meeting, the female actors in which, are often so carried away by their fervid feelings as to be totally insensible to the nature of what they experience. This I say of course, merely as a Medical Man, and from the number of patients I have had who have been the victims of these exhibitions, 1 feel fully justified in making the observations I have. Hysteria, and other nervous affections, Palpitation of the Heart, and irregular menstruation are a few of the evils that I thus find produced, to say nothing of the liability to affections of the brain, and Chlorosis.

One of the most remarkable circumstances connected with the experience of the sexual feeling, in females, is the fact that it will often be felt with one companion, even to excess, but not with another, though there may be nothing like dislike or disinclination. This shows how much it is under the influence of the mind with them, and to what an extent it is modified by other emotions. Some little matter, perhaps a mere association of ideas, may be sufficient to prevent excitement entirely, or raise it to the highest pitch.—This also shows that there is a natural *adaptation* required between married persons, and that marriage is never precisely what it ought to be unless that adaptation exists. It is not easy, however, to say in what that adaptation is to be found, nor can its absence or presence be known precisely, except by experience. To a certain extent, however, it may be known whether it subsists or not, before marriage, but only by those who have made it a matter of special study and observation.

In addition to its other uses, sexual excitement is undoubtedly beneficial, in various ways, to the organization generally. It serves as a wholesome stimulus to the Nervous system, at ordinary times, and a means of expending surplus energy when the Vital Functions are too active. It is very seldom the case that there is perfect health without it, and scarcely ever is there an exemption from severe nervous affections. This accounts for the fact that married people are always longer lived, on the average than those that remain single, notwithstanding that they have more anxieties, and that married females are subject to so many accidents.—A celebrated Physician, (Pidoux,) who had been much employed in the Nunneries, assures us that almost invariably the Nuns are afflicted with flood ings, and with other uterine diseases, after they attain a certain age.

In short, marriage, or the union of the two sexes, is or dained by Nature, and this ordinance can no more be vio lated without evil consequences than can any other. The physical enjoyments appertaining to marriage, also form part of that ordinance, and are undoubtedly both proper and advantageous, within certain limits.

In all cases where the sexual system is mutilated, so that none of those feelings and desires are experienced, the in dividual remains ever after imperfect, both bodily and mentally. Proof of this is to be seen daily in our domestic animals, the nature and form of which are changed in the most remarkable manner, by *castration*, or *spaying*. The most remarkable effects of this kind, however, are seen among human beings, in those unfortunate creatures term ed *Eunuchs*. Stunted or deformed in body, imbecile in mind, and preverse in disposition, they drag on a wretched existence for little more than half the usual term of human life. Decrepid and decayed while yet young in years, old age comes prematurely upon them, and an untimely grave closes their imperfect career. Nature, in short, seems to say, that where the generative apparatus is absent, the res of the system is not worth preserving, and she, therefore leaves it to speedily decay.

Even in after-life, when all has apparently become per fected, the presence and proper action of these organs is necessary to maintain health and vigor. If any accident occurs by which they are destroyed, or their powers se riously impaired, every thing else suffers, and the whole system speedily goes to decay; without them, every thing else seems to be abandoned.

The sexual system is, therefore, necessary, at first, to effect the full development of the whole organization, and it is equally necessary afterwards, to maintain it in healthy and vigorous action. On this subject, however, see my book on *the Male Organs.*

Perfect continence, in those who have natural sexual tendencies, is always attended by a variety of evils, some of them of a serious character, showing that temperate indulgence, so far from being hurtful, is both necessary and beneficial. Perfect continence in the male leads to Spermatocele, Spermattorrhœa, and even insanity. In the female it leads to Ovarian and Uterine diseases, Hysteria, and mania, and in both it originates the most singular and distressing vagaries of mind and thoughts. In severe cases, it leads to Erotomania, Satyriasis, or Nymphomania.

An instance occurred in England, of a young female, who became insane, from not being allowed to marry —though the true cause was not suspected—and who was confined in a private asylum in consequence; while there, one of the keepers noticed certain peculiarities in her conduct, and abused her for his own gratification. The result was, however, that she perfectly recovered her reason, though at the expense of her honor.

In short, it is with these as with all other organs, a temperate and proper use of them is conducive to health, and creates happiness, but abuse or destruction of them leads to misery and death.

In connection with this subject, there are a few remarks in my work on *the Male Organs* that may be advantageously referred to, and as they may not be seen by many of the readers of this book, I will quote them:

"Constant and healthy exercise of the whole *muscular* system is also of great importance to the preservation of sexual power. It is true that if a man takes little exertion—particularly if he lives high—he will be apt to exhibit an unusual tendency to amorous indulgence, because, as before remarked, gluttony and idleness lead to licentiousness. This effect, however, is only a temporary one, and, sooner or later, the individual finds that he has *permanently exhausted* his vital energy, and that his health and strength is seriously impaired. The vital power that may be *safely* expended in sexual indulgence, is only the *surplus*, after every part of the system has appropriated its due amount, and if more be so expended, some part must suffer. In other words, we may suppose that every healthy man has a certain stock of vital energy, which we will call his *capital*, to which he keeps adding more or less, by the function of nutrition; this addition may be compared to *interest*, which may be expended without any loss of capital, and, of course, without making him any poorer. If, however, by any *excess* he expends more than this addition, the capital is proportionally diminished. *ana permanently too, for it can seldom be made up again.*

Now, the idle man does not expend enough vital energy on his muscular system, to keep it healthy, but at the same time gives a superabundance of it to the sexual organs, so that they are over-stimulated, and suffer from excess. They become habituated to great indulgence, and are constantly causing a drain on the vital power, that soon exhausts both principal and interest, and leaves the individual completely exhausted.

The philosophy of this has been frequently alluded to in the course of the present work, but it is so important that I wish to present it in a strong light. I am fully persuaded that there is no case of precocious or excessive sexual propensity, unless caused by disease, that cannot be easily subdued by *muscular exercise.* No matter how vigorously the seminal glands may act, in a state of leisure, they *must* become less active if the body be exhausted by active exertion, and to this rule there is scarcely any limit. One of the Reports of the Massachusetts Lunatic Asylum strongly impresses this truth, and shows conclusively that we have, in *hard labor,* a *certain means* of subduing this propensity to its proper limits under any circumstances. The application of this truth to young persons is obvious, numbers of whom are made licentious only by bodily inactivity and over-feeding.

The invalid, or the man whose powers are impaired, must, of course, husband his strength, because he does not require exhaustion, but only sufficient exercise to ensure health.

Exercise of the *mind* is also equally important as exercise of the body. The man who is mentally idle, is nearly certain to experience too strongly the force of the animal propensities, and licentious thoughts are too often indulged merely from the absence of better ones. It must be recollected, however, that too much mental exertion, particularly if attended with care and anxiety, is most destructive to the sexual power, and frequently leads to impotence, as many of our cases have shown. Those who wish, therefore, to preserve their virility, should endeavor to maintain a happy medium, laboring with the mind sufficiently for health and utility, and endeavoring to preserve perfect calmness and equanimity."

One singular circumstance may be mentioned here, in connection with the Genital Organs, which is both curious and important. They appear to possess, in an eminent degree, the power of retaining animal fluids in their substance without those fluids becoming decomposed. Thus in many cases *sacs* of water, blood, and other fluids, have been formed and retained in these parts both in males and females, for months and years, and yet no change has taken place in these fluids. Now in all cases where such accumulations take place in other parts of the body decomposition speedily ensues, an abscess forms, and perhaps serious wasting disease commences. The Genital Organs, therefore, possess a preservative power greater than any other part, and this is doubtless owing to their great vitality, and vigorous circulation.

CHAPTER X.

INFLUENCE OF THE BRAIN OVER THE GENERATIVE
POWERS.

It is important, in connection with sterility, that the direct influence of the Brain upon the Generative Organs should be noticed, especially as it is manifested in cases of injury. My Book upon the Male System contained a number of instructive cases of this kind, a few of which will serve our present purpose.

§ INFLUENCE OF THE BRAIN ON THE GENERATIVE
POWERS.

In a former part of this work a number of instances were narrated in which impotency followed injuries of the head, and we will now narrate a few others, because this is a most important fact, in many respects.

About five years ago I was consulted by a married man who had totally lost his sexual powers from striking his head against a beam. The blow had stunned him for a time, but did not lead to any serious symptoms afterwards. He found, however in two or three days after that he was perfectly impotent, and had so remained for eighteen months when I saw him. There was but little loss of desire, with no wasting of the Genital Organs, nor any other indication whatever of his deprivation. He had previously been a man of temperate habits, and at the time of the accident was as vigorous as most men. The blow, it may be as well to remark, was received on the *top* of the head and was not followed by any swelling or pain in the Cerebellum or neck. When I saw him he was in perfect health, and in good spirits, in fact nothing was complained of but this unfortunate impotency, which he was very desirous of having removed.

The great point was to ascertain, if possible, in what way the concussion of the brain had suspended the transmission of nervous power to the genitals, and how it could be restored. I recollected that in several cases where injuries to the head had paralyzed particular muscles, or limbs, their power had been restored by *Galvanism*, applied so as to pass along the course of their Nerves from the spine. It seemed to me as if the blow had impaired the proper connection between the spinal marrow and these nerves, at their roots, and that the passage of the electric current in some way or other restored that connection. It was similar in fact to starting the Electric Telegraph again by mending the wires, or making the connections perfect, after they had been destroyed by violence. I therefore applied the Galvanism, passing the current from that part of the spine where the Spermatic Nerves originate, to the pubes, perineum, and neighboring parts, applying also a stimulating liniment, and occasionally using the congester. The result was highly satisfactory, and speedily obtained. At the third application he experienced a decided *tingling* about the perineum, and along the penis, and the next time a partial erection occurred. After persevering for five weeks, using the Galvanism daily at first, and then every other day, and finally but twice a week, he was fully restored, without any apparent tendency to a relapse. In this case it will be observed that the injury was not received at the *back* of the head, on what the Phrenologists call the Organ of *Amativeness*, but at the top, nor did it in any way whatever affect the Cerebellum.

In another similar instance, Impotency, with complete loss of desire also, followed a fracture of the skull over the *left Temple* and no means that were used had the slightest effect in restoring it. In a few months the Testes began to waste, and eventually almost totally disappeared, but the general health was only slightly affected.

In the American Journal of the Medical Sciences, for February, 1839, Dr. Fisher relates a curious instance of a gentleman injured in a railway car. He was looking out at the moment when a collision occurred, and the shock threw the back of his head against the edge of the window with such force as to stun him; he, however, recovered his senses and was taken home, but suffered great pain in the back part of the head and top of the neck. His right arm was numbed a little and some difficulty was experienced in passing the urine, but in two weeks he was able to walk out with no other inconvenience than a slight dimness of sight. About the fifth week he discovered that he was impotent, and had lost all sexual desire. The means used to restore his genital powers were only partially successful, nor was his memory so perfect as before, but all he other difficulties disappeared under proper treatment.

In the Lancet for August, 1851, is an account of a medical student who received a blow on the face, in a quarrel, which knocked him down so that he fell on the back of his head. He was totally unconscious for eight or ten hours, but gradually recovered, and on the following day even resumed his studies which he continued unremittingly for the next six weeks. He, however, became exceedingly irritable, with a feeling of general uneasiness, and after the first week he observed the genital organs begin to waste, and desire to weaken, till he finally became nearly impotent, but afterwards recovered under proper treatment.

Many instances have been observed of soldiers being wounded in the head and suffering afterwards under the same disability, some of which were given in a former article. It is perhaps proper to remark, however, that this is not the only nor even the most frequent result of such injuries, as many patients so hurt suffer no deprivation of their genital powers but have some other functions impaired. Thus some lose their sight, some their hearing, and others become paralytic in their limbs.

The prospect of recovering the sexual powers when lost from injuries of this kind is very small, especially if the parts have really begun to waste. The treatment at first must be that best calculated to subdue the irritation which is probably existing in some part of the nervous system, and afterwards, if requisite, to rouse the spermatic nerves to more energetic action. Every case, however, will require something peculiar to itself, which can only be discovered by a patient and careful attention to all its symptoms and influences.

A further corroboration of the facts above stated may also be found in certain physiological indications observed in those who have died from strangulation. It is well known that in very many men who have been hung, erections and even seminal emissions have occurred, and experiments upon animals have often led to the same result. This is attributed to the pressure of the rope on the back of the head, which in some way or other excites the spermatic nerves. I have even known pressure made on that

region purposely, in a particular manner, in order to excite erections, and *frequently with perfect success.* Some
of the females in the Turkish Harems understand this, and
they habitually chafe, or *shampoo,* the back of the neck of
their companions of the other sex, for this very purpose.
I have frequently made an application of this important
fact in my practice, in cases where there was merely a
suspension of that sympathetic influence which the brain
ordinarily exerts upon the sexual organs.

The particular mode of doing this, though well understood to eminent medical men in the old world, is I believe
totally unknown here. An explanation of the process,
and the apparatus employed, would require to be extended
beyond the limits of the present work, to make it practically understood, and as after all it would not be available
for the patient's own use it is not necessary to enter into
it. I have often astonished persons both by its singularity
and its unexpected effects.

A full consideration of all the facts and arguments
bearing upon this influence of the brain over the sexua
functions, have left the subject, so far as I am concerned,
in great obscurity. That a singular influence is *often* exerted by the brain in this way, sometimes beneficially, and
at others the reverse, is undoubted, but whether *such influence* emanates from a *particular part* of the brain, or
from the whole organ is uncertain. The Phrenologists
affirm that only a particular part of the Encephalon is
concerned in this phenomenon, namely, the lower part or
Cerebellum, which rests upon the spinal marrow.

But after a careful consideration of all the reasons
brought forward in support of this affirmation, I am no.
yet convinced of its correctness. That many facts favor
such a theory I am willing to admit, but it is also certain
that many others militate against it, and, as a searcher
after truth, I must consider everything that bears upon
the question, even though opposed to my previous opinion.
I set out with firmly believing that the Cerebellum *was* the
organ of the sexual propensity, and my investigations
have made me doubt it. It is not true, I am convinced, that
the strength of a man's propensity can be estimated by the
development of his Cerebellum, nor is it true in regard to
animals either. If it were so, we ought to find that organ
largest in those who exhibit the propensity most and in
numerous cases it is not so, though in others it is. A cele

brated German physiologist made some investigations bear
ing on this point, of an interesting character; he had nu
merous opportunities of dissecting horses, and curiosity in
duced him to weigh the Cerebellums of these animals, some
of whom had been castrated when young, and others left
entire. Now if the Cerebellum be truly the organ of Amativeness, it ought, of course, to be largest in the entire
orses, who have always exhibited that propensity, and we
hould expect to find it almost disappeared in the others,
seeing that they could *never* have felt anything of the
kind. The result of the experiment was, however, on taking the average of an equal number of each, that there
was scarcely any difference, or if any at all, the castrated
ones had the *largest* Cerebellums. In observing idiots
also, some of whom were notoriously licentious, and others
directly the reverse, I have not found that the development
of the Cerebellum correspond to the phrenological system.
Neither can it be contended that the size of the Cerebellum
in the castrated animals was only the result of disease, for
no difference could be detected in it between them and the
others. All that can be said, therefore, is, that certain
agencies acting on the Cerebellum, *sometimes* cause sexual
manifestations, and at other times check them. The same
agencies also acting on *other parts* of the brain will sometimes produce the same results, and sometimes when the
Cerebellum is acted upon, it is not the Generative Organs
that are affected, but the sight, hearing, or speech, which
might, therefore, just as properly be considered under its
exclusive influence.

It should also be stated, as bearing on this subject, that
certain influences operating on various parts of the body
will often affect the Generative Organs in a decided manner. I have known a blister *on the leg* cause the most uncontrollable sexual desires in one man, and the application
of caustic *to the throat* do the same in another. In applying blisters to the top of the neck also, though it is followed
by erections in some, yet in others no such effect takes
place, and occasionally it will produce a nervous twitch-
ing, like St. Vitus' Dance, in the arms. Flogging the
back, it is well known, will frequently cause erections and
emissions, even when very severe, as has been observed in
soldiers when undergoing that brutal punishment. Rousseau tells us, in his confessions, that flogging boys at
school, in the disgraceful manner formerly practised i

sometimes followed by similar results, and he remarks that the pain of the punishment may be forgotten under the powerful excitement it leads to, a fact of deep moral importance. In short, there seems every reason to believe that the strength of the sexual propensity is dependent upon some peculiarity of the sexual organs themselves, though it may be often modified by various mysterious sympathies emanating from other Parts. If the semen be never formed, there will never be any sexual desire, and will be proportionally great, independent of all other influences. In those who feel desire without having any semen, as is sometimes the case in impotency, or even after castration, it is only *the remembrance of a lost pleasure.*

In treating disabilities of the Generative Organs, however, the possible influence of injuries to the head, even at former periods, and long ago, should always be borne in mind.

Similar facts I have also noticed in Females, showing that the influence is similar in both. Some have never conceived after receiving a blow upon the head, and others have always miscarried after. In some it has entirely destroyed all sexual feeling, and in others it has, for a time, excited it to a most uncontrollable height.

CHAPTER XI.

By *Continence*, is meant a voluntary abandonment of sexual indulgences, in those who are capable of, and who have a desire for them. When a person abstains simply from want of inclination for such pleasures it is called *Chastity*, which differs from continence inasmuch as it requires no effort.

Chastity is a natural condition for many, owing to peculiarity of constitution, and is therefore both proper and beneficial. Continence on the contrary, is an unnatural struggle, against one of the strongest animal instincts, and is always more or less injurious, as every attempt to evade the laws of our being must be.

Every living thing, *Vegetable* as well as *Animal*, has, at some period or other of its existence, a desire, or tendency, towards the opposite sex, and this desire or tendency should be gratified, both for the purposes of procreation and also because it is necessary to the individual's own well-being.

To praise and recommend absolute continence as a *Virtue* is a great mistake, and to suppose that it can be really practised, by those who are *physically perfect*, is equally a mistake! It is true we hear of it, and possibly some persons think they really are absolutely continent, but most assuredly they deceive themselves. Some of these persons are really *Impotent*, and give themselves credit for Continence, when in fact, they are only *powerless ;* others who forswear natural indulgence, either abandon themselves to disgusting habits, a thousand times worse, or suffer from unnatural pollutions.

There is a period of life, in all perfect organizations, when sexual indulgence becomes an actual *necessity*, as much so as food or drink. In some organizations this necessity is of course much stronger than in others, and the consequences of not obeying it are in them proportionably increased. In such persons we often observe the most singular Mental eccentricities, and sometimes even moral perversity, carried to excess, and not unfrequently ending in mania, melancholy, suicide, or crime. The physician often sees, in cases of forced continence, the most hideous exhibitions of Nymphomania, Satyriasis Priapism, and Erotomania, not unfrequently terminating in Insanity or Death.

Besides mental and moral perversions, Continence also originates many physical derangements, such as various infirmities of the Genital and Urinary organs, softening and inflammation of the brain or spinal marrow, with wasting of the flesh, and fever.

The celebrated Esquirol remarks, that most of the insane persons who come from *Convents*, exhibit morbid amative tendencies. And Mathieu gives us an instance, in his *Etudes Clinique sur les Maladies des femmes*, of a young girl who was attacked with Nymphomania after a fit of religious fervor, and probably from previous undue restraint. Many of the so called *Perfectionists* in religion, especially those who exhibit the phenomena of TRANCE, or *Convulsions*, have confessed that during their fits of excitement, they experienced the liveliest sexual emotions. And I have heard similar confessions made to me, by those who have been excited in the same way at *love feasts*, and *protracted meetings*.

In short, in all cases where the natural propensities are unduly restrained, especially from mistaken religious views, there is a constant liability to such exhibitions of Erotic furor, which are often mistaken, even by the individuals themselves, for genuine devotional fervor.

Those who are curious about details of this kind should read the writings of *Hecquet*, who had many opportunities of becoming acquainted with these religious enthusiasts. In my own practice, I have had similar facts communicated perhaps equally curious and equally instructive, some of which will be given in another place.   In all my experience, and it has been extensive, I have never known a female who was subject to fits of intense religious excitement, such as we often see at *Camp Meetings*, but who either had *some uterine disease*, or was naturally of an ardent amative temperament.

I have often seen the characters of these *Devotees* change in the most extraordinary manner, under a proper course of *medical treatment*, so that their church friends accused them of *backsliding*, and attributed the change to the influence of *Satan!*   Many others I have also seen changed in a similar manner, on being *married;* and in one such instance the husband was accused of leading his wife *from religion.*

The old *Ascetics*, who swore to practice perfect continence, have left us many records of their daily and nightly struggles against nature, and of their remarkable *amative hallucinations,*—for which, by the way, they often were called *Saints.*

This is particularly seen in the records left by Ascetic Females, whose lucubrations are curious compounds, half pious, half erotic, betraying either uterine disease or intense warmth of sexual feeling.

Many Medical writers have testified, after long and careful observation, that *uterine furor* is very general among those females who resist all amative impulses from religious motives.   And not unfrequently, in spite of all their severe chastity, nature overpowers conviction, so that the poor victim of a so called *virtue* is constrained, in spite of herself, to betray her real condition.   In more than one instance, during uncontrollable erotic furor, exhibitions, and advances, of the most libidinous character have been made unwittingly, by those renowned for having conquered all *fleshly lusts.* So much so in fact is this the case, that, in France, it is a common proverb that *the Convent and the Confessional are the Parents of Hysteria and Nymphomania!*

The terrible struggle which many estimable females maintain in this way is most extraordinary, and not unfrequently terminates in Insanity or death,—though those around them have no idea that any unusual effort has been required on their part.

In short, sexual approach is a necessity of the organization, and those who practice undue continence will always suffer a variety of evils from which those who do not are free. It is also the foundation of *Marriage*, one of the fundamental Institutions of civilized society, and equally beneficial to individuals and to the community at large. Continence is of course opposed to this institution, and should therefore be discountenanced by all well-wishers of our race.

Statistics prove that married persons on an average, are longer lived than single ones, and my own observation has convinced me that they are more exempt from disease. So well convinced were the ancients of this, that they erected a statue to Hymen, the God of marriage, with this inscription " *To Hymen, who prolongs youth!*"

According to statistical reports it appears that while, in a given time, among *single* men between 25 and 45 years of age, 28 will die out of every hundred, among *married* men of the same age only 18 die out of the hundred!

It appears also that for every 78 married men who attain 48 years of age there are only 40 single ones who do so, and as we advance further in life the difference is still more striking. Thus out of every hundred married men 48 will live to be 60 years old, but in a hundred single men only 22 will attain that period of life. And at 80 years of age we find nine married men, to only three single ones.

Among females the difference is still greater in favor of the married, notwithstanding the many dangers of maternity, and they are also less subject to disease.

As a further proof of this important truth, it is found that out of every hundred *suicides*, sixty-seven are single, and only thirty-three married! And in seventeen hundred and twenty-six Insane, also nine hundred and eighty are single, and only seven hundred and forty-six married.

It is true that the unmarried state may not necessarily

be a state of *Continence*, but it must either be that or a state of illicit or unnatural indulgence, either of which is injurious.

Many of the diseases and infirmities arising from Continence are attributed to other cases, both by people generally and also by Medical men, who have not made these matters their study.   This is especially the case with young females, whose natural modesty induces them to carefully conceal the truth, even if they fully perceive it themselves.   A crowd of hysterical and nervous derangements are originated in this way, besides various uterine diseases.

In describing *Chlorosis*, or the green sickness, which is often the result of forced Continence, a celebrated French writer gives us the following touching picture, true to the Life.—" See that young female with pale wax-like cheeks, languishing sunken eyes, and tottering steps, hanging her head like a withered flower, her heart palpitating and her breathing interrupted by heavy sighs.   Her digestion is bad, her appetite capricious, and she has an unnatural tendency to eat strange unusual substances, which she often craves in the most urgent manner.   If allowed to remain in this state too long she will continue to languish, and at last descend prematurely to the tomb.   Let her *marry* however, to the being she has constantly seen in her dreams, and health returns like glorious day at the rising of the sun.   The roses soon return to her cheeks, happiness brightens her eyes, and a pure wholesome blood rushes gaily through her veins."

Such pictures are daily to be seen, though none but experienced eyes detect their meaning.   In the other sex also we have similar experience but not so frequently, owing to less innate modesty, and more facility for gratification.

In history also, as well as in modern experience, we find numerous instances of the evil effects of undue Continence, some of which are worthy of being referred to.   Hippocrates saved the life of a young Prince, who was fading away from some unknown cause, by advising his marriage with the young female he loved, and the same service was also rendered to another young Prince by Era sistratus. The celebrated Galen likewise, being called to treat the daughter of a noble house, who was pining away, detected at once that she was a victim of forced continence, and he assured her father that nothing but marriage could save her life. Much against his will he had to consent, his daughter refusing to marry any other than a young *plebeian*, with whom she was in love. The result proved however, that though pride was sacrificed, health was repaired and life saved.

In that interesting work the *Physiologie des Passions*, we find a curious instance of the same kind. The subject, a young lady, was intended by her parents for a *Nun*, but having an ardent *Uterine Temperament* the idea was extremely distasteful to her, and she became seriously sick from grief and apprehension. At first she fell into a dull stupor, from which she roused only to pass through all the stages of Hysteria, and Nymphomania, till her reason seemed almost gone. That skilful physician Alibert, being called in, he saw at a glance what was the cause of her sickness, and promptly told her parents that she must marry or *die!* Their love for their child was fortunately stronger than their fanaticism, and they consented to her marriage. She at once recovered and became a happy healthy wife and mother.

In such cases, the natural action of the Genital organs is indispensable to the health of all other parts of the system, and their forced inaction is highly prejudicial.— The Physiological reason for this, and also the rules by which indulgence should be regulated will be found in the " *Marriage Guide.*"

The evil consequences of Celibacy, whether it be accompanied by actual *Continence* or not, are as great perhaps to society as to the individual, a fact which many lawgivers have recognized. In the sacred writings of the Persians, the Hindoos, the Chinese, the Hebrews, and the Turks, we find Celibacy expressly condemned, and in some of them it is even stated that the souls of those who die in a state of Celibacy will not enter heaven, but will wander eternally on earth. To avoid this it was customary to marry the *dead*, before they were burnt. The old Romans, and the Greeks, had express laws against Celibacy, and so harrassed those who practised it, that the offence was quite rare.

Lycurgus excluded those who practised Celibacy from all civil and military employments, forbade them attending the public amusements, and branded them as infamous. At certain solemn fêtes they were also exposed to the ridicule of the populace, who promenaded them around the public places with shouts and laughter, while the women tore their faces and struck them with small whips.

A curious instance of the contempt which was shown for the unmarried is found in Spartan History. It is well known what extreme reverence these people had for their old men, who were invariably saluted with respect by the young whenever they met. On one occasion however, an old man was refused the customary mark of respect by a youth, of whom he accordingly complained, to the magistrates. The youth on hearing the accusation admitted its truth, but replied, " this old man has never married,— how then can he demand marks of respect from me when he will leave no children to show them to me, when I am old ?" The reason was deemed good, and the old man was sent away with contempt.

The Laws of Plato tolerated Celibacy in men only til the thirty-fifth year, and in females only till the twenty fifth,—after these periods they were socially outlawed.

A Roman Citizen could not testify in any case till he replied in the affirmative to this question—" on thy soul and conscience art thou married ?"

Under Julius Cæsar, and many of the other Emperors, laws were passed to degrade those who did not marry, and to reward those who did.

Even in the Romish Church, among the Priests, Celibacy is comparatively a modern Institution, and except in as far as it makes the Church itself more powerful, it has always been objected to.

In fact, Celibacy is an unmitigated evil to society, as Continence is to the individual. A forced abstinence from natural indulgence leads to disease or unnatural abuses while a neglect of marriage leads to licentiousness and prostitution. In all cases where a nation has become vitiated by luxury and vice, it has disregarded marriage, as we see in the decline of the Roman Empire, and of the Grecian communities.

In giving these remarks I presume no apology is needed, at least not to those who *think*, because their *utility* must be apparent. I will now proceed to give some cases from my note book, confirmatory of the statements above made.

To the prudish, and to those who are governed by old prejudice against such discussions, I recommend the following passage from Montaigne.

" What is there then in the Genital act, necessary and natural as it is, which should cause it to be proscribed as a subject for rational conversation ? We pronounce commonly enough the words *kill, steal, filthy,* and *Adulterous,* but must not name the act by which our lives begin, and by which the race is continued ! Oh false modesty !—oh shameful hypocrisy !"

CASES FROM MY NOTE BOOK,

UNDUE CONTINENCE, FROM WORLDLY PRUDENCE.

THE first case which I extract from my notes is a good type of a large class,—those who are continent from *prudential* motives, and who think to avoid complying with the requirements of nature without suffering permanent inconvenience.

CASE I.—The subject of this case was a Lawyer, aged thirty-one, of good constitution, and of active Temperament. When he applied to me his general health was not much affected, but from various unusual symptoms he had begun to be somewhat alarmed.

I found on inquiry that he was naturally very amative, but at the same time *very prudent*, and uncommonly fond of money. He had made up his mind not to marry till he had secured a *fortune*, and was able to support a family in *good style*. This he expected to do before he was forty, and in the meantime sexual gratification was to be foresworn.

His fear of consequences, and of exposure, kept him from illict intercourse, except very rarely, and he had too much good sense to practice self abuse, except when quite young. He entertained the notion, as many others do, that his reproductive powers could be held in abeyance as it were, and yet be found ready when he could *afford* to employ them. In fact I have no doubt but he promised himself extra indulgence then to make up for his prudential restraint.

The only serious inconvenience experienced up to his twenty-eighth year was nightly emissions, which somewhat affected his mind, making him, as he expressed it, not quite so bright as usual. This however, became gradually less frequent, but the effects *increased!* His memory especially began to fail, and also his *power of application*, so that he had to *drive* himself to his work, instead of making it a pleasure, as formerly.

At times he would feel nearly as well and energetic as ever he did, but then would follow a period of terrible depression and languor, which he was strongly tempted to relieve by using stimulants, but fortunately did not.

His consolation was in thinking that he could keep on at least as well as he was, until the hoped for period of his retirement, when all would come right again. The symptoms had however become so much more strongly marked, and his periods of depression, or fits of the *horrors* as he called them, so much more frequent, and so much longer in their duration, that he began to fear he might be *too far gone* to recover.

In this state he called upon me, and I found he had a tolerable idea of his condition, though unwilling to do what nature demanded. " I know," said he, " that I *ought* to marry for my health's sake, but my business is not yet in a satisfactory state, and I *cannot* be troubled now with domestic matters, they would unsettle my mind, though I have no doubt I should be very happy with a wife and family."

In vain I argued with him on the folly of such a course, and tried to show him of how much more conse-quence his health and happiness were than any amount of mere money; he tacitly agreed with me, but unfortunately had the idea that he could still hold over by *the help of Medicine!*

I told him unhesitatingly that this was a vain depend-ance, and that I should only deceive him if I made him any promise that would favor it. The utmost that could be done, I fully assured him, was, to correct the evil al-ready done, sufficient to make *marriage* proper, so that nature herself might have a chance to work. His sexual powers had become considerably impaired, but still were capable of renovation, by judicious treatment and con-duct, if such renovation were advisable. It would how-ever have been useless to restore his powers unless they were to be naturally employed, because they would other-wise fail again worse than ever.

In spite of all, however, he determined to try his pow-ers of endurance still further, and accordingly procured a *Nervous stimulant* which was recommended to him and kept on as before. I lost sight of him for about nine months, and then receiving a letter dated from a celebra-ted water-cure establishment, informing me that he was *worse*, and that he would shortly come on to consult me again.

The Letter states—" I found myself so much worse about four months ago, that I was compelled to leave my business, and abandon the medication I had to then per-sisted in. In my despair I came on here, to try the *cure-ill* treatment, but to my sorrow it has failed also. I am worse, and *growing worse!* You can have no idea my dear sir what I have suffered, and yet with little or no bodily ailing, at least none that is very apparent. Day after day have I sat in my office trying in vain to *fix my mind* on a case. I could not do it to save my life.— My mind would fly to the stars or to the depths of the sea, or even lose itself altogether, but *would not* fix upon

what I wished to study. After hours spent in these vain
attempts I would rush out in a state of absolute despair,
and conceal myself, from very shame and vexation. And
then oh ! who can imagine the torture I underwent? You
may, my dear sir, from having seen so many similar cases,
but others I am sure cannot, and I would rather die than
ttempt to explain my condition to my friends.

My head has also begun to pain me, especially in the
back part of it, and is constantly *full* and heavy, as if
packed with *lead*,—my eyes often become dim, and a
rushing sound fills my ears, till I become quite confused.
Latterly also I have suffered considerably from palpitation
of the heart, and my bowels and stomach are quite irregular in their action. The emissions I have not seen now
for six months, and this I think must be a good sign. I
am however troubled with a very frequent desire to urinate, and my water is often thick and cloudy.

Now, my dear Doctor, I am determined to follow your
advice, *providing* you can sufficiently restore me ! There
however is a new apprehension, my sexual powers and
desires have decidely lessened, especially since I have
used the cold water, and I begin to fear I never *can*
marry,—in which case I say solemnly, *I do not want to
live!* You must therefore be candid with me when I
come, and tell me the *truth*, as nearly as you can, for I
wish to know the worst at once. As for the *fortune* let
it go to the dogs ! Only let me be again a *man*, and I
care not what labor or privation is before me, nor what
station I occupy. Remember, therefore, your decision in
my *fate*, but do with me, and direct me, as you choose.
I shall be with you in two weeks. Yours, &c."

On seeing this Gentleman, I found he really had, as he
remarked, gone *down hill* at a rapid rate, and I by no
means felt sanguine of his recovery. From his excellent
constitution however, and from his not having been exhausted by excesses of any kind, I did not despair, but
put him at once under proper treatment.

The *worst* sign was precisely that which he thought the
best, namely, the stopping of the *nightly emissions*. I suspected at once that the discharges still occurred, but in

another and unseen form, much more dangerous. I explained to him how, in such cases, the semen began at last to flow out *with the urine*, by which means so much was lost that the ordinary emissions ceased altogether. This was a new light to him, and he at once called to mind a number of symptoms which seemed to prove my position. To make it certain however, I at once submitted a portion of the urine to microscopical examination, as is my custom, and the result left no doubt as to the existence of the trouble. The urine in the morning contained an immense quantity of semen, and I found that more or less escaped every time the bladder was emptied.

On reading my book on *The Male Generative Organs*, which he had not seen before, the truth broke at once upon him, and he remarked that if he had perused that work earlier, particularly the part referring to *seminal losses*, he should not have delayed as he had done.

The first thing to be done was to remove the irritability and relaxation of the seminal Ducts, which was the immediate cause of the semen flowing out with the urine. This was effected by *Cauterizing*, the case being one which properly admitted of that operation. The result was perfectly satisfactory, the urinary losses ceasing entirely, so that the old nightly emissions again commenced, at intervals, and his desires and powers evidently began to return. The administration of my Aphrodisiac Remedy with strict attention to diet, and general hygienic measures, made the improvements still more manifest, but it was necessary for him to abandon *business* altogether, and live perfectly at ease.

In six months he was decidedly *restored*, to a very great extent, though not fully to the condition he enjoyed originally. I saw however, that the system could recuperate its energies, to a great extent, sufficient in short to allow of his marrying with *physiological* propriety, providing he continued in the proper course, which he was determined to do.

In ten months after my seeing him he did marry, and the result was very satisfactory. He is now the happy Father of two healthy children, and in the enjoyment of very tolerable health himself. His sexual powers however are inferior to what they ought to be, and to what they would have been had he married earlier, but still, as he expresses in one of his Letters, sufficient for the mutual happiness of himself and partner. His mind has, to a great extent, recovered its powers, but he is net even now capable of any continued mental efforts, as in former times.

Here then is the result, under *favorable* circumstances. If this man had not been properly instructed in regard to his case, in time, he would have become incurably, hopelessly, powerless and probably insane, unless his bodily deterioration had terminated his existence. As it is, he has now a reasonable prospect of existence and of considerable enjoyments of life, though probably in a much less degree, and for a *shorter time* than he otherwise would.

UNDUE CONTINENCE, FROM MISTAKEN NOTIONS OF RELIGION.

This was a minister of the Gospel, a man of earnest piety, and of the most perfect self-denying character. He conceived the idea that it was his duty to fly from all *fleshly lusts*, and devote himself entirely to his religious ministrations. This he did most scrupulously, till he was twenty-seven years old, though with hard struggling against the promptings of sin. " I have," said he, " passed entire nights combatting my evil thoughts, and resisting those physical manifestations which indicate our earthly longings. In spite of all my efforts however, I realise too forcibly how weak we are, and what an empire the old Adam has over our souls. Of myself, I see too well I can do but little, and my sole dependence is upon assistance from above."—

With this man it was much more difficult to deal, owing to his peculiar notions about *sin*. I could only tell him that, in his circumstances, the sin really lay, according to my notions, in what he considered his only *virtue*, and that both his well being and his power of doing good depended entirely upon his obeying the laws of nature.

His principal reason for applying to me was the singular state of his feelings, and a peculiar distress in his head. He was subject at times to fits of excitement of the most violent character, without any apparent provocation, and even when quite alone. At such times he could not rest, but seemed impelled to move quickly about in spite of himself, while anger and rage, he knew not what for, filled his mind. At other times on the contrary he fell into a state of *dreamy* languor, or mental torpor, so profound that he was scarcely conscious of his own existence, and utterly indifferent to anything that occurred.

Before any of these attacks he usually experienced a buzzing in the ears, with a throbbing in the large veins of the neck accompanied by a redness of the eyes and a kind of *whirling* in the brain, which occasionally even made him feel quite giddy.

In all respects the life of this man was irreproachable. He was strictly temperate in eating and drinking, took plenty of exercise in the open air, and cultivated a cheer ful contented tone of mind. His general health too, until quite recently, had been quite fair, with the exception of a constipated state of the bowels.

His Genital development was perfect, and his amative propensity quite strong, or, physiologically speaking, he formed a large quantity of Semen, the excess of which nature intended to be expelled according to the laws of his organization. This natural expenditure not going on however a constant struggle became necessary, the organs trying to retain the fluid with which they were overburdened, but being compelled at times to allow it to escape, in the form of nightly emissions. This overcharged con dition of the Seminal organs kept the *brain* also in a constant state of excitement, from the powerful efforts required to overcome the feelings and desires engendered by the Seminal stimulus. And in this way was produced the different moral paroxysms into which he was plunged.

It was with difficulty I could make him see and admit his actual condition, and on no account would he admit that the natural remedy I advised was necessary. He had made up his mind to a life of Celibacy let the consequences be what they might, and he merely wished me to give him medicines to palliate his troubles and to deaden his sexual feelings, so that they would not require so much effort to overcome them.

This I of course refused to do, because it required more or less injury to the organs themselves, and my duty was to *heal*, not to *hurt*. I candidly told him, that as long as his organization remained perfect those feelings must be experienced, and that as long as he persisted in his celibacy he would always have the same trouble in struggling against them. As to injuring the organs, or *checking their action*, as he expressed it, I of course refused to do any thing of the kind.

Finding that my views of duty would not allow me to treat him as he wished he left, and for a time I heard nothing of him. Afterwards I learnt however that some of his admirers,—and he had many of them,—sent him on a voyage to Europe, in the hope that change of scene and air would benefit him. This however did no good, and finally he died in a private Lunatic Asylum, in France, after suffering intensely both in body in mind.

A VICTIM TO BUSINESS.

This was a mercantile Gentleman, who remained un-married till his forty-fifth year, when he retired from busi-ness, with a hundred thousand dollars, and married a young Lady with whom he had kept company for nearly fifteen years. For the previous six or seven years he had suffered more or less, in the same way as the Gentleman in the first case, but as his business was well regulated, and he had excellent agents, his own deficiencies were not so apparent, neither to himself nor to others. His stomach and bowels had become very irregular, and he was troubled with an almost constant desire to urinate, but other wise his bodily health was quite passable.

In regard to his sexual powers he admitted that for the last three years he had experienced a sensible diminution so much so in fact that he scarcely ever felt any desire at all Formerly he was accustomed, at irregular intervals to have illicit indulgence, which had doubtless delayed his decay considerably, but when about forty-one years of age he unfortunately attended a Lecture on *Amativeness*, by a Phrenologist.

In this Lecture he was told that all sexual connections, except for the purpose of *procreation* was improper, and that the true way to preserve the generative powers was not to use them, except for that purpose. He accordingly practised the strictest continence after this, and found that his amative propensity became gradually weaker, till at last it seemed almost entirely extinguished. He consoled himself however by thinking that all would come right at his marriage, and that his present state of *rest*, would only give him greater power afterwards.

Neither he nor the Phrenologist, whom he consulted, were aware that *Urinary Spermatorrhœa* had taken place, in consequence of his continued Continence, and that his sexual organs had nearly become powerless. Such however was the case, and to his horror he found on his marriage that he was nearly *Impotent !*

The state of mind of a man so circumstanced may be better imagined than described. " Here I am "—said he to me, " *a poor, wealthy, imbecile wretch !* In my senseless pursuit of riches, I have lost that which all the wealth in the world cannot recompense me for. Had I known ten years ago what I have since learnt from your book, ('The Male Organs,) I should now have been fifty thousand dollars poorer in *money* perhaps, but a healthy perfect *man :* I might also have become a proud and happy *Father*, which alas I now never expect to be."

This was one of the most unpromising cases I ever had to deal with, as I candidly told him, but still I undertook to do the best I could.

By means of a good tonic regimen and diet, sea bathing, Champooing of the Genitals, and the use of the Aphrodisiac Remedy, he began in three months to have some slight indications of power, and in six months much . stronger indications. It was not possible however to make a *permanent* restoration, because the Testes were considerably *wasted !* They were not so far gone as to be totally inactive, but it took them a long time to form any considerable quantity of Semen, which of course made his periods of power and inclination very rare.

Even what he did gain, small though it was, was much more than he ever expected, for he fully believed he was incurable and totally impotent. Had I seen him two years before I would have answered with my life for making him comparatively perfect, for I gathered from what he told me, that no wasting of the Testes had then taken place, and till that occurs *no case is hopeless*.

In addition to these, I could quote a large number of other cases, to show the evils of undue continence, and especially some very curious ones in young females, who were brought to me as being *Chlorotic*, and *Hysterical*, but these are quite sufficient for my present purpose. I have had a *Priest,* who declaimed against sexual indulgence as improper, and who adduced his own case as a proof that Continence was possible, came to me to be cured of a loathsome infirmity which that very continence had caused.

CHAPTER XII.

THE CONSEQUENCES OF SEXUAL EXCESSES AND ABUSES

THESE consequences are much more frequently seen than those of Continence, and people are more generally aware that they are of a hurtful character, though the actual extent and nature of the injuries resulting from them are not suspected.

From a variety of causes, many of which are but little known, a majority of human beings are addicted to excess in sexual indulgences, and to various unnatural modes of gratification. The *reason* for this is a matter deserving

of . earnest investigation, though unfortunately it has hith·
erto received but little attention. The Theologian is con-
tent to ascribe these, in common with all other human
frailties, to *Original Sin*, and seeks their source only in a
depraved soul. But the enlightened student of human
nature as it really is, recognizes various direct and indirect
influences, some belonging to the individuals own Organization, and others to the objects and circumstances by
which he is surrounded. These influences often impel
man to that course of conduct which his reason condemns,
and which produes untold misery and pain.

Among these influences may be mentioned **Hereditary**
Tendency, Excessive development or morbid irritability
of the Genital organs, vicious associations, stimulating
food and drink, and various social institutions more or less
opposed to nature's requirements.

In those persons who have little or no knowledge of
the consequences of sexual abuse these influences operate
almost unchecked, but in those who have such knowledge
the fear of those consequences operates more or less as a
restraint. The influence, however is frequently so powerful as to overcome all such restraints, and the victim falls
into the gulph with his eyes wide open, but still impelled
by a force from which he has neither the power nor the
desire to escape. There is good reason to believe that
sexual excesses and abuses produce, directly or indirectly,
by far the largest part of human suffering and disease,
much more in fact than all other causes that can be enumerated. People generally only observe the more palp-
able and direct consequences of these vices, while the indirect results of them are lost sight of, or attributed to
other causes.

The sympathies of the sexual Organs are both extensive and complicated, in consequence of which their derangements often affect remote parts of the system, and in
many different ways, appearing like so many different diseases. This is especially exemplified in *Venereal diseases*,
and particularly in *Syphylis*, the different stages and *here-*
ditary modifications of which, extending as they may do
over several generations, are only just now being under-

stood even by medical men.   (On this point I would refer
my readers to my Treatise on *Venereal Diseases*, in which
all this is fully explained.)

The connection between the Sexual Organs and the *Ner
vous System*, especially the *Brain*, is another important
matter, also but little studied or understood, and yet it is
of the most overwhelming importance.   Not only may
the bodily health of human beings be affected by peculiarities in the action and development of their Sexual
organs, but the tone and ability of their *Minds*, and also
their *moral tendencies* are under the same influences.

It is requisite, for the welfare of society, perhaps even
for its very existence, that certain *actions* should be called
virtuous, and be held up to praise, and that others of an
opposite tendency, should be called *vicious*, and be condemned.   Every one is interested in the maintenance of
that *moral order* which experience has shown to be most
productive of human happiness, and we must therefore,
as rational beings, approve of whatever is favorable to
the maintenance of that order, and disapprove of whatever militates against it.   It may be requisite, with this
end in view, to condemn, or even to punish, in many cases
where our consciences so far from *blaming*, see only cause
for pity and regret.   The regulation of society must have
for its end the *general* good, and to secure this it is often
the case that *individuals* are sacrificed to *expediency*.

Thus, for instance, a particular *crime*, or immoral
action, is punished the same in all who commit it, though
we know that it must have been much more *criminal*,
properly speaking, in some than in others.   Thus for
instance, in sexual immorality the degree of culpability,
properly measured, must be infinitely varied for the same
offence, though all are punished for it alike.

Some human beings are strongly impelled to *seek* sex
ual indulgence from the peculiarity of their organization
from disease, or from hereditary tendency, while others on
the contrary are but slightly impelled, and others even
avoid it, except at rare intervals.   It is therefore evident
that, under the same circumstances, the effort of self-denial,
or resistance to temptation, is required to be *much greater*

in some cases than in others, and of course the *possibility* of successfully resisting the temptation is proportionably less.

Society however cannot consider the distinctions, because it is impossible to ascertain the relative degrees of criminality, and therefore similar criminal acts must entail similar penalties on all alike.

The institution of *rewards* and *punishments* has become such a fundamental principle in our social order that, whatever we may, in many cases, think of its *abstract justice*, we cannot consent to its being abolished. Till better motives than *fear*, and the hope of *reward* can be generally instilled we must not do away with these, for if we do we shall have nothing to fall back upon.

The Philosophic mind, which traces *cause and effect*, and which draws its conclusions from *reasoning*, and not from *passion*, must often pity the criminal as a *victim*, and conscientiously exonerate him from all *moral blame* even when admitting the necessity for his *punishment*,—so true it is that our Social duties and requirements are often at variance with our conscientious convictions. As *Individuals*, in our own hearts we must often have *charity*, or even *commiseration*, for those that social duty compels us to condemn; and, in fact, with reflective minds this is ordinarily the case.

These remarks I have made to prevent the possibility of my being misunderstood, or misrepresented. In the course of this book I shall show numerous causes disposing, or even impelling, human beings to immoral acts, and which causes many cannot escape from. I do not wish it to be understood however that I advocate, on this account any radical change in our *conduct* towards these persons, for such acts, but merely that we think of them justly and charitably *in our own minds*, and that we strive to remove, or modify such unfavorable causes, and so prevent others being equally unfortunate. As men become more experienced, the science of *preventing* evil will be generally studied, and then such inconsistencies as I have alluded to will gradually cease. The present little book, I trust, will do something towards attracting attention to these matters, and lead those who read it to *reflect* and *eason* on human frailties as well as *condemn* them.

Sexual abuses commence at a much earlier period of life, in many cases, than is usually supposed, and their injurious effects are also much earlier experienced. A precocious development of the Sexual organs, or a tendency to preternatural exaltation of the genital instinct is by no means uncommon, and from either cause the most injurious habits may be practised even in Infancy. Many persons suppose that such manifestations never commence till the age of *puberty*, but this is a mistake, they are sometimes observed, unmistakeably, while children are yet in their Nurse's arms.

It is an error to suppose that no injury can result except from a *loss of Semen*, for long before that fluid has begun to be formed both mind and body may be irretrievably ruined, by nervous excitement and exhaustion. This is of necessity the case with females, who form no Semen and it is also equally the case with males, though few persons are aware of the fact.

One of the most obvious principles of Animal Physiology is, that no vital action whatever, can occur except through the agency of the *Nervous power*,—whether we *think, eat, digest, walk*, or *speak*, every muscle is moved, every secretion is produced, and every idea is eliminated by the stimulus of the mysterious *Nervous fluid*, the grand excitant and moving power in all Organic or Vital processes.

If the Nervous power be deficient in any organ, that organ will work imperfectly, to a corresponding degree, and if it be absent altogether the organ cannot work at all, any more than a Steam Engine can work without Steam. Any cause therefore which decreases the requisite amount of nervous energy in the system causes imperfect or inefficient action, either locally or generally, and thus predisposes to disease and premature decay.

We require so much Nervous power to think, so much to digest, so much for muscular exercise, and so much for all the other organic processes, and in a healthy condition of the system there is always enough for the proper performance of them all. If however any one function be performed in an exaggerated degree, so as to exhaust more of the nervous power than properly should be expended upon it, the others must of necessity receive less than they naturally should do, and must be imperfectly performed.

Instances of this kind are often seen among *Business men,* who expend so much of their nervous power in intense *mental exertion,* owing to pressure of business, that they have not enough left to effect *digestion, nutrition,* and all the other processes necessary to the maintenance and continuance of the system. In consequence of which they become *Dyspeptic,* debilitated, and *Impotent,* and after living miserably they at last *drop off,* in an orthodox business way, long before they naturally might be expected to do so.

Such men suppose that *Pills, Bitters,* and *Stimulants,* or a day or two or relaxation once a year or so will make all right,—but they too often find out their mistake, and become *first rate patients,* always on the *Books,* and calculated upon for so many " *hundreds* " a year, by their physicians, with as much certainty as his Bank is calculated upon by the Banker for his *Dividends.*

In the same way other men think they can expend most of their nervous power in *Sexual excesses,* and yet perform sufficiently well all the ordinary organic functions at the same time, but they likewise discover their error, and frequently too late to retrieve it.

The performance of the Generative act requires more Nervous power than perhaps any other organic function, and of course it exhausts in a corresponding degree. So also does mere Sexual excitement, and therefore indulgence in either should be regulated on proper Physiological principles, such as are laid down in my Book called " *The Marriage Guide.*" Excesses of this kind are the most injurious of all, and the evils resulting from them are amongst the most irremediable.

Different periods of life, as also different conditions of the system, require different amounts of Nervous power, and also to have it differently *distributed.*

In Adults the Body is only required to *Maintain itself,*

or to hold its own, but in Youth it must not only do this but also *increase*, or *grow*, to perfect itself. There is therefore required, at this period an *extra amount* of nervous power, and if it is not supplied the body becomes, in consequence, imperfectly formed. •Anything therefore which causes great nervous exhaustion is peculiarly hurtful in youth, and its evil effects are seen afterwards throughout the whole of the individual's life.

This is the reason why *Sexual abuses* are so very injurious in young persons, and why their effects are so often irremediable. Numbers have their *growth arrested* in this way, and remain more or. less dwarfed, or weakly developed, while in others the *internal organs* are imperfectly formed, and in consequence always *act* imperfectly, thus causing a liability to *Disease*, and to *premature old age*, or *untimely death* '

Such instances come every day under the notice of the observant Physician, and are in fact every where to be met with, though there are few who understand them aright. Those however who bear in mind the Physiological principles/above laid down, will be able to explain them, and to comprehend why our efforts to *cure* such evils so often fail.

No matter in what form Sexual abuses are practised during youth, the same consequences to a greater or lesser degree, may be expected to follow, and, generally speaking the *earlier* the abuses are practised the more serious are the after consequences, because of the more imperfect stage at which the system is arrested. This is the reason why *Infantile Masturbation*, in both sexes, is so hurtful. There is nothing similar to the *loss of Semen*, of later years, but there is an equal, if not greater amount of *nervous excitement*, and *exhaustion*, and for want of the power thus wasted the system cannot perfect itself.

In like manner Sexual abuses are extremely hurtful in the decline of life, because then there is a less amount of Nervous power eliminated, owing to the decaying energy of the system, and anything which unduly exhausts it still further hastens the period of its final extinction. Many old men have experienced this to their cost, in expanding as much vital power in one Sexual act, imperfectly performed, as would have sufficed for the ordinary purposes of existence for a month.

In short, it is only after the system has perfected its growth, and before it begins to decay, that Sexual indulgences can be practised with impunity, except in the most prudent and temperate manner. In the prime of life, with a perfect healthy acting body, there is *more* nervous power produced than the system requires merely to *live* with, and this *surplus* may be safely expended in Sexual indulgence.

But even at this age, if exhausting labor have to be performed, whether bodily or mental, or if sickness makes an extra drain upon the nervous power, or lessens the quantity of it produced, Sexual indulgences must be correspondingly abbreviated.

These are the true principles which should regulate the conduct of human beings in these important matters, and just in proportion as they understand, and act upon them, will they be able to avoid those evils which ignorance, or inattention of such things are sure to entail upon them.

I shall now proceed to detail a series of CASES, in illustration of these matters, taking them mostly as I find them in my *note book*, and making such comments, and explanations, as I may think requisite. They are not arranged systematically, so as to apply only to certain topics, but are taken promiscuously, to illustrate *all* though I shall endeavor to make some of the first ones refer more especially to the principles just laid down.

PART III.

FACTS FOR THE FEEBLE!

OR PROFESSIONAL NOTES OF

CURIOUS MEDICAL CONSULTATIONS

RELATING TO THE VARIOUS PECULIARITIES, DISABILITIES, AND FORMS OF DECAY OF

THE SEXUAL SYSTEM

BEING THE RECORDED EXPERIENCE OF MANY YEARS SPECIAL PRACTICE IN SUCH CASES, AND SHOWING THE ACTUAL EFFECT OF THESE NEW REMEDIES, AND MODES OF TREATMENT NOT SO GENERALLY KNOWN EVEN BY MEDICAL MEN.

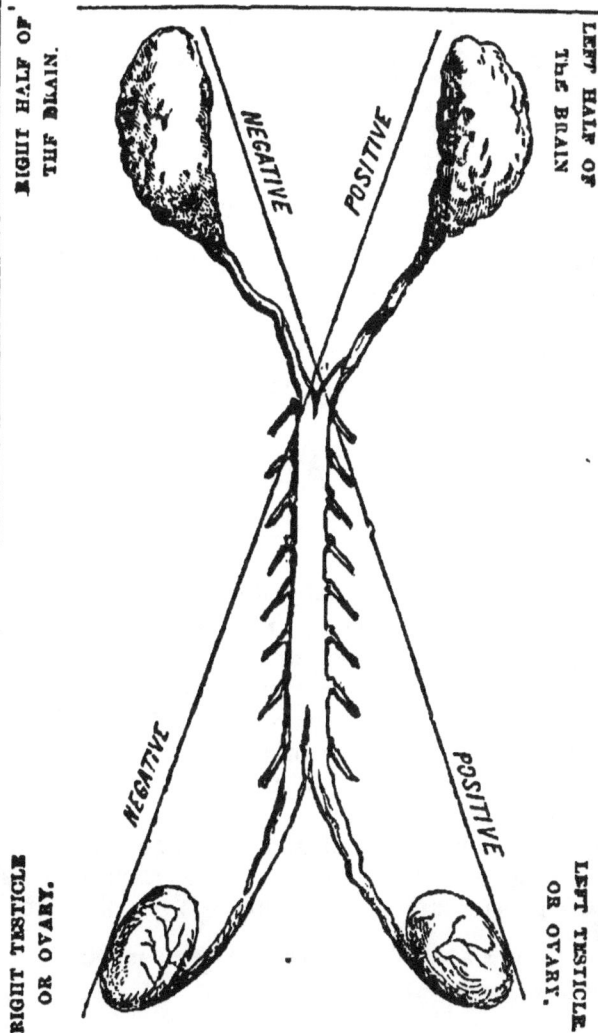

CONNECTION BETWEEN THE

BRAIN AND THE SEXUAL ORGANS.

RIGHT HALF OF THE BRAIN.

LEFT HALF OF THE BRAIN

NEGATIVE

POSITIVE

NEGATIVE

POSITIVE

RIGHT TESTICLE OR OVARY.

LEFT TESTICLE OR OVARY.

The two halves of the Brain are separated, to show they are distinct from each other, and to show their connection with the Sexual Centres. (See page 46.)

MISCELLANEOUS "CASES,"

WITH

NOTES AND EXPLANATIONS.

RETARDED DEVELOPMENT

THIS was a remarkable instance of *Retarded develop-ment* from Masturbation, which, fortunately was partially corrected, by the subject of it having his attention awak-ened in time. I shall first let the individual speak for himself, and make my comments, and explanations, when I think most useful.

To DR. F. HOLLICK,
*New York City, N. Y.**

" MY DEAR SIR,

" A short time ago I attended your Lectures on Parental Pysiology, in Philadelphia, and from hearing them I have determined to address you. I am one of those truly pitiable creatures of whom you spoke, in the early part of your discourse, when referring to *Infantile Masturba-tion,* and I am perhaps as painful an instance of the awful effects of this practice as you ever saw. When you first spoke upon this subject, and portrayed the terrible *after consequences,* I was plunged in despair, and truly felt desir-ous to ' shuffle off' this mortal coil' as soon as possible, for to *live* as I am is impossible. Your final remarks

* This Address will always find me, at any time

however gave me some hopes that possibly it might not be too late for me to recover, at least to some extent, and it is for the purpose of having your opinion on this point that I now address you. On your opinion depends *much*, I assure you ;—I will not however say further on this point, but proceed to my *statement*, which shall be *full*, nd *truthful*, in every particular, though it has cost me a evere struggle to make such a confession, and it never would have been made had I not heard you *Lecture* ' From your excellent discourse however I felt full confidence, both in your skill and in your kind sympathy, and I therefore reveal to you what I have hitherto concealed from every human being, and which, had I not met with you I should have carried a secret to the grave.

I am the son of Parents well to do in the world, and who have always, to the best of their knowledge, striven to do what was best for me. Unfortunately however their kind attentions were but imperfectly realized, owing to their want of proper information.

In early childhood I was very stout and robust, full of animal spirits, and active to an unusual degree. Everything seemed to promise that I should grow up a well developed man, but alas all such expectations were doomed to be disappointed.

My parents kept a female help expressly to attend upon me, whose whole time was occupied in playing with me and taking me about. One day she took me with her to see some of her friends, who lived in a very low part of the City, (Baltimore,) and while engaged gossiping she left me play with the children of the neighbour's, who were swarming all around. They were as depraved, miserable, and vicious perhaps as could be found, and child as I was, being not over four years of age, I could not help thinking their conduct and language very strange It was new and exciting however, and that was enough to make it interesting, so that in a short time I cast off all restraint and became fully initiated into many of their habits and sayings, which I thought especially excellent, no doubt. Among the rest was one precocious ragamuffin, older than the rest, who undertook to explain to them various mysterious points in physiology and Parentage, and the uses of certain parts of their bodies, to which my attention had never before been directed. This was done *practically*, there being both girls and boys present, and none having the slightest objection to any kind of exposure, but rather courting it. The revelations which I then heard, given in the grossest manner, and the sights I saw, have never been effaced from my mind, but, young as I was at the time, they are as fresh and vivid now as if it occurred but yesterday.

Among other things we were all of both sexes, taught the habit of *Masturbation*, to the pleasurable feelings from which I was peculiarly liable, owing to my temperament I suppose, and from that time I began to give myself up to the habit. I had command enough of myself to keep it secret, from my parents, because I felt instinctively there was something in it they would condemn, though I know not why. My attendant knew, and rather encouraged it than otherwise, because it often relieved her of the trouble of attending me. In fact the whole group, at the time of the *initiation*, were surprised, in the very midst of their proceedings, by my nurse and one of her female friends, who seemed to consider it a capital joke, and highly amusing, by the way they laughed about it when describing the scene to their companions. She however frightened me out of telling any one else about it by assuring me I should be severely punished if I did, and besides this I did not want to do so—it was *my secret*, and in my way I felt quite important about it.

From this time on I continued more or less, almost constantly, to practice this habit, in various ways, till it became a perfect furor, and at six years of age I have kept awake for hours together, in the night in this way.

The immediate consequences were, that I became puny and weak, and irritable in my disposition, to such an extent that I was both wretched myself and a source of constant discomfort to those around me. To add to my misfortune, my Parents placed me under the care of a *Physician*, who drugged me, and sent me to the sea side but all to no purpose, for I did not improve in the slight est degree. Study I could only pursue at intervals, and in a very *flighty* manner, so that I was behind with my education, and as my memory was bad I fell far behind my schoolmates.

Things continued more or less in this way till I was fourteen years of age, when puberty became established, and I began to form Semen. In consequence of this, I suppose, my Sexual desires and feelings grew stronger, or perhaps I should say they then first became natural, and I indulged more frequently than ever. I have frequently expended the Semen four and five times a day, for several days together, till I became so weak I could scarcely walk, and quite childish in my mind. My friends all thought I was in a Consumption, and none of them ever expected me to live.

From that time till now *I have never grown,* and I am over *twenty-one!* Neither do I seem in any way further *developed.* I am no heavier,—my voice has the same sound, and my Sexual Organs are quite as small as they were at fourteen years of age. In some respects, however I am better than I was, and I attribute it all to this circumstance. I was one day passing down the street and looking into a Bookstore window, I saw your Book on "*The Male Organs,*" and from curiosity went in and bought it. The perusal of that book first opened my eyes, and made me begin to think that my weakness and sickness was caused solely by Masturbation. It is true I had partially suspected this before, but the impression was not strong enough to make me leave off the habit. Now however I determined to do so, and by hard striving I partially succeeded.

At times I had felt, for a year or two past, much better, and my mind became a little stronger, and more settled, so that I made up a little for my past deficiency, and began to reflect upon my situation. While in these favorable moods I did pretty well, and conquered my fatal inclinations, but when the mood past off I fell back again.

It was in my seventeenth year when I purchased your Book, and from then till now I have been struggling in this way, and on the whole perhaps I have gained, but still very little, and latterly I have begun to fear I should never be much otherwise than I am. This fear began to haunt me continually, and I had made up my mind to come to New York to see you, when I noticed the Advertisement of your Lectures here, and to my great joy had an opportunity of hearing you. After I left the Lecture room I determined, in the first place to write to you, and then, if you thought there might *possibly* be anything done for me, I would visit you personally. I am rich enough in this worlds goods, having inherited considerable property, and am both able and *willing* to recompence you to any extent you may think requisite, within a reasonable amount. Money I value no more than the dust under my feet, for unless I can be *made a man* I shall not need it, and if I can be, I shall be quite glad to give it to *my saviour.*

I have thus my dear sir, made a sufficient confession, I hope, to enable you to judge of my case, and I trust you will render me your reply as *promptly as possible*, for you may well imagine the agony of suspense in which I am. Excuse my long and rambling Letter, which is, I fear, like my mind, very confused,—and accept the enclosed check as a retaining fee.

" Yours, most truly,

———— ————."

Upon fully considering this Letter, I concluded it was *possible* that the subject of it could be helped, though to what extent was uncertain, and so I informed him. The result was an interview, in which I found him, as his letter described, *half developed, puny, and weak minded,* but still with indications that *originally* he had been possessed of a good constitution. There were also indications that nature was even now endeavoring to recover her lost ground, and some little growth, with occasional increase of mental power, gave *hopes* for the future.

At his earnest request I at once commenced to advise and to treat him, his circumstances fortunately being such that he could live as I choose to direct. In the first place I prescribed such a regular course of diet, daily exercise,

bathing, and friction of the skin, as I thought mos likely
to promote his general health and bodily growth. With
that I also commenced to treat the *Genital Organs*, in the
most active manner, feeling assured that their develop
ment would stimulate the whole organization, and add to
the power of both body and mind.

The *Congoster* was used daily, with shampooing, and my
Aphrodisiac Remedy was also used, though very carefully.
The result began to be obvious in less than *three months!*
The Genital Organs increased in size and power. The
Semen was *secreted* in greater quantity,—and the Sexual
desire became strong and natural. The whole body also
soon began to develop most obviously, so that his friends
made remark of it, and his mind became more *manly* in
its tone, and more *steady*, so that he was capable of more
continued mental exertion, and soon extended his acquire-
ments considerably. One difficulty however arose which
I had forseen, but could not altogether prevent. His continued practice of *Masturbation* had of course both *weakened* and *irritated* the Genitals, so that when the Semen
began to be secreted in greater quantity it could not be
retained, and he suffered from *Spermattorrhœa*. To such
an extent did this evil prevail, especially in the *urinary*
form, (as described in my book on " *The Male Organs*,")
that I feared it would counteract all I could do. By degrees however it was overcome, by *Cauterization*, and then
the real advance commenced in earnest.

In the course of the next *two years* he seemed almost
to *leap forward*, so rapid was his growth, till I feared he
would become sickly and weak from it. By good Tonic
treatment however, and constant care, this danger was
avoided, and he continued to advance, so that in his *twenty-
fifth* year he was fully up to the average standard of
young men of that age, in size, weight and strength. His
mind was also quite active, and of good ordinary capacity,
though not capable of very powerful or long continued
efforts. No one who had known him formerly ever supposed it possible for him to become what he was, and he
himself felt so elated, that he entirely overlooked the

actual deficiencies which still existed, and thought himself perfect enough.

His greatest pleasure was in writing regularly to me, and constantly noting the different stages of advancement, and speculating as to the future. I never knew a patient more gratified or more grateful. In one of his Letters he remarks, " such as I now am you have made me, for without your assistance and advice I certainly should not have now been in existence!"

The *Sexual* powers of this young man became quite good, though irregular in their manifestation, and he was fully capable of the duties of Married Life, but not sc frequently as in the generality of persons at his age.

On this case I shall make but few comments, because it tells its own tale, in most respects, and the instruction it conveys must be obvious. The principal facts indicated by it are the *arrest of development*, caused by the loss of nervous power, from sexual abuse, and the recommencement of growth when the sexual power became restored. If the Sexual Organs had not grown, and become active, *no other development* would have occurred to any useful extent, and if their weakness and irritability had not been overcome he would soon have died from *Spermattorrhœa.*

It was also fortunate that proper attention was bestowed *in time*, before the period when growth is possible had passed. In several such instances I have been consulted *too late*, when that time had gone by, that is for the body generally, though the *Sexual Organs* may often be much perfected until nearly the *thirtieth year*, and of course the *energy* of the system,—especially of the *mind*,—along with them.

The *Moral* Lessons which such a case conveys, particularly respecting the patient's *childhood*, must. I think, be clear to all, and do not need special remark. There are more children exposed to *similar* evils than is usually supposed.

Unfortunately this individual was *killed*, in one of those *steamboat accidents* which are unfortunately so frequent out West, or he would now have been a remarkable instance of what proper Medical and Hygienic means can accom plish, even in the most unpromising cases, when employed on correct Physiological principles.

Similar cases to the above I often have communicated to me, not only by Males but also by *Females*, many of whom are taught such practices by their domestics, or at school.

In one such instance the patient was perhaps the most wretched victim of alternate excitement and depression of the Nervous System ever seen. At times she was subject to fits of almost frenzied agitation, and was so restless, both bodily and mentally, that she could not sit down, nor sleep, nor speak on the same subject two minutes together. At other times she would be perfectly listless, and almost as if suffering from Congestion of the Brain. Indifferent to all about her, powerless and torpid she seemed altogether too low ever to rally again.

All that could be ascertained about the origin of her suffering was that she had been taught the practice of Masturbation by a female domestic, when about ten years old. She had never Menstruated, though nineteen years of age when I saw her, and she had many peculiar imperfections in her organization. The Pelvis, and internal Organs were unusually small, while the external Genitals were remarkably large, and singularly irritable. Her head was also small, and her muscular system lax.

The case was interpreted easily enough by these signs. Her *development* was imperfect and irregular, from the nervous excitement and exhaustion she had undergone just previous to puberty, from the habit that had been taught her.

Every means was tried to lessen the irritation of her system, and to perfect her development, but all failed. She died before her twentieth year, almost a maniac.

CASES SHOWING THE USE OF THE MICROSCOPE.

IN DETECTING THE ABSCENCE OF THE SEMINAL ANIMALCULES.

THOSE who have read my Marriage Guide will be aware
that the Semen can impregnate only when it contains living and perfect Animalcules, and that many men may be
able to have connection, and even appear Vigorous, in
whose Semen there are no perfect living Animalcules.
Such men of course can never become Fathers, though
they may be totally unware of their imperfection, and
always ascribe the fault to the female.

This state of things can only be detected by microscopical examination of the Semen, which in the course of my
practice I am often called upon to make, frequently with
very unexpected and curious results.

Some years ago I was waited upon by a married couple,
of high standing in society, to get my advice in regard to
their being childless. They had been married nine years,
both were young, and apparently perfectly healthy. The
Gentleman informed me that, independent of the gratification to their own feelings, which were intense for offspring, it was of the utmost importance they should have
a child on other accounts. It seems a large property was
so left that their child would inherit it, if they had one,
or themselves as its heirs even if it died, while if they
died childless it would go to a distant connection of the
family, who was already enormously rich, and a very un-
deserving personage into the bargain.

Here there was both happiness and wealth at stake
and I was requested to do or suggest anything in my
power.

The parties were fully communicative, and disposed to
hear anything, or to discuss anything that I thought necessary. The result was that I became fully convinced the
Lady was in no way whatever imperfect, but fully capable
of Conception, and consequently the fault was with the
Husband. On stating this to him he was amazed, and

quite incredulous, for, said he, how am I wrong ? I enjoy
the same feelings, and the same powers as other men, and
have even a copious Seminal Secretion. I then explained
to him in what I thought the difficulty consisted, and a
Microscopical examination of the Semen was at once in-
stituted. My surmise proved to be correct. 'There were
only a few, very imperfect animalcules contained in it,
utterly inefficient for the purpose of impregnation. The
examination was of course frequently repeated, to make
sure that this was the normal condition, and always with
the same results.

On the true state of affairs being made obvious to him
he became unusually thoughtful, and evidently brooded
over the matter most intensly. At last he remarked, in a
half abstracted manner, " Well, it has always been my
strongest desire that Maria, (his wife,) or her children,
should inherit this property, and it shall be so,—if possible ! So now Doctor *what can be done ?*"

I told him at once that I believed the case was hopeless, for the imperfection, in his case, was not the result
of weakness, disease, or over indulgence, such as can often
be recovered from, but was evidently *constitutional*, and I
therefore could hold out no prospect of its removal. He
made me the most liberal offers if I could succeed in making him capable, but I told him at once I could not deceive him.

Soon after this they returned to Europe, where the
property lay, and I heard no more from them for four
years, when one day the Gentleman again called upon me,
and after stating that they had been travelling for some
time, requested me to call and see his wife, who was some
what indisposed, and desirous of seeing me. On enquir-
ing after his health I found him just about the same as
usual, only much stouter, as is often the case with such
constitutions on approaching forty years of age. He was
unusually cheerful however, and on leaving remarked, in
a matter of course way, and with an evident effort to be
unconcerned—" by the bye Dr. *our little one* is not very
well either, and I shall be much obliged if you will pay

particular attention to him, for you know how much depends on his life!"

The announcement took me quite by surprise, and he probably saw by my look that it did so, for he at once apologized for not having told me of their good fortune before, knowing how I should be interested in it. But, said he, it is now three years old nearly, and I forgot that you had not been informed of the happy event. I of course made no remark, but paid my visit, and found the mother and child only a little inconvenienced by the journey, and change of air. In a short time they were quite well again.

A happier couple I have seldom seen than they were. The child was adored by both, and fortunately seemed likely to live to reward them for their care and affection.

There was however a little awkwardness and restraint in their manner to me, and an evident avoidance of the subject of our first conference. Only on one occasion, just on the eve of his departure for Canada, did he allude to it. He then remarked, "Doctor, could any one else find out what you told me four years ago?" No sir, said I, only by the same means, and there are perhaps not two other men in the world who would think of using them. "Oh well," said he, "I am glad of that, though its of no consequence now, because matters have turned out right at last you see, and Maria's property will not go to those who had no right to it." To this I replied not, and he went away. Six months after he died of Apoplexy, quite suddenly, to the great distress of his wife, who was sincerely attached to him. Her grief in fact made her quite sick, and for some time her life was despaired of, but finally she recovered, apparently more from love to her child than from a desire to live on her own account. In fact her whole existence seemed devoted to her son, whom she watched with unremitting care.

One day that he was somewhat indisposed, I was called to see him, and found with her an old female friend, one of those who always say whatever comes uppermost, without thinking of consequences. I had just assured the mother that nothing serious was the matter with the child, as

indeed her family Physician had stated just before, when
the female friend, an old Lady, remarked, that the child
had a *thick neck*, and " what a pity it would be if it took
after its Father, and was Apoplectic !" I could not for
bear looking toward the mother, whose eyes met mine,
and I saw at once that she detected my after-thought in
a moment, when I gravely said I thought there was *no
danger !*

Some days after she requested to see me, on the eve of
her final departure for Europe. A candid admission was
made to me that my first judgment had not been invalid-
ated by what had occurred. Suffice it to say, the Husband had determined, with her concurrence, that *her* child
at least should inherit the coveted wealth, even if one of
theirs could not,—and hence what had followed. They
had thought I might imagine a change had occurred in
him, and that matters were perfectly natural, which was
the reason why our first consultation was never referred
to. The old Lady's remark however, and my manner of
replying, showed the mother that I was not deceived, and
hence the confession. Of course it was no concern of
mine, and I could only assure the mother that the secret
was perfectly safe. He had been, I fully believe, almost
as happy as if really a parent.

On another occasion I had for a patient a married Gentleman, but Childless, who had unfortunately got entan-
gled with an intriguing Mistress, who was perpetually ex-
torting money from him. Being rich, however, this was
not of serious moment, but at last the Lady became Pregnant, and in due time was safely delivered of a son. My
Patient was now informed that he must make ample provision for this new comer, and its mother, for Life, or
some very disagreeable disclosures should be made. I
was not aware of this event till the child was ten months
old. The Gentleman then mentioned it to me to explain
the great embarrassment and trouble under which he
labored, and which was acting very prejudicially upon his

health. I was then treating him for Spermattorrhœa, which had begun to weaken his powers and to affect his mind. My Microscopical examination had shown me that he was naturally imperfect, like the Gentleman in the previous case, and I at once saw that he could not be the Father of the young stranger. He however had no idea of this, and was really desirous of settling upon it a handsome annuity, but some unexpected embarrassments had made it difficult for him then to do so. Being my Patient I considered it my duty to tell him the truth, to prevent his being imposed upon. He was both astonished and indignant on learning this unexpected fact, and would at once have had a final, and not very friendly interview with the Lady, but the fear of consequences deterred him.

Now here was a terrible state of embarrassment for a man, with no apparent means of getting clear. He must either be plundered and imposed upon to maintain the offspring of another man, or he must be disgraced. and his domestic happiness destroyed, by a disclosure of his own improper doings. What was to be done ? In his despair he was almost driven to suicide, but by degrees his mind was calmed, and I induced him to consider his predicament in a proper manner, with a view to his extrication.

After consideration I told him I thought I saw a means which might be successful, and though not called upon to do anything of the sort, as a Medical man, yet out of consideration for an old and liberal patient, I consented to try. At my suggestion the Lady was induced to visit me, as a patient, she being a little indisposed. I saw at once that she was a designing *intriguante*, but evidently not overburdened with information, and readily impressed by a confident manner of speaking.

After attending with all due consideration to her own case, the conversation was gradually turned towards the Gentleman her friend, who, I remarked, was one of those peculiar beings, that Medical men like myself occasionally met with, whose *bodily imperfections* would never be suspected ! This piqued her curiosity, as I intended it to do, and led her to inquire more closely what kind of imperfections I alluded to ? The matter being thus entered upon, I at once told her, in an off hand manner, that it was impossible for him *ever to be a Father!* The announcement seemed to come upon her like a clap of thun der, and for some time she remained silent. Finally how ever, putting on a show of offended dignity, she remarked that perhaps I was not aware of the relation in which the Gentleman and herself stood? Excuse me madam, said I, but I am aware of your *liaison* perfectly well. Oh! said she, that is not what I mean, you do not know then, it seems, that he is the Father of my son, now ten month's old? No madam, said I. Nor can such be the case ;— it is *an utter impossibility!*

This assertion brought on a perfect *scene* of rage and assumed grief at being *suspected*, but finally the tempest cooled down, and she began to talk more coolly. I told her that I had no wish to give offence, and was entirely ignorant that my friend was accused of being the parent till just now, and that in all probability she was deceived herself. Finally she seemed to change her tactics, doubt less from a consciousness of being in the wrong, and at last asked me, with evident interest, if the peculiar imper fections which I spoke of in the Gentleman could be *proved?* I assured her it could be, and that if called upon in evidence I could readily prove it, beyond a doubt. This evidently put her completely to a nonpluss, and she went off, quite crest fallen.

At my suggestion the Gentleman entirely discontinued his visits to her, and treated her in quite a cool manner, as if he no longer had any fear. This created a disposi tion on her part to come to terms, and by the agency of a legal friend, who visited her for the purpose, and hinted something about a possible prosecution for attempted *im position*, matters were finally arranged, and for a reason able consideration she and the child went away, and my friend was relieved from his embarrassments.

On another occasion I had a Patient who died of Con sumption at the age of twenty-eight, leaving a widow, and a son aged three years. It had been what the French call a marriage *de convenance*, in which there was neither affection nor even respect on either side.

This Gentleman made one of those unjust wills by which his widow had the enjoyment of a handsome income for life, *providing she never married again*. The disposition of considerable property also depended on the life of the child being preserved till he became of age. Now the widow had no desire whatever for another marriage—probably from her experience of the first,—and was quite satisfied with her condition. She almost idolized her child, and devoted every moment to his care.— He was perfectly robust, and no apprehension whatever crossed her mind in regard to his health till in his fifth year. She visited a part of the country where lived the connections of her late husband, with whom she had never been at all acquainted. The marriage had been altogether the work of so called *friends* on both sides, and respecting the family or antecedents of her husband she knew very little previous to their union, and cared nothing about after.

Being now however quite free from all restraint, and in the neighborhood, she naturally sought some further information respecting him that was gone. To her great Consternation she learnt that his whole family had always been noted for their tendency to *Consumption*. Very few of them were then left, the majority in every Branch, having died quite young, and not one having been known to live over *twenty-eight* years, which was the age of her husband at his death. It was in fact generally called *the doomed family*, and an old Nurse thoughtlessly remarked, as a matter of course, that little Charley, strong as he looked, would never see his *thirtieth* year, even if he passed childhood. The mother became at once almost frantic with despair. She looked upon her darling boy as doomed also, and thought with horror of the day when he would be taken away from her, perhaps when just bursting into manhood and promise.

I have never seen a woman so entirely possessed by one idea as she was with this. She left the neighborhood at once where she had learnt this fatal news, and began resolving numerous plans to escape the threatened evil, but with no confidence in any of them. Finally she came to me, to ask my advice as to the probable success of a removal to another part of the Globe. Our consultation was of course confidential and full in every respect, because I felt it necessary to arrive at the true cause of her evident terror and apprehension. I had previously been her medical adviser, as well as her husband's, whom I had also known before his marriage.

Now it so happened, that he had consulted me immediately after their marriage, in reference to his Sexual powers, which were rapidly failing, as I discovered, from Urinary Spermattorrhœa. This was arrested and he partially recovered, but only imperfectly. In the course of Microscopical examinations I discovered that he was then totally impotent, there being but a very few animalcules in his Semen, and all *imperfect*, though he had, to a certain extent, the ordinary Sexual powers.

This fact I had intended to make known to him in order to explain better his real condition, and also why he had no family. To my surprise, however, he announced to me one day that his wife was *pregnant!* Of course I did not then feel called upon to state what I knew, more especially as the expectation of an heir seemed to give him great pleasure. His health also was evidently failing, and I expected his death from Consumption even before it occurred. This secret therefore was mine alone, and would have been buried with me, but for the present state of affairs. I *knew* that this man was not the father of the child whose mother was then suffering from such terrible apprehensions. I felt perfectly assured in making the assertion I afterwards did, and I had no doubt but that my accusation would both be admitted and pardoned, for the sake of the consolation it would bring. I therefore said at once, in the most decided and emphatic manner, that the child was in no danger whatever *from his connection with the family of the late Mr. ———!* The way in which I said this evidently caused both surprise and interested attention, and in a somewhat confused manner she asked me to explain what I meant? I then remarked without any comment, and as a matter merely of professional interest, that the boy was perfectly safe from that source, because it was *impossible* Mr. —————— could have been, at that time, his Father !

It is not necessary to attempt a description of the confusion, shame, and pretended anger which at first followed. Suffice it to say all this passed off, and in tearful humility, but with eager earnestness I was asked if this was *beyond doubt*. I assured her it was so, and that her child run no risk of inheriting the Consumptive fate of her late husband. Of course I could not say what risk he might run from his real *father*, because he was unknown to me.

The peculiar mental condition of this woman, at this time, was one of the most curious perhaps ever known. Consternation at the discovery of what she had no doubt thought past discovery, and shame at thinking I had known it so long, was intermixed with real joy and thankfulness at the escape of her child I of course assured her that the secret was as safe as if it really rested with her alone, and that to me it had no other interest than a professional one, and would never have been disclosed even to her, but under such circumstances.

Immediately afterwards she departed with her child for France, where she intended to bring him up away from all the associations of her own previous life.

On the eve of her departure I received anonymously a handsome present, with these words—" I had never dared or wished, to think it might be as you said, but now *know* it must have been so, and feel that I ought to make you this acknowledgment."

SOFTENING OF THE BRAIN.

Thus is a much more frequent disease than most people have any idea of. Medical men are only just beginning

to appreciate its importance, and to be aware of the fear
ful destruction of intellect and life, which is caused by it.
Softening of the Brain is the same disease, essentially, as
that called *Spinal Consumption*, of which the old writers
tell us so much.

The causes of this justly dreaded disease were till lately
unknown, or but vaguely suspected, and a variety of
Theories were invented to account for it. Lately however, its connection with Sexual derangement, in the majority of cases, has been established conclusively, and to
make this clear, we must give a little Anatomical and
Physiological explanation.

The substance of the Brain, and of the Nervous System generally, is essentially different, both in its structure
and composition, from all the other parts of the body, and
therefore it requires to be nutrified in a different way, and
by different material, from any other part. All the Vital
Organs may be perfect, and the Muscular system well developed and supported, owing to the special nutrition
being complete, and yet the Nervous System may be in a
state of decay. It is true that decay of the Nervous
System is soon followed by decay of all the other parts,
but it may commence independently of any imperfection
in them, and even while they are as perfect as usual.

The actual material, or substance, of the Nervous System, as elsewhere remarked, is almost identical with that
of the *Seminal fluid* in Man, and the *Ovae* in Woman,
and its composition is also very similar.

In all probability, the same vital effort which calls forth
the Generative Elements also creates, at the same time,
the Nervous substance. Whenever therefore the produc
tion, or nutrition, of the one is imperfect, so is that of the
other. There is therefore not only a close sympathy, but
a real coincidence of origin, and mutual dependence of
existence between these two most mysterious portions of
our being. The Brain and the Sexual Apparatus are
placed at the opposite extremities of the body, like the
two poles of a Galvanic Pile, each being connected with
the Spinal marrow, which unite them. When one of
these Poles is overcharged with vital power, the other is

undercharged, and when one is exhausted the other is soon in the same condition.*

This explains at once why excessive mental exertion is often followed by Sexual importance, and why, on the contrary, Sexual abuse so frequently destroys the intellect. Softening of the Brain is caused by an actual deficiency of some of the substances composing it, and these substances are precisely those that are carried off by the Seminal discharge. When a man expends too much Semen therefore he does the same thing as if he really destroyed a portion of his brain, because he takes away that which is necessary to nutrify it. Nature will not produce enough of these substances to make Brain and to allow of licentious indulgence at the same time. In this way arises softening, or chronic decay of the Brain, a disease which may be very slow in its progress, but every step of which weakens the intellect more and more, and which eventually causes either death or idiocy.

It is not wilful Licentiousness alone however which leads to softening of the Brain, but more frequently it arises from Urinary Spermattorrhœa, or loss of Semen in the urine. This is a most destructive and insidious disease, but little known to Medical men, and almost totally unsuspected by the people at large, numbers of whom are its daily victims. The first, and only full account of this disease, in the English Language, was given in Dr. Hollick's Treatise on "The Male Generative Organs," to which the reader is referred for fuller particulars.

In treating softening of the Brain, or the Sexual difficulties from which it arises, it will readily be seen that quite a different course is required from that which is pursued in other diseases. It is not only necessary to arrest the Nervous decay, and Seminal loss, but also to supply such substances as will make more new brain, or new Generative elements, and this none of the ordinary Medicaments will do. There are but few things in fact that are suitable for this purpose, and it requires an accurate knowledge of their real properties, and of the true Chemical composition of the Nervous and Seminal matters, to know

* See Frontispiece.

how to properly combine and apply them. The ordinary *Cordials*, and *Invigorators*, are mere excitants, or stimulants as elsewhere explained, and only excite for a time the little Nervous or Generative matter that is left, but do not stop its decay, nor cause a new production of it.

The effects of softening of the Brain are worse even than those which follow from Urinary loss of Semen, because they effect more generally, and quickly, the whole system. It is also a more hopeless disease than Spermattorrhœa, unless taken very early. Its extent cannot always be judged of however by the apparent effects, as some patients will suffer much from the first, while the Disease is but slight, and others will hold up for a considerable time against it till they give way at once.

The condition of a person suffering from Softening of the Brain is, in the main, much like that of one suffering from confirmed Spermattorrhœa, and it requires careful Microscopical examinations to tell which of the two troubles is being experienced, or if both exist together. Usually however there is more *mental imbecility* in Softening of the Brain, with a greater *change of character*. The patient *feels* that his *mind* is passing away. He *cannot think clearly*, and has a sensation as if his head were really *empty*, and as if he would like every moment to close his eyes and *go off!* There is no possibility of *rousing* a man in this state, nor of doing him good in any way, till the waste of the Brain is arrested and the process of renovation recommences.

Many patients remark, after their recovery, that they used literally to *lose themselves*. and forget *who* and *where* they were. One Gentleman assured me that on waking in the morning he would frequently be half an hour or more, before he could make out who he was, and what he should do. It would partly come in his mind and then go out again, till he got some *stimulant*, and then, for a time, he would gradually come round. The fact was, that his ideas were previously only *half formed*, and imperfect, owing to the imperfect condition of his Brain. He could no more *think* perfectly than a man can labor hard who has weakened muscles.

NERVOUSNESS.

It is scarcely necessary to remark that Nervousness is very general, and spoken of as something which all people are supposed to be acquainted with, but still it is something which no one can describe or define. The term *Nervous* is applied to such a variety of bodily and mental derangements, combined so differently in different people, that it is scarcely possible to find two nervous people whose experience is the same. This however, need not surprise us, when we reflect upon the functions of the nervous system, and its associations with every part of the organization. Itself the source of all organic power, upon which every part depends, and by which alone the whole is maintained in action, it cannot experience the slightest derangement without affecting all that is dependent upon it. If the integrity of the Brain and Spinal Marrow be impaired, we not only experience mental imbecility, or moral perversity, but derangement of the Vital organs also, though in their *structure* they may be apparently as perfect as we could wish.

Even a slight affection of the great Nervous centres causes *sympathetic* derangement of everything else, which is the reason why *nervous people* suffer from such a complication of symptoms, without perhaps having a single organic disease they suffer the peculiar effects of almost every disease known. Once correct the vitiated condition of the Nervous System in these cases, and all the symptoms vanish at once, so that the patient passes in a single day almost from the extremest misery to well ·being and happiness. Uninformed people either ridicule such cases, or else attribute them to mere deception or wilfulness, but those who know their nature look upon them as among the most interesting that can be met with, and eminently deserving of true sympathy.

A deranged condition of the Nervous system arises either from actual decay or change, in the Nervous matter itself, as in *Softening of the Brain*, or else from sympathetic irritation, as in various derangements of the Sexual Organs. In fact the nervous system becomes deranged through the influence of other parts in nearly every instance, and seldom suffers from any disease originating within itself. In the majority of cases *Sexual* derangement precedes or accompanies *nervous* derangement, and must be corrected before the Nervousness can be overcome.

In Nervous *females* the Womb, or Ovaries are affected, and in Nervous *men* the Testes or Prostate Gland, almost invariably, and to those who are acquainted with the Physiology and connections of these different parts of our organization, this mutual action and reaction will be no mystery. Those who have not yet become acquainted with these matters are referred for a full explanation, to *the Marriage Guide.*

The great misfortune for Nervous people is, that they are seldom treated for the disease under which they really labor, but only for the *secondary* derangements to which it has given rise. The *effects* only being observed, while the *cause* remains unnoticed. This is owing to the general inattention among medical men, of all matters relating to Sexual Physiology and sympathy. Now for instance, a female will have chronic irritation of the Womb, or Ovaries, giving rise to the most curious train of nervous derangements and symptoms, and will be treated with the utmost skill as a *Nervous Patient*, without the slightest benefit, but once remove the Ovarian or Uterine irritation and the *Nervousness* ceases at once. Numbers of men also lose their judgment, and memory, and become wretched to the last degree, from Urinary loss of Semen, which must be stopped before any assistance can be rendered to them.

Severe Sexual derangement will even cause actual *wasting* of the nervous substance, as before experienced; and on the other hand any serious disease, or exhaustion, of the nervous system, reacts upon the Sexual organs and deranges them. In the *great majority of cases* however, the Generative Organs are the first to become impaired, and the Nervous system follows, in both sexes.

The intimate mutual relation of the Nervous and Sexual systems will be made more evident by an inspection of the Plate of the *"Nervous and Sexual Centres."*

The Brain is composed of two perfectly distinct halves, either of which may act, or become diseased, without the concurrence of the other,— the same as either Testicle or Ovary may act perfectly, or become diseased, independently of any action, or affection of the other.

The *Testicles* in the Male, and the *Ovaries* in the Females, are precisely similar, both in their organic functions and in their symathetic relations. In fact they are identical in every respect, in the earlier stages of development. The Testicles are merely more fully developed Ovaries, in the same way that all the Organs of the Male Generative system are merely more perfect developments of corresponding parts in the female.

The two Sexual Centres, and the two Nervous Centres, stand to each other in the relation of *Electric Poles*, being Positive and Negative reciprocally. If an undue amount of power be concentrated, or expended in a Sexual Centre, the opposing Nervous Centre must be proportionably deficient in power, and on the contrary, if the Nervous Centre be over excited the opposing Sexual Centre must become torpid.

This will make the true nature of all cases of Sexual or Nervous derangement evident, and will also show the reason why all past treatment of them has been so useless. Dr. Hollick has found out, from his experience, that all the old ideas on these subjects were fallacious, and he has been compelled to study out the true explanation of them from actual observation and experiments. These views therefore are entirely new, and are now for the first time laid before the public. In a short time they will be more fully elucidated in a work which Dr. H. is now writing exclusively upon the Nervous system.

PERFECT RECOVERY FROM IMPOTENCE,

BROUGHT ON BY EXCESSES.

In this case we have an example of a very large class Persons naturally of *powerful Sexual Organizations*, capable, in the first vigor of virile power, of the most continuous and exalted enjoyment, but, *from ignorance alone,* becoming *dispirited, debilitated,* and *impotent.* It also shows that, in even the worst of such cases, it is generally possible, *by the use of proper remedies,* to recover most of what had been lost, and to *rejuvenate* the Sexual Organs after their functions are thought to be entirely extinct.

The individual living at a distance communicated with me by the following Letter.

————

To Dr. Hollick,
       New York City, N. Y.

" My dear Sir,

A fortunate chance having thrown in my way your Invaluable and unique Book on " The Male Generative Organs," I have determined to address you in regard to my case, feeling fully assured that if any mortal man can assist me it is you.

Not to lose time, or to occupy you unnecessarily, I will make my statement as brief as possible.

I was born in affluent circumstances, well brought up, and well educated, and at twenty-one years of age found myself the uncontrolled master of quite a respectable income, and in the enjoyment of a large circle of friends and acquaintances. I had never been much addicted to the usual vice of young people. *Masturbation,* though constantly in the midst of it, neither had I ever been intemperate, and at twenty-one I was healthy, full of animal spirits, and capable of the most perfect physical enjoyment. About my eighteenth year, my Sexual desires became very strong, but my position and prudential considerations, prevented me from running into excesses. Besides this I looked forward to my majority as a time when I could indulge as I should wish, without any control, and thus repay myself for past restraint.

Had it not been for my Guardian I should have married as soon as I was of age, and had I done so it would have saved me incredible suffering, and a broken down constitution. He however, dissuaded me from it from *pecuniary* motives, and ignorantly sacrificed my health and happiness to filthy lucre.

I formed several attachments of an illicit character, and being led away by my powerful Sexual propensities, I indulged to excess. How much I need not perhaps specify, but suffice it to say, that till my twenty-fifth year it was almost my sole occupation, and till that period I felt no diminution of power, but soon afterwards my *appetite* for these indulgences began to lessen, and by degrees my *powers* also. I had neither desire nor capability so often as before, and frequently for a considerable period would be totally indifferent. This falling off in my Sexual powers was also followed by a lassitude and debility, both bodily and mental, which unfitted me for any active exertion whatever. I became dull, listless, peevish or morose, my appetite failed me, and all the symptoms of confirmed dyspepsia set in. My condition in fact became so bad that I consulted a Physician, but only about my general health, for I dared not then speak on other matters He gave me directions as to my diet, and directed some Tonics, with cold bathing. These did me some good, for a time, but I rapidly fell off again, and became worse than before, especially *Sexually*. In fact I was nearly Impotent, and in my despair I resorted to many of the *Cordials* and *Antidotes* which I saw advertised, in the hopes that they would restore me. Some of them did stimulate me for a time, and I began to hope I was going to recover, but alas it was soon over, and I felt that I was worse than before, and that my general health had also been much injured by these remedies. I then gave up all hope nearly, and came to the melancholy conclusion that I must drag out a short-lived miserable existence in the best way I could. This has continued till now, my twenty-ninth year, when a gleam of hope has been awakened by perusing your book.

Now Doctor I want you to deal candidly and honestly with me, and tell me plainly if a person in my situation has *any prospect* of *recovery?* I don't wish to be deceived, and would rather know the worst at once.

I will tell you plainly, I am as nearly Impotent as man can be, not being capable of Sexual communion more than once in two or three months, and that in the most imperfect manner, with no enjoyment, and scarcely with any Seminal flow at all. My Organs are wasted, and my desires for the other sex are almost extinct—in fact I am becoming *a woman hater!* Of my state of mind I can scarcely trust myself to speak. Doctor, I am perhaps the most utterly wretched being that lives! I sit and mope for hours together, with the most gloomy images crowding upon me, and black despair hovering over all. Fearful apprehensions constantly haunt me of some impending evil, and I distrust every one who comes near me. This I know is wrong ; but *I cannot help it!* A dark cloud seems constantly weighing upon me, and casting a gloom on all my thoughts. Reason I cannot, for my judgment and memory are nearly gone, and my mind is not under my control.

Of my bodily sufferings I will not now speak, though they are severe enough I can assure you. Suffice it to say here, that my system is thoroughly debilitated and run down, and that scarcely a single function is perfectly performed.

Doctor, I am a mere *wreck*, and I fear too much broken and shattered to be ever repaired. Perhaps I am only showing my imbecility by indulging even in a hope, but I could not resist the impulse to address you. Had I read your book, Doctor, when I was twenty-one, oh what might I not have been. It maddens me to think how terribly I have paid for my ignorance. But I must now stop. I have written this, Doctor, under the influence of stimulants, I confess it to my further shame, but I could not have made the effort without. The effect of the stimulant

Is now passing away, and oh the sinking which I feel coming on is horrible to think of,—but it is done, I have written to you, Doctor, and earnestly pray you will speedily reply. Tell me if it be *possible* for me to be *helped*, I will not dare to say *recovered*, and if you will take me under your care. The expectation of your answer will somewhat buoy me up till I hear from you,—but what this answer may do I dare not even imagine. Write soon, Doctor, and let me known my doom.

" Yours, despairingly,

— —— ——.."

On receipt of this Letter, I at once wrote for him to come to see me, as I considered a personal interview desirable. On his arrival, I certainly found as unpromising a case as could be well imagined, but still I did not despair, and without making any definite promise I agreed to advise him.

In conjunction with appropriate general treatment, I commenced giving him the Aphrodisiac Remedy, and carefully watched the result.

In a short time it became evident that he was recovering, and I gave him leave to return home, having first arranged to correspond with him regularly, and supply him with the Medicine.

In *six months* he was so much restored that no further treatment seemed called for, and I requested him to send me a full account of his condition at that time, to put on record, as a contrast to his first statement. The following is what I received :

To Dr. Hollick, New York.

" MY DEAR SIR,

" According to your request I send you a report of my present situation, as I feel I ought to do, if it will be either useful or interesting, for there is nothing, it seems to me, which I can do for you but what gratitude calls on me to do. I merely request that if you make use of my

Letter it will be in such a way that no one who knows me can recognize them.

I am now, my dear sir, I verily believe, *the happiest man living!* I am quite well in health, in every way, my mind is clear, my spirits buoyant, and my strength greater than I have ever known it before! In fact, I am quite *gay,* and instead of moping at home, as I used to do, afraid to see any one, and thinking life a burden, I am constantly on foot, whistling, or singing, as I used to do when a boy My friends wonder what has happened, and can scarcely think it is really me. I dare not tell them the cause of my happy change however, because it would expose the secret of my former misery, and that I could not bear.

The greatest change however, is in my *Sexual Organs,* whose functions I had thought lost. I am now *nearly as powerful as ever I was,* and am evidently gaining still, every day. In fact, I intend, if you think it proper, to *marry,* which at one time I never dared to look forward to! It is now the dream of my life, and if you give me leave, it seems to me there is little else I can ask for. Please be plain on this point, and tell me candidly if I may, and how soon?

That Medicine of yours seems almost magical, and I wonder you do not make it generally known. The good effects of it were manifested on me *the third dose,* and so convinced did I feel of its good effect that I would have given *all I was worth in the world* for sufficient of it, if that had been necessary! You must, if you can, let me have some to keep by me. The cost is no object. I have not taken any for the last two weeks, because I felt powerful enough.

How evident it now is to me, as you explained, that all my other troubles arose from decay and derangement of my Sexual Organs. Immediately they began to improve. and gain strength, I became better in every way, just in the same proportion. How silly the practice now seems of giving tonics and stimulants for the Stomach, or Liver, to try and cure them, while the sole cause of all their disease is left untouched.

In conclusion, my dear sir, I am a perfectly *well man,*

and I firmly believe that your advice and medicine would make any one so.

May you enjoy as much happiness as I do. I cannot wish you better,—and may I be able to show myself as grateful to you as I ought and wish to be.

"Yours, ever truly,

———— ————."

Being satisfied that he might marry with propriety, I gave him leave to do so, and he is now the happy *Father* of two healthy children, and younger by *Ten Years* than when I first saw him !

This case I have been more particular in describing, in detail, because it is a good example of a large class that come under my care, nearly all of whom are equally benefitted by the same means.

———— ✦✦ ————

RESUSCITATION OF THE SEXUAL POWER

IN AN OLD MAN.

THIS individual was aged *sixty-six* when he called on me, and had been for some three or four years almost entirely *Impotent.* In fact, he had begun to think that his powers were really gone, from *age,* and he scarcely ever thought of their being in any degree restored. His health was very good. and his years had evidently affected him but little in other ways, which made him sometimes wonder why he should fall off in this respect alone, and disposed him to ask my opinion.

I told him without any hesitation, that proper treatment would act favorably upon him, out I could not judge to what extent. He accordingly commenced following my advice, and in three months afterwards sent me the following Letter

To Dr. Hollick,
New York City, N. Y.

" My dear Sir,

" I wish you to send me a fresh supply of the Apho-
disiac Remedy. I still have some, but wish to be sure of
not getting short.

In regard to the *effect* of your treatment, it has worked
a real miracle ! I am almost as young, in one way at
least, as I was at *Forty*, and I assure you that were I not
prudent, I might easily be led into some folly. What surprises me most however, is my not suffering in any way
from my indulgences. I was somewhat afraid, when my
powers were first revived, of using them, for fear it might
do me an injury, but incredible as it may appear, I feel no
ill effects whatever afterwards. In fact, I feel less lassitude after Sexual indulgence than I used to do, and it
seems as if my organs were really stronger.

To say how much my happiness has been increased, and
how much I feel indebted to you, is unnecessary.

" Yours, truly,

————— —————." "

I'his old man I knew when he was past *seventy-two,*
and there was then no indication of decay in his powers.
He merely required to take a little of the remedy occasionally, and decay seemed totally arrested. I have known
some instances of even older persons being much benefitted in a similar manner.

- ———•••———

BARRENNESS IN A FEMALE

OF THIRTY-SIX, CURED.

In many instances Barrenness is caused simply by a
torpid condition of the Genital Organs, which prevents

the absorption of the Seminal fluid, as explained in my "*Marriage Guide.*" The Lady referred to was an in stance of this kind, and the result shows the power of the Aphrodisiac Remedy alone, in such cases. Her husband had obtained some of the remedy from me without saying definitely for what purpose he wished it; the Letter will tell why.

＜　———

DR. HOLLICK, *New York*.

" DEAR SIR,

" You will recollect probably that I requested you, as a personal favor, to let me have some of your Aphrodisiac Remedy. I will now tell you what I wished it for, and what has resulted from its use.

I had been married nearly Twelve years, and with no prospects of being blessed as a Father, when I read your book, " *The Marriage Guide.*" The perusal of that work led me to think that our childless condition was owing to my Lady's extreme *indifference*, she having always been perfectly cold in her temperament, and I thought possibly your remedy might change this, and cause her to conceive. I accordingly procured some from you and she agreed to take it.

The effect has been as surprising as satisfactory. I need only say, that she is *entirely changed in her temperament*, and is now, our Doctor tells us, *five month's Pregnant*, for the first time !

If any one had told me before this, that any remedy could effect such a change I should have laughed at them, but such is the fact, and I inform you of it because I know it will both interest and please you, and because I think you are justly entitled to know what your remedy has d ne. I advise all my childless friends to read your ' *Marriage Guide.*"

" Yours, truly,

———　———.＂

GREAT LOSS OF SEXUAL POWER,

AND SEVERE NERVOUS DERANGEMENT IN A MERCHANT CURED.

This Gentleman, like a great many more of his class, had completely exhausted his nervous power by intense application to business. He had *made* his fortune and *lost* his health. The following is a part of the incoherent Letter he first addressed me.

To Dr. Hollick, *New York.*

" My dear Sir,

" Will you be so kind as to tell me at once, if you can do me any good? I am a Merchant, age forty-one. Good constitution naturally, fully grown, and formerly of excellent health.

About seven years ago I began my present business, which required me to exert all my energies, and to apply myself unremittingly. For the first two or three years I held out well, but gradually my energy began to fail, my digestion became disordered, and I felt miserably weak, low-spirited, and dejected. In fact, I became a perfect hypo, and had I not been blessed with a good and trustworthy agent, my business must have utterly failed, for I could not, during half my time, pay proper attention to it.

I found it utterly impossible to apply myself regularly or to stick to anything,—my mind wandered away in spite of me, and the smallest forcing of attention to any thing threw me into utter confusion.

For the last two years this has been much worse, and now I have many bodily ailings too. I cannot sleep well and wake in the morning with difficulty, and feeling as I

I had been intoxicated the night before, which I never am.

Besides all this, I find myself *Sexually Impotent.* My powers have been getting less for the past three years, and are now almost extinct. In fact I have a repugnance to the association, and am utterly incapable either of giving or of receiving enjoyment.

Doctor, I cannot say more,—this has required great effort, and I feel weary. Your experience will probably show you exactly how I am, in all that is not here told Try what you can do for a wretched debilitated man, to whom money is no more than the dirt under his feet if he can but get well. Tell me at once if you can help me.

"Yours, &c.,

———— ————."

I made no hesitation in promising this Gentleman that he could be helped, providing he could fully relax from his business. This he did effectually, by selling out, and investing his money.

He commenced at once using the Aphrodisiac Remedy, and observing proper rules of *regimen* and *diet* which I gave him. In two months he was a new man, and by the fourth month he wrote me a Letter from the country of which the following is an abstract.

———

* * * "Doctor, I don't need you any longer now, nor do I think I ever shall again, if you will only let me always have some of that Medicine by me. Don't think this ungenerous. I mean it to be *complimentary.* From the very first dose *I felt* it would cure me. It seemed to *satisfy* as it were, my nervous system, like food does a *hungry stomach.* All my anxiety and apprehension left me, I felt calm, cheerful, able to apply myself, and disposed to be active. My mind cleared up as if the sun had suddenly broke in upon it, and I began to digest so heartily that I gained flesh rapidly.

My *Sexual powers* also are *fully restored !* I need say no more on this point, except to assure you that your

caution as to being *temperate* shall be faithfully observed,
though I am free to confess *it requires an effort now!*

How many of my brother business men lose their health
and powers in the way I did,—but how few of them
are so fortunate as I have been in restoration. Doctor, you must try to announce that remedy publicly.
Why, my dear sir, it would save many a man from ruin,
and not a few from insanity and suicide, to say nothing
of mere suffering and imbecility. So far I have said nothing about it, as you requested, though I have often been
sorely tempted to do so when seeing an old friend suffering, and hearing him demand—*'what makes you look so
well?'*

Please accept the enclosed in addition to your account.
I can never repay you, for I verily believe had I not met
with you I should not now have been alive."

* * *

NOTE.—I do not wish it to be supposed that a similar
result would follow in *all* apparently similar cases, by
simply following the same course. In many instances
there are other matters to be attended to, and other derangements to be corrected, before the remedy can act
This was a case of simple Seminal and Nervous exhaustion uncomplicated.

CURE OF SEXUAL IMPOTENCE

AND INDIFFERENCE, IN CUBA.

SOME two years ago, a Gentleman from Cuba called
upon me to see if I could render him any assistance. He
was only thirty-five years old, but *quite Impotent*, and altogether indifferent to the other sex. He had been *originally* of an unusually warm temperament, and had indulged

to excess, till his powers became so exhausted that he could do so no longer. His general health had held out pretty well. though latterly it had begun to fail, and he suffered from severe attacks of nervous depression.

His desire for a restoration of his Sexual powers was so great, that nothing seemed too dear to pay for it,—indeed he assured me he would not care to *live* as he was. Unfortunately, before I saw him, he had injured himself by taking a stimulating *Cordial*, which he saw advertised. and I had in the first place to overcome the ill effects of that. I then commenced treating him, and in less than a month he experienced such evident indications of restoration that he arranged to return home, taking sufficient of the Aphrodisiac Remedy with him to perfect the cure.

He also begged me to let him have a little besides to try the effect alone, on some of his companions, who were like he had been. The following Letter shows the result.

To Dr. Hollick, *New York*

" DEAR DOCTOR,

" I send this by the Brig ———, just to say that I am now as good as ever, and am too busy *enjoying myself* to write much. You know I have much *lost time* to make up for.

The medicine I brought here, except what I wanted for myself, I gave to several Gentlemen about here, whom I knew to be in want of it, and it has been *fully successful in every case!*

This has made a most extraordinary sensation about here, and I am almost worried to death by others. In fact, I have often regretted giving any away, and to save me in future you must really send some more. I could sell any amount for you, if you wish to sell it. Some of *my patients* have been known hereabouts as perfect *Impotents* for many years, and their *resurrection* is regarded as little less than a miracle. Some of their unexpected *gal*

azure. are most amusing, but I am afraid that in the ex
uberance of our new-born strength we shall be apt to
need your services again. It is hard to *restrain* ones-self
when all seems to prompt to indulgence, in spite of your
caution. To give you an idea of how I am now, I will
give you an account of one of my Adventures.

*   *   *

REMARKABLE CURE OF IMPOTENCY

AT NEW ORLEANS CURED

This Patient, like numerous other high spirited and im
petuous young Southerners, had thoughtlessly delivered
himself to unrestrained Sexual indulgences, till he had become completely exhausted and powerless. In this predicament he was strongly urged by his friends to marry,
as a most advantageous opportunity of doing so presented itself, and they knew no reason why he should not.
He was also extremely desirous of forming the Union, the
young Lady and he having become ardently attached to
each other, but alas, his condition forbade it. He thus
wrote to me, in describing his case.

---

*   *   *   *   " Sexual Union is scarcely possible at all
At times I have imperfect indications of power, but they
never come when I will them, and they disappear in spite
of all my efforts to perpetuate them. Oh! how mortified
I have been at my vain attempts with females lately, and
how wretched I have felt at the thoughts that it must always be so. Doctor, I cannot live in this way,—I don't
care to do so. And then in regard to this proposed marriage, what can I do, what can I say, how can I possibly
excuse myself? Oh Doctor, this is misery indeed,—help
me and name your reward."

*   *   *

After being treated for *six weeks* he felt so far restored as to arrange for his marriage, and in *three months* from the time of his first consulting me that event took place. He then wrote to me another Letter, from which I extract the following.

———

* * * * " All my fears are dissipated, I have no apprehensions as to the future, and feel myself *in every way* as capable as I could desire, and much more so than I deserve to be perhaps. No *failures* have occurred, nor have I any reason to dread them in future. In fact, it is rather *restraint* that I need now! Doctor, what is that you gave me? By Jove its effects are scarcely credible, and I certainly should be skeptical about them had I not experienced them in my own person. But for that, I should now have either been dead or a poor miserable wretch, instead of the healthy happy *husband* I am. There are thousands in this part of the country who need such a remedy, and who would give their own weight in Gold for it." * * *

———•••———

●

CURIOUS CASE OF LOSS OF SEXUAL POWER

IN A MARRIED MAN, CURED.

This was one of those curious cases occasionally met with, in which the Sexual power suddenly fails a man without any previous warning, and from no very obvious cause.

The individual was forty years of age, had been married fifteen years, and had four children. His health was good, his habits regular, and his Sexual powers naturally quite strong. He had never been addicted to Sexual excesses at any period of life, and had never felt symptoms of decay come on.

All at once he found himself quite indifferent to the

caresses of his partner, and quite incapable of Sexual association. To use his own expression " the parts seemed *dead*, and utterly refused to perform their office." His alarm and mortification at this unexpected occurrence may be conceived, and the most gloomy apprehensions took possession of his mind. He not only thought that his Sexual powers were totally and unaccountably gone, but c also feared that it was only the beginning of complete bodily decay, and visions of premature old age and death loomed fearfully before him. Matters were also made much worse by the fact of his partner being naturally of a warm temperament, and of course chagrined at his impotent condition. Under such circumstances unpleasant surmises arose in her mind as to *the cause* of his indifference, which he was unable to dispel, and thus both were made wretched.

In this condition he sought me, and I commenced the investigation of his case. From his statement however, I could discover no very obvious cause for his sudden deficiency, and therefore concluded that it arose from want of sufficient *Seminal and Nervous Nutrition*, brought about by some unusual combination of circumstances. The Aphrodisiac Remedy was therefore given to him, with proper general advice, and with full confidence, on my part, as to the result, though he felt sorrowfully dubious.

After the third day, he felt *certain* that his powers were returning, and in two weeks, to use his own remark, he was " *a man again!*" It is now several years since this occurrence, and he still retains his usual vigor, though occasionally requiring a few doses of the Remedy, as he says, to keep him *quite right*.

' But for proper treatment he would have remained perfectly impotent, and his general health would soon have decayed also.

A CASE OF INVOLUNTARY, AND INSTAN-TANEOUS SEMINAL EMISSION,

WHICH HAD ALWAYS EXISTED, FULLY CURED.

THIS individual was a perfect Type of thousands of men that are daily to be met with. In his youth he had been much addicted to *Masturbation*, and in consequence, his Sexual Organs, and Sensibilities, were so preternaturally irritable, that Sexual union was utterly impossible. He had a plentiful *seminal secretion*, but the slightest attempt at connection, or even thinking about it at times, brought on *immediate emission*, so that he was in reality powerless, and had always been so. He had taken I believe every *Cordial* and *Tonic* that was advertised, but all to no purpose, and scarcely a hope of relief seemed left.

By some accident he fell in with the "*Marriage Guide*." and that induced him to seek me

The first thing I did was to *Cauterize* him, as explained in my book on "*The Male Organs*," and that at once stopped the *involuntary* emissions, but still any attempt at connection brought them on *too soon*, so that the act could not be consummated. For this trouble I gave him the Aphrodisiac Remedy, to *Nutrify* and *Tone* the parts, and improve the *quality of the Seminal fluid*.

The most perfect success followed this course, and in a short time his powers of *retention* were perfect, so that he married, and is now a father.

This trouble, of *too quick emission*, is very common, and is both annoying and hurtful, for it is sure eventually to bring on involuntary emission. I have never known a case that was not cured in this way.

HABITUAL AND SUDDEN CESSATION OF SEXUAL POWER, CURED.

THIS case was very curious, though not uncommon, in certain degrees. The patient was a vigorous, and healthy *sexually*, as any man, and *when alone*, his *feelings*, and *desires*, and the *development of his Organs*, were perfect, but always on attempting connection he became *powerless*, and without seminal loss! *Afterwards* he would become as perfect as he was before, but never could remain so *at the proper time*.

After taking the Aphrodisiac Remedy for *six weeks*, with general treatment, his condition improved so much that for the *first time* in his life his powers were *fully manifested*. The trouble however had existed so long, and had become so fully established that he is compelled even now, to use a little of the remedy at times.

Many men are troubled in this way, more or less, and I believe all may be completely relieved, unless too far advanced in life.

———•••———.

DISTRESSING CASE OF INABILITY AT THE

TIME OF MARRIAGE, CURED.

In this instance a young man found himself, at the time of 'his' marriage, perfectly impotent from inability to retain the Seminal fluid,—the emission occuring always on the instant of his making an attempt. His shame and despair may be imagined, and I verily believe that nothing saved him from committing *suicide* but the fact that he had read my book on the *Male Organs*, and thought that I could help him.

I advised him to feign sickness for a time, as a reason for his situation, while he underwent proper treatment. This he did, and before *two weeks* the difficulty was over and has never returned since

MISCELLANEOUS CASES.

BESIDES those aboved describe, and which are only specimens of hundreds which could be given, of the same kinds. There are numerous others of a different character, and which can only be perfectly understood by persons acquainted with the Physiology of Generation. Those persons who have read my " *Marriage Guide* "—or the " *Male Organs,*" will understand this at once, and will perceive that many of these cases are the most interesting of all that can come under a Physician's notice.

There are some men impotent because their Testes form no *Semen*, not having become *torpid*. Others form it but of an imperfect kind,—watery, and *without Animalcules*. In some men again, there is a peculiar loss of *Nervous sensibility* in the Organs, owing to which there is no *proper feeling*, and though there may be *desire* yet there is neither *enjoyment* nor efficient *capability*.

In the same manner, Females are often *sterile* from causes but little known or suspected. The *Ovaries* may be *torpid* the same as the Male Testes, and then they form no *Ova*, or *Eggs*, and sometimes these are formed, but *imperfectly*. In this case, they either cannot be impregnated or else they germinate into *monstrosities*, as shown in " *The Marriage Guide.*"

In the greater part of such cases, the Aphrodisiac Remedy, conjoined with proper treatment, usually effects a cure, unless there be virulent disease, or organic defect.

Numbers of *childless couples*, who have called on me, have had their dearest wishes fulfilled, who otherwise would have had no hope whatever. In such cases however, it is necessary first, to know *in which party is the deficiency* and this can always be told, by a careful consultation.

The beneficial effects of similar treatment have also been equally apparent in numerous cases of the most distressing NERVOUS DEBILITY and *Irritability!* In these the Aphrodisiac Remedy acts in the most beneficial manner, soothing the *excitable*, giving strength to the *debilitated*, and new power to the *imbecile*.

Many men, unable to attend to their business, from *Nervous Debility*, have been completely cured in a very short time, and others have had their mental powers so much improved as to be much more capable than ever they were before. The common expression of these men is, that their minds seem " *to clear up*," or " *brighten*," so that mental labor is a pleasure instead of a burden, and application does not distress them.

DR. HOLLICK'S

APHRODISIAC REMEDY,

THE ONLY SURE AND RELIABLE AGENT

FOR THE

PERMANENT CURE OF

IMPOTENCE, STERILITY,

AND

NERVOUS AND SEXUAL DEBILITY,

IN EVERY FORM;

BEING THE CELEBRATED REMEDY USED FOR SO MANY YEARS IN

DR. HOLLICK'S EXTENSIVE PRACTICE,

DEVOTED EXCLUSIVELY TO SUCH CASES, AND NOW FOR THE FIRST TIME, OFFERED

TO THE

PUBLIC.

GENERAL DESCRIPTION OF APHRODISIACS,

AND HISTORY OF

DR. HOLLICK'S APHRODISIAC REMEDIES

MEDICAL REMEDIES are classified and named according to the mode in which they act. Some affect one part of the system, and others affect other parts. Those which act upon the sexual organs, so as to preserve or restore their powers, are called APHRODISIACS. Remedies of this kind have always been eagerly sought, and paid for at any price: even gold itself has not been more eagerly prized, and at this hour will be given in profusion for a good Aphrodisiac, though begrudged for anything else—for nothing does a man more crave than sexual power, and nothing does he more fear or regret to lose.

Numerous remedies, called Aphrodisiacs, have been in use in different parts of the world, for ages past, with more or less repute; but their employment never resulted in much good and often in much positive injury. It is the same at the present day—the greater part of such remedies now in use have no effect at all, and those which do act had better be left alone. This arises from the fact that they are administered only empirically, and without any knowledge of their true powers or of their variable effects under different circumstances.

When I first began to use the common remedies of this kind. I found that they were, for the most part, only traditional compounds, often dating back to the dark ages, and given merely because the physician did not know what else to give. Some of them, it is true, acted as powerful *stimulants*, giving temporary power

at the cost of future debility, but the greater part were
either utterly inoperative or else acted only on other
parts of the system : in short, they were *not* Aphrodisiacs!

I, therefore, set to work to investigate the whole
subject of man's sexual nature, and the action of all
Aphrodisiac Remedies upon it, for myself. For years I
experimented with them, in thousands of cases, both
simply and variously combined, carefully noting their
effects, and thus by degrees finding out the true value
of each, and how and when to use it. No one else, I
really believe, ever went into this subject so thoroughly, or with such extensive opportunities for experiment
and investigation. My lectures and my books made
me so universally known in connection with this subject, that cases of every kind came to me in abund-
ance, from all parts, and I was thus enabled to study
practically what had been before only speculated
upon.

The result was, after endless trials, the formation
of a compound possessing TRUE APHRODISIAC POWERS!
which, when judiciously employed, invariably increases
and maintains sexual power, or restores it when lost.
This remedy, from its constant success in all cases of
impotence, sterility and natural deficiency, became
very celebrated, and my practice—which comprised
only such cases—rapidly extended. Every day the
demand for my Aphrodisiac increased, and I soon
found a difficulty in procuring enough for my professional use, on account of the limited supply and great
cost of many of the ingredients.

Many of the most powerful and reliable Aphro
disiacs are among the rarest of Nature's products, and
are obtained only from the least known and most inac-
cessible parts of the world ; MUSK, for instance, which
is a powerful Aphrodisiac, and of which I use a large
quantity, is always *worth its weight in gold*, and often
much more. There are, however, other substances
still more valuable, for which I have often given hundreds of dollars for a few grains. Some of these are

natural and some artificial products, obtained by chemical means, and which can be produced only at immense cost. The great power of most of these articles fortunately makes a small portion go a long way in use, or they could scarcely be employed at all. In my Remedy, there are altogether *thirty-three* different ingredients, and of some of them not more than *the hundredth part of a grain* can be used at a dose. Each of these ingredients has some peculiar power of its own, or is necessary to the full development of the power of some other ingredient, so that the whole act together in producing that wonderful effect for which this Remedy is so celebrated.

At the same time, however, that it acts so energetically as an Aphrodisiac, it has no effect in any other way, and is perfectly harmless to all parts of the system.

It will be readily seen that such a remedy must necessarily be costly, and can never come into common use : it must, in fact, ever remain a special luxury for those who have been favored with Fortune's golden gifts, or for those who are willing to make great sacrifices. As a natural consequence, my constantly increasing demand for these rare articles made them still more scarce and dear, till, finally, I began to fear that my supply would run short ; I, therefore, sent agents to all those parts from which they are obtained, with instructions to regularly buy up and pre-engage all that could be procured. This, of course, took a long time to accomplish and entailed an enormous expense, but it was the only sure course, and was crowned with success. A supply has thus been ensured, which enables me not only to provide all my patients with sufficient, but also leaves a surplus, so that I can now prepare the Remedy FOR PUBLIC SALE, as I have constantly been importuned to do, but for the reasons given was unable to do previously.

In this way originated the Aphrodisiac Remedy, the most remarkable medicine perhaps ever compounded, and the most wonderful in its effects. No advertising, or other means for disposing of it, are necessary, for its value is so well known that the difficulty will rather be in supplying all who want it Numbers of my patients always keep as much by them as I can spare to one person, for fear of running short, and many of them would give thousands of dollars rather than run any risk of ever being without it.

As regards the obtaining of this Remedy, or any similar one, I may as well remark here that no one else but myself can possibly supply it! Not only because the proportions of the various articles comprising it, and the manner of combining them, is a secret only known to myself, but because the whole quantity pro duced, of many of the most valuable articles, is in my hands, or secured to me alone, by always paying large sums in advance, so that no one else can obtain a grain. This I was compelled to do in order to secure a sufficient supply, and to make sure that my patients would not be disappointed. Many of the artificial products are not made for public sale, and, to obtain them, I am obliged to purchase all that certain skillful chemists can produce, and at a rate, too, which offers inducement enough to them to keep up the manufacture for me alone : besides this, some of the articles are made by myself, by a process which I have never disclosed.

It is, therefore, impossible for any one else to supply a true Aphrodisiac Remedy, containing the rarest and most effective agents, because no one else can obtain them. All other Aphrodisiacs can be formed only of the more common and inefficient remedies, such as are to be found in most apothecaries' shops, but they in no respect resemble mine.

The subtle and apparently mysterious way in which this Remedy operates, surprises most people, and it is therefore necessary to give an explanation of its physiological action. Medical agents act in different ways, some as stimulants to particular parts of the body, some as alteratives, and others again as special excitants of particular organs : thus some act on the bowels, some on the kidneys, some on the heart, and others on the skin. A few act on the nervous system, through the brain, like alcohol and opium. Usually, they excite in the first place, and afterwards act as sedatives, or *stupify*. The Indian Hemp, or *Haschisch*. is of this class, and usually forms one of the main ingredients in all common *Exhilarants* and *Aphrodisiacs*. It is a dangerous drug when so used, and utterly valueless for any such purpose, but when properly combined with the other articles which I have described, it becomes a valuable auxiliary.

Woe to those who use it and opium for the purpose of intoxication! Alcohol is harmless compared with them!

The true Aphrodisiac, as I compound it, acts upon the brain and nervous system, not as a stimulant, but as a *Tonic* and *Nutritive* agent, thus sustaining its power and the power of the *sexual* organs also, which is entirely dependent upon *Nervous Power*.

A man's sexual vigor represents merely his excess of nervous vigor. All the functions, both of body and mind, are carried on only by nervous power, which enables each organ to perform its peculiar function. The heart, stomach, lungs and every other organ, act only from the stimulus which the nerves bring to them from the brain and spinal marrow. Cut these nerves through and stop the supply, and they act no longer.

Now, every man only possesses a certain amount of nervous power, which varies in quantity according to the health and natural vigor of his system; if, therefore, too much of this power is employed in one of the functions, the others must run short, and, of course, be imperfectly performed. Thus, if a man *thinks* too much, his brain uses up so much of his nervous power that he has not enough for other purposes, and some organs must act imperfectly. Most likely his *stomach* will be one of these, and then he becomes *Dyspeptic ;* or he may have Heart Disease, or Liver Complaint, or any of those numerous diseases which we commonly see—all of which spring originally from impaired nervous action.

An imperfectly acting stomach again re-acts on the whole system, because it prevents proper *nutrition*, and thus causes general weakness or debility. No act, however, exhausts more of nervous power than the *sexual act!* and this is why its too frequent performance is so terribly injurious, and why the votaries of Venus so frequently become debilitated, weak-minded and impotent.

(NOTE.—Those who wish to see this subject fully explained, should read my books, "*The Marriage Guide,*" and "*The Male Organs,*" in which the whole subject is fully gone into.)

Whenever the system generally, or any particular part, becomes debilitated, and performs its peculiar function imperfectly, we use some medicine to *stimulate* it or improve its action. Thus we employ various bitter tonics to help the stomach, in Dyspepsia, and use Aphrodisiacs in Sexual Impotence. The way in which they really act has only lately been found out, and I will, therefore, now explain it.

CONNECTION BETWEEN THE NERVOUS AND SEXUAL SYS-
TEMS, WITH AN EXPLANATION OF THE MEANS WE
POSSESS FOR THEIR NUTRITION AND RENOVATION.

IT has long been known, as a general truth, but very vaguely, that there is an intimate connection between the Nervous and Sexual systems, but it has hitherto been thought to be merely *sympathetic*. Physiologists have, however, recently discovered that the composition, and mode of production, of the Nervous substance and the Seminal fluid are almost identical- that, in fact, they are essentially the same thing. It has also been ascertained that, in all cases of severe Nervous or Mental derangement, the actual *substance* of the Brain and Nerves either *wastes* away or undergoes a destructive *change*. And in the same way, in all cases of confirmed loss of Sexual power, the seminal substance either *wastes*, or becomes *destructively changed*, in a similar manner. But, what is still more important, the destruction or injury of either one of these elements of our systems brings on inevitably a similar evil to the other. Every man, therefore, who becomes *Impotent*, is in imminent danger of becoming *Insane*, or at least of weak Intellect, and every one whose nervous substance is seriously impaired will almost certainly lose his sexual powers. The two are intimately dependant, the one on the other, and are affected, for good or for evil, by the same external and internal causes.

At the present time, a number of causes are in constant operation, on most men, exceedingly destructive both to their Nervous and their Sexual powers, causing an actual waste of Brain and Seminal substance, and entailing bodily suffering and mental deficiency to an unknown extent.

This has, of course, originated plenty of *remedies*, as they are called, which are put forth as infallible, by those who know nothing of the nature of these evils, and who care nothing for the effect which follows after the remedy is sold.

In all such cases, it is requisite, in the first instance, to arrest further change, or waste, and then effect a *Restoration*, if that be possible. To effect this Renovation, we must, of course, use such means as will really *create new Brain, or Seminal Substance*. The same as we create new *Muscle* in cases of muscular weakness. That this can be done is undoubted, for each portion of the organization draws the elements of its nutrition from peculiar sources, and when we know what those elements are, and whence they can be obtained, we can supply them. It is not possible to nourish and renovate the Nervous and Sexual systems by the same elements alone that nourish and renovate the muscular system, though these are necessary as adjuncts; there is needed in addition certain *rare elements* that are found only in the Nervous and Seminal substances, and which can be supplied only by the *Aphrodisiac Remedy.*

This preparation is not a Stimulant or Excitant, nor a mere Tonic, but a real *Renovator*, supplying precisely that kind of material and influence, that is needed to produce *New Brain* and new *Seminal fluid!* I have myself often been amazed at its effects, and seldom despair of any case in which it can be used; in fact, it is almost infallible, except where there is some Organic Defect, or some primary lesion which requires correcting first. In proof of this, I need only refer to the "Cases."

It is, of course, equally useful in all kinds of *Nervous debility and derangement*, because they depend upon precisely the same causes as the sexual ones which have been described, namely, want of proper nutrition of the Brain and Nervous Substance.

Especially will it be found effective in that terrible, and too frequent disease *Softening of the Brain*; hitherto deemed *incurable!*

The reader will now understand the Nature of this Remedy, and will see the footing on which I place it. It is not advertised in the manner of the Quack Cordials and Invigorators of the day, nor will it be so, but can always be obtained by those who require it.

In short, it will be found, I venture to assert, as nearly infallible, and self-sufficient, as any medical remedy, in the nature of things, can be! If *it* fails, the patient should at once seek Dr. H.'s advice, for he may rest fully assured there is some Organic or functional derangement which imperatively and urgently requires Surgical or Mechanical aid.

For convenience, I have it so put up, in a dry form, air and water tight, that it can be kept uninjured, for any length of time, in any climate, and under any cir cumstances. It can also be taken without the inconvenience of *measuring*, using *Liquids*, or any other troublesome requirement, thus ensuring secrecy and facility of use, let a man be situated however he may. A gentleman can keep it in his vest pocket without the fear of detection from smell or appearance. It will go anywhere *by Post*, with perfect safety, and in such a *form* that no one through whose hands it passes would ever suspect its *nature*, or that it was anything *peculiar!*

The price for a package is FIVE DOLLARS! and if ordered by Post it will be sent *free*, to any part, with full directions. There are *no Agents* for it anywhere, at present, nor will there be except they are specially mentioned in my Books, so that it can only be obtained from me personally, by addressing through the Post to " DOCTOR F. HOLLICK, *New York*, Box 3606." I do this to avoid trouble, and also to prevent *Counterfeiting*, which would be sure to be practised if it were generally sold through Agents. One package is usually sufficient in all ordinary cases of simple debility, from excesses or imprudence ; but, in severe cases, it will, of course, require to be used longer, according to the severity of the derangement. Old persons, and those who are much broken down, should use it regularly, at intervals : but, in every case, one single package will prove its power.

It is scarcely necessary for me to repeat that there is nothing whatever in this preparation that can be in any way hurtful, under any circumstances. It is applicable to cases of *Female Sterility* and torpor, as well as to derangements of the male System or Nerves, as will be seen by some of the "Cases" in my Books.

Persons sending for DR. HOLLICK's APHRODISIAC REMEDY, should be careful to send the address *mainly* and in *full!* naming the Post Office, County and State, and be sure to address—

"DOCTOR F. HOLLICK,

"Box 3606, Post Office,

"*New York City.*"

For the *Five Dollars*, it will *be sent free anywhere* !

EXTRACTS FROM LETTERS FROM MY AGENTS IN VARI-
OUS PLACES.

ADEN, Arabia, *at the mouth of the Red Sea,* }
October 3, 1861. }

TO DR. HOLLICK, New York, U. S. A.:—Box, 3606.

DEAR SIR—In accordance with your directions, I proceeded from Egypt to this place, and have now been here three weeks. I find, as you supposed, that this is the best place at which to secure many of the articles you have commissioned me to purchase: but it is much more difficult and expensive to obtain some of them than I had supposed.

The ———, though brought to this place, really comes from the interior of Africa, and reaches here by way of Abyssinia. The Somali, a most wild and blood-thirsty tribe, possess the country where it is produced, and they will take the trouble to procure it only in exchange for arms and certain kinds of cloths. I shall therefore be compelled to keep here a stock of these articles constantly on hand, sufficient to exchange for all they may bring. I do not suppose there will be more than you will need, but if there is, it must still be bought, both to secure the monoply, and to give them encouragement not to neglect gathering it.

The ———— comes to this place from the interior of Arabia—where, I have not yet learnt. The caravans that bring it arrive only twice in the year. I have seen the only merchants who deal with it, and have arranged with them for the purchase of the whole supply in future, so that no one else can procure any. The other articles I shall also ensure in the same way, and stay here till I have done so.

Respectfully yours,

ARNOLD HUFER.

———

ASSAM, *in the interior of Hindostan,* }
March 3, 1861. }

To DR. HOLLICK, New York, U. S. A.:

DEAR SIR—I have now been at this point five weeks, and have been very successful in the objects for which I came.

In regard to *Musk.* I find that it can be obtained purer and in larger quantities, at the southern borders of Hindostan, than anywhere else. It is not produced here, but on the other side of the mountains, in Thibet, South-east China, and some parts of Tartary; there is, however, an active trade carried on across the mountains to those regions, from these parts, and this is the way it comes. It is far purer than what comes from China, but is much dearer, owing to the long and dangerous journey which the traders have to take. I am told it occupies seven months to go and return, and through a most lawless, inhospitable region. I have already arranged with the principal merchants to whom it is always consigned, to take all that comes, at each trip, so that it is useless for any one else to come here after Musk. It is necessary, however, to make large advances and run considerable risk of loss, but that is unavoidable.

The ————, I find, comes only from Northern Burmah, and is never openly sold. The despotic rulers

of the districts from which it comes, prize it so highly,
that they utterly forbid its exportation, under penalty
of *Death!* Like everything else here, however, it can
be obtained if you go the right way to work, and give
plenty of money in the right quarter. It will cost
some lakhs of rupees to obtain the quantity you name,
besides heavy fees to the officials, but you may depend
upon it, and may also rest assured that, no one else
will have any out of this country. Merchandise cannot be brought here, so that all has to be paid for in
silver, and you must, therefore, be careful always to
keep a sufficient supply at your agents in Calcutta.

This region is quite healthy, and I shall stay here
till the necessary arrangements are made permanently.   Yours, etc.,

                                      JAMES HOXTON.

———·

Cuzco, *in the Andes*, South America, }
                     May 15, 1862. }

To DR. HOLLICK, New York City, U. S. A. :

DEAR SIR—Now I am here, I find no difficulty in
procuring all the articles you need. They can be obtained only from the Indians who gather them, and
who never take them to the cities. My own experience has shown me the astonishing virtue of the *Coco*-
leaves most conclusively, and I now know that the
statements of Tschudi, Stevens and others, are not at
all exaggerated.

An Indian, at least 50 years old, carried me on his
back up the mountains, in a kind of chair, at the rate
of twenty miles a day, without a particle of food for a
whole day at a time, and yet showed no signs of exhaustion. At starting, he placed his ball of Coco-
leaves in his mouth, with a little lime, as a taster, and
this sustained him thoroughly; in fact, he seemed as
fresh at the end of the journey as when he began. In
the same time, I required three good meals, and ye'

was tired enough, though walking with another man's legs. They both chew it and make tea of it, and I am beginning to use it regularly myself. It is certainly harmless, as all experience proves, and its power of preventing bodily and mental fatigue is amazing. I have been busily occupied for a whole day, and yet at night, by using the Coco—could sit up all night, if necessary, writing, with scarcely a symptom of fatigue. It seems to suspend the waste of nervous power almost entirely.

You will receive a regular supply, both of the Coco and other articles, from Lima City.

Yours, etc.,

ARTHUR LE ROY.

(*Translation.*)

LEIPZIG, Germany, October 9, 1861.

DOCTOR HOLLICK:—P. O. Box, 3606, N. York, U. S.

DEAR SIR—I can arrange with Mr. ——, the well-known chemist, to prepare you the articles you name; but he will require to build a special apparatus for the purpose, and will require you to give security for all the expense. and also to take all the produce at the price agreed upon. He is the only man who will undertake the manufacture.

Yours, etc.,

HERMAN BLUM.

These few extracts will show what an expense and labor it has been to procure a certain and sufficient supply of these rare articles, and also why it is that no one else can possi! ly provide an article like the *Aphrodisiac Remedy!*

F. HOLLICK.

MICROSCOPICAL EXAMINATION OF THE URINE.

No. 1. Represents the appearance of the Semen when perfectly healthy, as seen under the microscope. It was a portion lost in consequence of straining at stool, from constipation, as is *very often* the case.

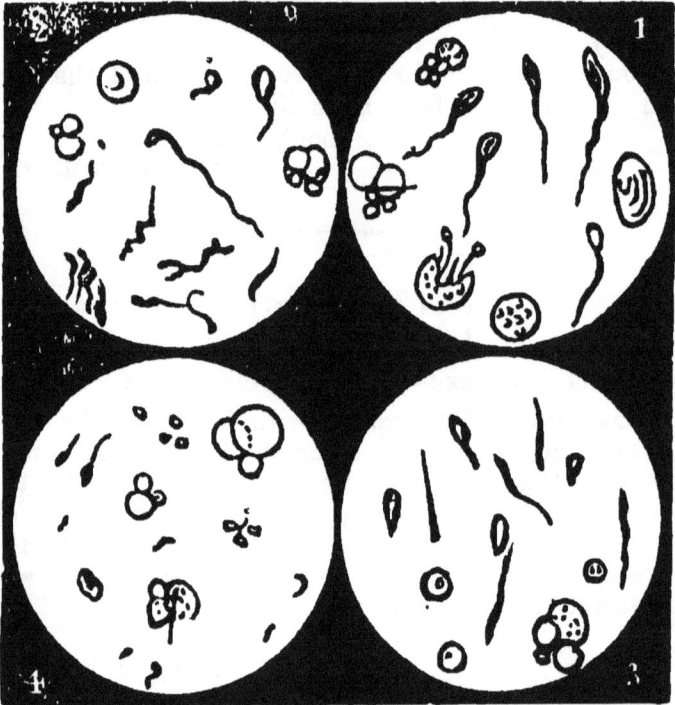

The *Seminal Animalcules*, those minute *living beings*, always found in that fluid, and without which it is *imperfect*, will be seen perfect in their form, and active in their motions. While this state of the vital fluid exists, a man will retain his powers, but if it continues to be *lost* to an undue extent—and especially if it passes *in the urine*, a change occurs—the animalcules becomes less abundant, imperfect in form, and with very feeble powers of motion. This is shown in No. 2.

No. 2. This was a portion of Semen contained in the *urine* of a person who had debilitated himself by masturbation, in early life. There are a few animalcules, but they are imperfect and very feeble. This individual had but faint amative desires, and but little power. It is possible that a man so circumstanced may be capable of *association*, to a limited extent, and may even become a *parent*, but his *children*, if he have any, are sure to be either *deformed*, *still born*, or *constitutionally weak !* Most usually, however, there is no impregnation, or if there be, *miscarriage* takes place.

The reason for this is obvious enough, to those who know the part which the Animalcule performs in originating the new being, and it is fully explained in " *The Marriage Guide.*"

No. 3. This was also taken from the urine of a man who had long suffered from Urinary Seminal loss, and who had become nearly *impotent*, with great decay of his mental powers, gloomy feelings, general debility, and all those distressing symptoms of *constitutional decay*, which invariably follow this disease if it is not checked.

In this case the Animalcules are all *dead*, and the parts of the body detached from each other. Impregnation from this semen could *never take place*, though the person might still at times, retain slight powers of association. Many men are circumstanced in this way—especially those long addicted to excesses of any kind, and also business men, exhausted by too much anxiety and mental labor.

No. 4. This view was taken from a man wholly and hopelessly *impotent*, and in the last stages of decay, bodily and mental. Of course, at this stage, there is neither power nor desire. The Semen is utterly destitute of animalcules, and almost substance. It passes almost constantly in the urine, and is merely like gum water. During the *second* and *third* stages, a man may recover, with proper assistance, but in the last stage there is *no hope*. There are many married people without children, owing to these imperfections in the male, though it is generally thought that it *must* be from the female. Some men are even *naturally* imperfect n this way, and never can be parents, though, *apparently*, like other men. The true reason for weakly and deformed children, and also for frequent miscarriage, is also often in the male, though not suspected.

Dr. H. is daily making *microscopical examinations* of this kind, both for those who call upon him, and for others.

Persons at a distance, who cannot possibly pay a personal visit to Dr. H. need not give up all hopes of receiving proper treatment in any of the above affections. Dr. H. can suggest a means by which the necessary examinations can be made perfectly, without their coming, so that he can advise by regular correspondence, as he does constantly with hundreds. All the peculiar medicines which he uses are so prepared as to go by *post*, without fear of injury or detection.

In short, Dr. H. attends to all those derangements which are connected in any way with the *parental system*, in both sexes, and those peculiar nervous affections which arise from them. His practice is, therefore, different from that of any other medical man of the day, and he does not interfere, except incidentally, with those diseases that ordinarily engage professional attention.

The success that has attended his efforts, and the public confidence and patronage that has been so extensively awarded him for many years past, and which is daily increasing, make it utterly unnecessary for him to adopt any means for extending his practice ; nor is this statement published for any such purpose. It has merely been issued at the request of many former patients, to let those persons know, who are suffering from these peculiar causes, that there is now one upon whom they can rely, who devotes special attention to such derangements, and thus rescue them from the despairing and hopeless condition into which they are too apt, naturally enough, to fall.

It is scarcely necessary to add that the strictest *confidence* and *secresy*, is observed in all communications, personal or otherwise, and that the most careful attention is bestowed upon every case. Dr. H. has numerous testimonials from those who were formerly impotent, debilitated, or childless, but who were fully restored to health, happiness, and parental enjoyment.

APPENDIX.

Notices of Dr. Hollick's Lectures.

DR. HOLLICK AND PHYSIOLOGY.—The second of a series of Lectures, by this gentleman, on human physiology, and the all important truths connected with our physical constitution, was attended by a full house, in National Hall last evening. The time was well spent, and so appeared to think the audience. On the delivery of the first of these Lectures on Tuesday evening, the speaker in a comprehensive and well-digested exordium, placed himself and the subject right with the public. His manner, language and style, did the first ; his sound logic, his argument, his candor and research, accomplished the second. Apart from the interesting and apposite details of the wonders of reproduction, the illustrations of the immutable wisdom of nature, which teem in the animal and vegetable worlds—which

> " Glows in each stem, and blossoms in each tree ;
> Lives through all life, extends through all extent,
> Spreads undivided, operates unspent."

Apart from all this, Dr. Hollick's Lecture was excellent as a defence of truth, a vindication of the right of free and unshackled inquiry, and as a convincing refutation of that silly, but far too prevalent opinion that there are truths of which it is better to remain in a state of ignorance. Had nothing else been imparted in the forcible and well defined exordium of Dr. Hollick, than this judicious demolition of that fallacious, silly, and injurious twaddle which would forbid research to pass in advance of the old landmarks prescribed by custom, ignorance or a spurious morality—even that would well deserve the public patronage. Truths, well set forth, will make an impression, whether their investigation be fashionable or not. There is an affinity between the capacity to learn, and the truths to be learned, which always results, when a fitting opportunity is presented, in a free inquiry, and the gentleman who is bringing, in a judicious and elevated manner, a knowledge of these fundamental principles of our corporeal existence which are abused because unknown, will accomplish more good than half a dozen teachers of higher pretensions, and lower ability. It was gratifying to observe the decorum—the sense of respect for both speaker and subject, that was observed throughout the evening, which evidently shows that those who go there are actuated by higher motives than mere curiosity ; by desires more ennobling than a passing gratification ; in a word, it was clear that those who composed Dr H's hearers, were men who know and dare to think, and who will profit by these most useful discourses.—*New York Herald, August 7, 1844.*

At a Meeting of the Class attendant upon Dr. Hollick's Select Lectures on the Physiology and Philosophy of the "Origin of Life" in Plants and Animals, held at the Lecture Room of the Museum, Wednesday evening, December 1, 1844, George G. West, Esq., was called to the Chair, and Samuel W. Black appointed Secretary.

Resolved, That we have listened with unfeigned pleasure and interest to the Course of Lectures delivered by Dr. Hollick, and now brought to a close, and that we deem it an act of justice to him and the community, to express our entire confidence in his character, ability, and the manner of illustrating his subject, which to use the words of a daily journal, "is couched in such delicate as well as perspicuous language, that the most fastidious could find no fault, nor the idlest curiosity go away unimproved."

Resolved, That a committee of three be appointed to tender to Dr. H. the thanks of the Class for his courtesy to the members in affording them every facility for obtaining information upon the subject of his Lectures, and that he be requested to repeat the Course at the earliest period consistent with his other engagements.

Published in all the Philadelphia daily papers of December 14, 1844, and signed by *one hundred and forty* of the most respectable and influential inhabitants.

(See similar Resolutions, with *over two hundred names* attached in the Philadelphia daily papers of March 9, 1844 ; also of March 16 ; and on several other occasions.)

From the Philadelphia Daily Papers, Feb. 21, 1845.

At a meeting of the Ladies composing Dr. Hollick's Class, held on Wednesday afternoon, February 19th, in the Lecture Room of the Museum, the following resolutions were unanimously adopted, and ordered to be published in one or more of the city papers :

Resolved, That we have listened with great pleasure and interest to Dr. Hollick's Lectures, and we are happy to add our testimony to the many already recorded in behalf of such Lectures ; and regarding Dr. Hollick as a benefactor of his race, and especially of our sex, we cordially wish for him abundant success, and ample reward in the consciousness of doing good.

Resolved, That we will exert ourselves to induce our female friends and acquaintances to avail themselves of the great and rare privilege of obtaining the valuable instruction imparted in these Lectures in so chaste and dignified a manner.

Signed on behalf of the meeting by

SUSAN WOOD, *President*

SARAH WEBB, *Secretary.*

☞ With over 50 names attached thereto.

(See also similar Resolutions, with numerous names, on Feb. 27, 1846, March 20, 1846, and on April 10, 1846, with over *three hundred names attached*.)

A GOLD MEDAL TO DOCTOR HOLLICK.—The Ladies of Dr. Hollick's tians have presented him with a beautiful Gold Medal, enclosed in a handsome morocco case. The front of the Medal bears the following inscription :

"Presented to Frederick Hollick, M. D., by the Ladies who attended his Lectures on Physiological Science, delivered at Philadelphia, March, 1846, as an expression of their approbation of the knowledge therein conveyed, and as a testimonial of personal regard."

On the reverse is the Sun, and reflected by the rays of the luminary, a scroll containing the words

"To give light to them that sit in darkness."

Phila. Spirit of the Times, March 28, 1846.

———

"LETTERS FROM NEW YORK, NO. 11.

" ✱ ✱ ✱ There have been several courses of Lectures on Anatomy, this winter, adapted to popular comprehension. I rejoice at this ; for it has long been a cherished wish with me that a general knowledge of the structure of our bodies, and the laws which govern it, should extend from the scientific few into the common education of the people. I know of nothing so well calculated to diminish vice and vulgarity as universal and rational information on these subjects. But the impure state of society has so perverted nature, and blinded common sense, that intelligent women, though eagerly studying the structure of the Earth, the attraction of the Planets, and the reproduction of Plants, seem ashamed to know anything of the structure of the Human Body, and of those Physiological facts most intimately connected with their deepest and purest emotions, and the holiest experience of their lives. I am often tempted to say, as Sir C. Grandison did to the Prude—'Wottest thou not how much *in*-delicacy there is ir thy delicacy ?'

"The only Lectures I happened to attend were those of Dr. Hollick, which interested and edified me much. They were plain, familiar conversations, uttered and listened to with great modesty of language, and propriety of demeanor. The Manikin, or Artifical Anatomy, by which he illustrated his subject, is a most wonderful machine invented by a French Physician. It is made of *papier mache*, and represents the human body with admirable perfection, in the shape, coloring, and arrangement even to the minutest fibres. By the removal of wires it can be dissected completely, so as to show the locality and functions of the various Organs, the interior of the Heart, Lungs, &c.

"Until I examined this curious piece of mechanism, I had very faint and imperfect ideas of the miraculous machinery of the house we live in. I found it highly suggestive of many things to my mind." ✱ ✱ ✱

L. M. C.

[Extract from a Letter in the Boston Courier of Monday, June 24, 1844, by Mrs. L. M Child.]

DR. HOLLICK'S course of lectures at Washingtonian Hall on the Origin of Life, commenced on Monday, and were listened to with breathless attention till the close, when the audience in a body assembled around the speaker's stand, and congratulated him upon the excellence, novelty and utility of his discourse, and the vigor and felicity of his explanations. The manikin used by the Dr. to illustrate his remarks, is as large as life, and contains a fac simile of all the important machinery of the human body, and it is a treat to behold them and listen to the accompanying observations regarding their uses and buses. The advance of modern science is aptly illustrated by the declaration of Dr. H., that within the last two years there have been discovered greater facilities for teaching medical doctrines to the *multitude* than the two foregoing centuries furnished for the instruction of *medical men*. If then, modern days afford so much additional light, it is even culpable on the part of the community if they do not avail themselves of knowledge so indispensable to health and happiness. Dr. Hollick's remarks are unexceptionable, easily understood, and have all the force of philosophy without the learned jargon of the pedant.—*Boston Post, March* 23, 1848.

☞ Dr. Hollick's new series of Lectures which commence to-day for ladies in the afternoon, and for gentlemen in the evening, will no doubt prove a course of high gratification, and useful instruction, to all who can attend them. We understand each lecture will be quite complete by itself, and will embrace every topic of interest and every fact of value, that have the slightest bearing upon the subject discussed. The Dr. has a most admirable power of condensation, and never loses time with mere words, so that he puts more valuable matter in one of his discourses than is ordinarily scattered over four. The ladies' lectures are all to be of a strictly useful character, embracing the causes of their various complaints, and how to avoid them, &c. It was remarked by many, who were there last week, that such knowledge would prevent more diseases than any medical skill could cure, and that they scarcely knew which to admire most, the value of the information itself, or the singularly pleasing, plain, and delicate manner in which it was communicated. The attendance will no doubt be large, and those who go late will probably be again disappointed, as hundreds were last week.—*Boston Bee, March* 7, 1848.

DR. HOLLICK'S NEW SERIES OF LECTURES.—At the request of many of our citizens, Dr. H. has arranged to commence on Monday next, a course for ladies and gentlemen together, on Physiology and Health and also one in the afternoon for ladies alone, illustrated by his celebrated models, paintings, &c. The great interest and importance of this subject, and the reputation of the lecturer himself, will no doubt cause a very large attendance, but the Doctor has properly made his arrangements, so that no more will be admitted than can be comfortably seated. These lectures will be quite a prominent feature in the next week's entertainments, and we should not be surprised if the Doctor is even better patronized than he was last winter, when hundreds could not obtain admission to hear him.—*Boston Times, November* 1848

Dr. P's style of lecture is exceedingly plain, lucid and intelligible. He relies on no mere artifice of art of oratory—no effort to surprise or startle—to obtain or keep up the interest of his lectures. But they are deeply interesting. They are listened to in silence and with enchained attention—an attention that would feel annoyed at any fictitious arts of the speaker. The reason of this is obvious. The entirely novel character of the lectures, the deep and pervading interest of the subjects discussed—subjects embracing all that is mysterious and of momentous importance in the matter of man's re-production and existence in this world—give to the lectures a solid and inestimable value as well as enchaining freshness and interest.

We believe Dr. Hollick is the only man in the country who has devoted years of study to this important but too much neglected branch of human knowledge, or rather of human ignorance ; and who is now trying to extend the lights of wholesome understanding on the subjects embraced, among the people.

In this matter, we recognize in Dr. H. a public benefactor, and we owe it to the welfare of our fellows to commend him as such in this decided manner. We give utterance to no formal or *paid for* puff in this matter. Our readers know us to be incapable of such a prostitution of our columns. The large numbers of ladies and gentlemen who have attended Dr. H.'s lectures, know that we do but speak of this subject as it merits.—*St. Louis Intelligencer, Feb.* 8, 1850.

We were most agreeably surprised and delighted. Highly as Dr H. came recommended, and thoroughly as were his lectures approved by men of intelligence abroad, we had no idea before hearing him, of the vast utility of his labors.

The subjects he discusses are of the highest importance to the well-being of the human race, and an ignorance of them is daily producing a degree of disease and death, the extent of which nothing but the astounding disclosures of eternity will reveal.—*St. Louis Era, Feb* 1, 1850.

He is certainly an admirable lecturer, being clear in voice, distinct in expression, and having a very felicitous manner of imparting instruction. We are persuaded his lectures must be productive of great good.—*Organ, St. Louis, Mo.*

DR. HOLLICK.—This distinguished lecturer had a crowded house at the Apollo last evening, and his delighted audience expressed their approbation at the close of his discourse by loud applause.

Dr. H. is indeed a most entertaining and instructive lecturer. We heard a medical gentleman say last evening, after listening to him, that he would not fail to hear the whole series even if he should have to sell his coat to raise the means. The information imparted by Dr. Hollick, must be truly invaluable to every one who possesses it.—*Louisville Journal, Jan.* 8, 1850.

Undoubtedly, he is the most eloquent, instructive, and impressive lecturer in the United States upon physiology and health. The people of Cincinnati were so delighted with him, that they prevailed on him to deliver four courses of lectures, and, when he was at length obliged to leave them, they obtained from him a promise to return.—*Louisville Journal, Jan.* 4, 1850.

ANOTHER COURSE.—Dr. Hollick, in consequence of the great success with which he has met, has concluded to repeat his course of lectures, as will be seen by reference to another column. His lectures impart information of such value, and are so highly interesting, that a person who hears him once, will not fail to attend the series.—*Times, Cincinn., December*, 1849.

DR. HOLLICK's Lectures have excited great attention and produced much benefit throughout the country. These lectures are strictly moral and highly instructive. There is nothing connected with them calculated to offend the most sensitive delicacy.—*Delta, New Orleans, February* 24, 1850.

In November, 1849, Dr. Hollick lectured in *Pittsburgh, Pa.*, to crowded audiences, and at the termination of his last course was publicly thanked and requested to return.

In December, 1849, he gave *four courses* in *Cincinnati, Ohio*, and then had to give a promise to return at an early period.

In January, 1850, after two crowded courses, the ladies of *Louisville, Ky.*, tendered him publicly a most flattering vote of thanks and requested him to visit-them again as early as his engagements would allow.

In St. Louis, Mo., February, 1850, he had crowded houses, both of ladies and gentlemen, for three weeks, and public resolutions, commending his lectures in the highest terms, were passed on several occasions.

On going down the Mississippi River, February, 1850, he was unanimously requested by the officers and passengers of the splendid steamer *Atlantic*, to unpack his Models and lecture to them *on the boat*, which he did on three several days. At the conclusion, the audience resolved itself into a meeting, Dr. Gibson of Mississippi, being called to the chair, and Dr. Clark of St. Louis, elected Secretary. A series of resolutions were then passed unanimously, returning thanks for the lectures, and commending them in the highest terms. These resolutions, headed,

"*Novel and interesting scene on board a Mississippi steamer.*"

were published in the Picayune, New Orleans, the inhabitants of which place, were strongly urged to attend when the lectures were given in their city, and which they did not fail to do.

During his stay in the West and South, Dr. H. was everywhere received in the most flattering manner, and his efforts to impart important physiological knowledge in a popular manner were fully appreciated. In every place the largest room that could be obtained was crowded at each lecture, and the number of applicants for consultations was so great, that on several occasions Dr. H. was obliged to postpone the lectures in order to attend to them.

WRITING DESK AND GOLD PEN PRESENTED TO DR. HOLLICK
BY ONE OF HIS LADY CLASSES.

DR. HOLLICK—*Dear Sir:* The members of your class, desiring the gratification of offering you some testimonial of their personal regard, and grateful appreciation of the benefits which you are conferring upon them and their sex generally, respectfully request your acceptance of the accompanying writing desk.

Were it necessary, we might repeat our assurances that your services to humanity will be, by us, long and gratefully remembered. The women of this generation have reason to rejoice that, by your efforts, a new and extensive field of information has been opened to them, whence they may derive treasures of knowledge, of immense importance to themselves and their posterity, hitherto concealed within professional enclosures.

Wishing you health and happiness, we beg leave to subscribe ourselves,

Truly your Friends,
Signed on behalf of the class, by
M. G
O. W B.

Philadelphia, March 20, 1845.

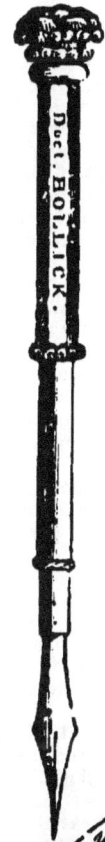

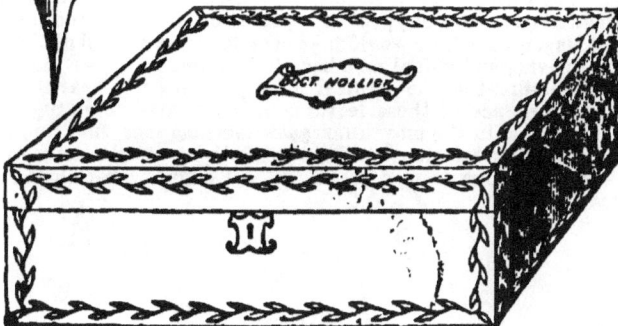

In the early part of 1852, Dr. Hollick lectured for *four weeks*, with the most unbounded success, in Philadelphia, and for four more in Baltimore, where his reception was enthusiastic, the ladies filling the room, and passing on the last day, a series of highly flattering and commendatory RESOLUTIONS, which were published in the daily papers. The following are a few of the Editorials given at that time :—

[COMMUNICATED.]

MESSRS. EDITORS.—The most scientific and useful lectures of the present day, which should claim the attention of every one, are now being delivered at Masonic Hall, by Dr. Hollick, on the subject of Internal Physiology and Health. The writer of this heard his first course delivered during the last week, and having been educated to the medical profession, is, perhaps, capable of judging of their usefulness. There is no doubt that the general feeling of the medical faculty, and of an enlightened community, towards itinerant lecturers, has been one of disapprobation and apprehension of quackery, but in the present instance there is certainly an exception.

Dr. Dunbar, (formerly Professor at the Washington College,) who attended Dr. H.'s last lecture, on Friday evening, was so pleased with the manner and matter of the lecture, that he came out openly at the close of the lecture and stated, before the audience had dispersed, that he had come there at the request of a patient, prejudiced against the lecturer, but on hearing him, he thought it his duty to say, that the lecture was perfectly fair, scientific, calculated to do a vast amount of good, and that every man, young or old, should hear, and would be benefitted thereby. His illustrations are complete and beautiful, and his explanations couched in such delicate language that the most fastidious can find no fault. Those of your numerous readers who may devote an hour to his remaining lectures will thank you for giving this publicity.—*Baltimore American*, March 2, 1852.

———

DR. HOLLICK'S LECTURES.—The distinction which Dr. Hollick has acquired as a most intelligent, judicious and salutary lecturer on the interesting and important subjects of human physiology and health, renders any commendation from us quite unnecessary ; yet, in view of the fact, that the course which he has lately delivered in this city, is, at the solicitation of many, to be repeated on this and the next two days, at Masonic Hall, we would take occasion to assure all of their great value to every individual member of the human family. Many of the most prominent of the medical faculty in this city bear testimony to the excellence of these lectures, as calculated to be highly useful, in imparting, in the most unexceptionable manner, that knowledge of human physical structure and the laws of health, the want of which now occasions so much calamity and suffering.—*Baltimore Sun*, March 1, 1852.

THE GOLD MEDAL PRESENTED TO DR. HOLLICK,

BY

Presented to

FREDERICK HOLLICK M.D.

by

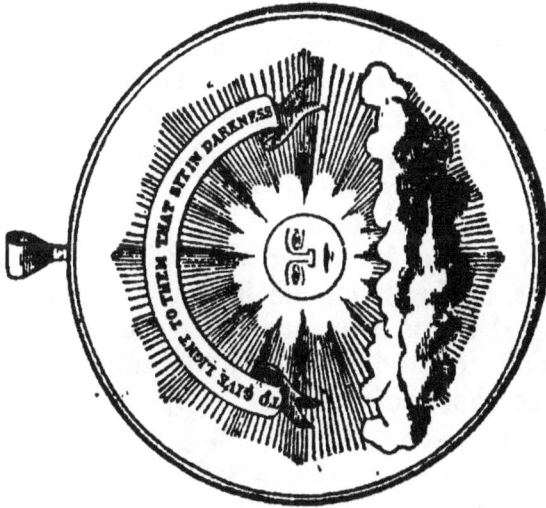

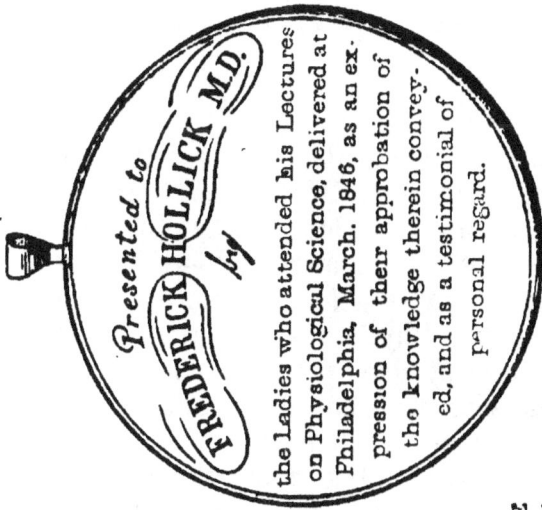

the Ladies who attended his Lectures on Physiological Science, delivered at Philadelphia, March. 1846, as an expression of their approbation of the knowledge therein conveyed, and as a testimonial of personal regard.

TO GIVE LIGHT TO THEM THAT SIT IN DARKNESS

THE

LADIES OF PHILADELPHIA.

CONCLUDING REMARKS.

From the Contents of this work, and from the references to other Books, and to my Lectures, the nature of my Practice and the object of my Public Lectures will be understood.—Circumstances have led me, for a length of time, to make a special study of the Physiology and derangements of the Generative system, perhaps more exclusively than any one else ever has done, and I have in consequence become familiar both with the subject itself and with the public requirements respecting it. Like all other branches of knowledge this is inevitably destined to become *popular*, though from its nature, and from the deficient information of professional men themselves, it has remained longer a mystery than many others. The *necessity* for a more general acquaintance with it, however, is becoming daily more evident, and more recognised, but still very few persons have liked to brave prejudice, and run the risk of being misconceived, or wrongly judged, by lifting the veil. My position, however, having made me independent of these influences, I felt it incumbent upon me to assume the task, and to study not only the subject itself but also the mode of making it popularly understood. The best interests of humanity require that this should be done, as the most obvious means of *preventing* both moral perversion and physical disease, which we now leave to originate unchecked, and vainly try to *cure*

Several years ago I commenced Public Lecturing on these subjects, and writing popular Books, in a more complete manner than any one else ever has done, and my success has been highly satisfactory. In some few cases I have been misapprehended, as might have been expected, but to so small an extent that the instances may well be lost sight of in the general tide of appreciation and approbation. Blind Prejudice and selfish interest have also striven to throw obstacles in my path, but their impediments have soon been swept away, and have only served to accelerate what they were intended to arrest.

The fact is, this subject is no longer *a professional mystery*, nor is it now esteemed a crime for a non-professional man to understand it, or for one in the profession to teach him, and I flatter myself that my own efforts have had an important share in bringing about this desirable result.

The people are now thoroughly aroused, and claim their right to understand these matters themselves, instead of being left in ignorance, as they have hitherto been, for the benefit of those who live upon their errors and misfortunes. No earthly power can now maintain at least not in our country, a monopoly of knowledge on these or any other subjects, and no sophistry can ever again persuade the people that ignorance is better for them than knowledge. The field of knowledge is now open for all to tread who choose, and none can make it *private property* again.

It is interesting, however, as a matter of history, to note some of the occurrences which have taken place while this great result was being accomplished, and to see how those who tried to prevent it have changed their Tactics.—At first the *monopolists of knowledge* stood upon their vested *rights*, as they termed them, and boldly asserted that no one else had any title to it. Finding, however, that their claim was indignantly disallowed, and that people *would know* in spite of them, they next took the ground that such knowledge was *improper*, and should be confined to them for safe keeping. This shallow pretext is equally disregarded however, and the old conservatives find that the people are bent upon running the risk of *being wise* in spite of all their warnings. This being the case they are slowly leaving off their opposition and will soon be putting themselves forward as *teachers*, though *grudgingly*, and in as niggardly a way as they can.

I wish especially to draw attention to this fact, and to remind my readers that in a short time our most eminent medical men will be striving against each other for popularity in this very way. The same men who now stand aloof from " *the vulgar herd*," and who affect to think their knowledge *too good* for *the common people*, will before long be proffering it those people for acceptance. As soon as they find that *the people* can obtain it *without them* they will want to give it, for fear of being left behind and forgotten.—Let this be borne in mind, so that when eminent medical professors write popular books on sexual Physiology, and eminent Publishers give them to the world, as they certainly will, though they now affect to be shocked at them, —it may be known how they have been *forced* to do so, and credit may then be given to those who did it *before them*, and *drove them to it*.

NOTICES OF DR. HOLLICK'S PUBLICATIONS.

" WE have just read a new work called ' *The Marriage Guide*,' by DR. F. HOLLICK, the well known Author of the ' *Origin of Life*,' and we are constrained to admit, that it is the most extraordinary Book that ever came under our notice. Thoroughly scientific enough for deeply read scholars, or for practical experimenters, it is yet plain and popular enough for the most ordinary understanding. Nowhere else in the English Language, can there be found such a complete and practically useful compendium of Physiological information, strictly adapted for the use of married people, or of those intending to marry. All the new discoveries of *Pouchet, Bischoff*, and others, are fully given, as well as many others by the author himself, never before made known. The engravings are also excellent, as well as curious. In fact, taking it altogether, it is beyond all question *the* Book upon these matters, and will probably become as popular in future, and as universally referred to as *Aristotle* has formerly been. One feature which peculiarly distinguishes this book from all others of the kind, is the peculiar tone of *morality* and *delicacy* which pervades it all through, and which makes it both proper and useful to be read by all persons, of both sexes, who have attained the age of puberty. A very eminent clergyman, authorizes us to say, that he deems it a duty to introduce it privately among his flock, as the best means he knows of preventing and overcoming those hateful vices, unfortunately so destructive to soul and body, which are at the present time so fearfully prevalent."—*Med. & Surg. Review.*

" THE MALE GENERATIVE ORGANS."—This book, by **Dr. Hollick**, the eminent popular Lecturer, and successful practitioner, should be in the hands of every man who values his health, and the preservation or restoration of his powers. It is complete in every particular, and is the only work in the English Language where that fell destroyer of thousands, *urinary seminal loss*, is fully explained, and its cure and prevention pointed out. How many thousands yearly die, or become imbecile from this cause, who have never heard it mentioned."—[*Med. Journal.*

DR HOLLICK'S BOOKS

THE

MARRIAGE GUIDE;

OR NATURAL HISTORY OF

GENERATION.

PRICE.—ONE DOLLAR.

A PRIVATE instructor for Married People, and those *about to marry*, both male and female, in everything relating to the Anatomy and Physiology of the Generative system, in both sexes, and the process of Reproduction. Including a full description of everything that is now known respecting the *prevention* and production of offspring, the cause of the difference in sex,—Parental influence,—Natural adaptation,—Philosophy of Marriage, &c., &c.

This is beyond all comparison the most extraordinary work on Physiology ever published. There is nothing whatever that *married people* can either *require* or *wish* to know but what is fully explained, and many matters are introduced, of the most important and interesting character, to which no *allusion* even can be found in any other work in our language. All the *new discoveries*, many of them never before made public, are given in full, especially those relating to *conception* and *sterility*.

No married person of either sex, should be without this book. It is utterly unlike any other ever published, and the matter it contains can be found nowhere else. It contains numerous *Engravings*, and *colored Plates*, designed especially for this work, and showing many of the new discoveries, as well as anatomical details and Physiological processes.

THE
MALE GENERATIVE ORGANS,
IN HEALTH AND DISEASE,
FROM INFANCY TO OLD AGE.

Price.—One Dollar.

A COMPLETE practical Treatise on the *Anatomy* and *Physiology* of the Male Generative System, with a full description of the causes, and cure of all the diseases and derangements to which it is liable.—*Adapted for every Man's own private use !*

This is not a treatise on *Venereal Diseases*, nor does it even refer to them, but to those derangements and difficulties, of all kinds, to which *every man* is more or less liable, and from which in fact but few entirely escape.

All the causes which lead to decay of the Generative system are fully explained, and the means pointed out by which its powers may be preserved *to extreme old age !*— More especially is explained that *unseen*, and usually *unknown* form of decay from which thousands become *diseased, insane,* and *die,* without ever suspecting what has destroyed them. Even medical men as yet know but little upon this important matter, which it is of the first moment every man should understand for himself. All the *recipes* are given in English, and the treatment is made so plain that all can practise it.

This work is also fully illustrated, both with *Engravings* and with *colored Plates,* and an introductory chapter gives an epitome of all the new discoveries respecting the *Female System* and *Generation.* No other work at all like this was ever published. *No man should be without it, young or old.*

THE
DISEASES OF WOMAN,
Their Causes and Cure Familiarly Explained,

With Practical Hints for their prevention, and for the preservation of
Female Health, intended FOR EVERY FEMALE'S OWN PRIVATE USE !—Illustrated with *Colored Plates*, and with numerous Engravings.

If all Females possessed this book in time, there would be incalculably less suffering and disease amongst them than is now seen.—Everything relating to female health is treated upon, *from infancy to old age*, and the most valuable *recipes* are given, together with practical directions, in the plainest manner. There is no known disease to which females are subject but what is here explained, and *so that all can understand.*

DR. HOLLICK has received piles of letters thanking him for writing this book, and has been complimented for it by many of his public audiences of ladies.

☞ *No female should be without it, especially if Married.*

THE MATRON'S
MANUAL OF MIDWIFERY,
AND THE
DISEASES OF WOMEN DURING PREGNANCY
AND CHILD-BIRTH.

A COMPLETE practical treatise upon the *Art of Delivery*, and upon all the accidents and diseases that may occur during these periods.

This work is especially intended for the instruction of Females themselves, and any one of ordinary intelligence, upon reading it carefully through, will be able to render the requisite assistance in cases of emergency. The description of all the various *Positions* and *Presentations* is on an entirely new plan, and is made both simple and intelligible. The management of new born infants is also given in full and the use of *Ether* and *Chloroform* during delivery is discussed.

This work contains over *sixty Engravings*, besides *Colored Plates*, showing the various periods, and how to ascertain them.—The different positions.—The progress of delivery, &c.

Price.—One Dollar Each.

*This List embraces the whole of the Works, which may either
be obtained singly or in the set.*

PRICE, ONE DOLLAR EACH,

All with Colored Plates.

PUBLISHED BY T. W. STRONG

599 BROADWAY. NEW YORK.

AND MAY BE HAD OF BOOKSELLERS GENERALLY

☞ They will also be sent by *Post*, Free, on receiving
the money and address.

TO THE TRADE.

☞ The Trade will find these works worthy of their
special attention, as the demand for them is unprecedented
and increasing, and the allowance most liberal. All whole-
sale purchasers will be provided with these descriptive
pamphlets free, and, on purchasing a certain number, with
their *imprint* upon them. ☜

AGENTS.

Agents are wanted to circulate these Books, and any
young man of good address and character, will find it extremely profitable; quite a large income being obtained
by many. Apply to the Publisher.

REMEMBER

These are books that any one can *confidently recommend*,
and which every one ought to read.

N. B.—The agent who leaves this will call again with
the Books.

DR. HOLLICK'S

APHRODISIAC REMEDY.

THIS is the celebrated Remedy so long used in DR. HOLLICK's extensive practice, for the cure of IMPOTENCE, STERILITY, and all forms of SEXUAL and NERVOUS DEBILITY!

For many years Dr. Hollick has been importuned to offer this remedy *for public sale*, but till now, has not been able to do so, on account of the SCARCITY and DEARNESS, of many of its ingredients, and the large quantity required in his practice.

Having at length succeeded after *immense cost* and *labor*, in procuring a larger supply, Dr. Hollick now *for the first time* offers it to the community at large, in compliance with the NUMEROUS AND URGENT REQUESTS that have been tendered to him *ever since its first introduction!*

This Remedy is THE ONLY ONE OF THE KIND which can possibly be obtained, because Dr. Hollick alone possesses the *secret of its composition*, and has secured the ENTIRE MONOPOLY of the *rarest* and *most powerful* of its ingredients. It is composed of THIRTY-THREE DIFFERENT SUBSTANCES; some so powerful that not more than *the hundreth part of a grain* can be used at a dose, and so dear that *a single grain* will often cost from two to four Dollars! It is however PERFECTLY HARMLESS, and may be safely used by all persons, and in any circumstances.

To the CHILDLESS, the IMPOTENT, the NERVOUS, the FEEBLE, both in BODY and MIND, the HYPOCHONDRIAC, and those who find themselves becoming OLD TOO SOON of BOTH SEXES; the *Aphrodisiac* will be found a SURE and PERMANENTLY EFFECTIVE REMEDY!

It is not a MERE STIMULANT, or INJURIOUS EXCITANT, acting *only for the moment*, but a true NERVINE and SEXUAL TONIC and RENOVATOR, *producing new Nervous and Sexual material*, when these have been *wasted* by *excess, abuse*, or *disease!*

Several of the articles which compose the *Aphrodisiac Remedy*, have been used from time immemorial, in a crude form, and separately, but no scientific combination of the whole was ever *possible* till now.

The celebrated DREAM DRUG of the East, the INDIAN HEMP, is often used as an Aphrodisiac, and will sometimes cause erotic dreams. This however is only occasional, and such an effect is always followed by unusual debility, terminating at last, if its use is continued, in complete sexual impotence.

In the Harems of Turkey, a compound is used called, in Arabic, "LOVES ASSISTANT!" It is composed of various stimulating spices, with opium and musk, and has some power, when first used, but at last it eventually causes general weakness and decay, both of body and mind. The late *Sultan of Turkey* used this compound till he was nearly an idiot; and at last died from sheer exhaustion.

In China they have a Pill somewhat similar to this, and which causes almost identically the same results. Sometime ago this *Chinese Remedy* was brought to France, and sold in Paris under the name of HONNEUR DE LA FAMILLE! (*Honour of the Family*) this being the Chinese name,—the evil results from its use however, soon caused it to be but little called for.

In some parts of Arabia and Africa, *an Aphrodisiac* has also been long employed, as we can see from allusions in old Chronicles, and in various Poems. Even in the Hebrew Scriptures the *Mandrake* is spoken of as being so used. The *Hindoos* have always been great lovers of Aphrodisiacs. and they possess some powerful ones, which however they use without knowledge, and consequently derive but little good from them, and much harm.

All these articles, after much trouble, time, and expenses, Dr. Hollick obtained and analyzed, so as to know exactly what they were.

The Aphrodisiac Remedy contains what is really good and effective in all of them, without any of their hurtful qualities.

The *Common Aphrodisiacs* are merely compounds of *Spanish flies, Opium, Strychnine, Arsenic, Phosphorus* and similar drugs; Most of them are *rank poisons!*

Among other names used for Aphrodisiacs, by the Turks, Arabians, and Hindoos, we find the following. PARENT OF PLEASURE!—DELIGHT OF PARADISE!—FAMILY MULTIPLIER!—YOUTH PROLONGER!—HOPE OF THE AGED!—BRAIN STRENGTHENER!—FOUNTAIN OF POWER! —STRENGTH GIVER!—And numerous others, all indicating the same powers. All of these various articles therefore, imperfect though they are, have still gained a reputation, and are eagerly sought. How much more valuable therefore must be a compound which combines the excellences of all, *without any hurtful qualities whatever!*

Although never advertised, and only known through the reports of those who had been restored by its use, the Aphrodisiac of Dr. Hollick has become known, and sought for in all the principal cities of Europe! Many persons of eminence have regularly obtained it, privately, and in more than one instance the *wishes* and *hopes* of married people of high rank, have been fulfilled through its means.

Its fame has even reached Turkey, and in *Constantinople* itself, the *Aphrodisiac* is rapidly supplanting the hurtful and inefficient drugs formerly in use.

No public announcement is needed therefore to *sell* the *Aphrodisiac*, but only to let those persons know they can now have it who have so long been wishing for it in vain.

In most ordinary cases of Sexual Debility, *One package* of the Aphrodisiac usually restores the virile power completely, and in all cases enough to show that entire restoration is only a question of time. When the system is much run down however, and the decay has existed for a long period, the remedy must be persisted in for a longer time, and several packages may be needed. Old persons, or those worn down by excesses, should take it *regularly*, to prevent further decay,—and so should those who *over indulge*, to ward off the consequences of their indiscretion.

If no sufficient restoration follows a *fair trial* of the *Aphrodisiac Remedy*, it may safely be inferred, that there is either a *natural imperfection*, or some *Organic Disease*, most probably there is *loss of semen in the urine!* In all such cases the person should at once consult Dr. Hollick, for the purpose of having a thorough *examination*, and a *full treatment* till the difficulty is removed.

FEMALES who are *Childless, cold in temperament, Nervous*, and *sexually feeble*, are as much benefited by the *Remedy* as males, and many a solitary hearth has been blessed with children through its use.

·
———

For those who cannot possibly visit Dr. Hollick, he will explain a simple mode of *examining* the *urine* by which the facts of the case can be fully ascertained, so that patients at a distance can be treated by correspondence with perfect success. All Dr. Hollick's Medicines are put up in the form of concentrated *dry powders*, to go by post, without any risk of detection. Hundreds of patients are constantly being prescribed for in this way, with perfect success.

☞ All letters are destroyed as soon as notes are taken of *the case*.

(See the Pamphlet accompanying each package—and also Dr. Hollick's Books on *Marriage*, and on the Male Sexual system.)

The APHRODISIAC REMEDY is put up in FLAT GOLD BOXES in such a manner that it will go anywhere by Post *like a letter*, without any risk of *Inspection* or *detection*. It will also *keep unhurt* for any length of time, in *any climate and in any circumstances!* It may be carried unobserved *in the vest pocket*, and requires no *liquids*, nor any measuring, or apparatus of any kind when taken; being in a *solid form*, divided into graduated doses, and *without* smell or taste.

PRICE FIVE DOLLARS PER PACKAGE,

For which it will be sent FREE BY POST, to any address.

☞ To PREVENT COUNTERFEITING, and to make sure that no one can be imposed upon by pretenders, *Dr. Hollick does not sell his remedy through agents*, (unless specially mentioned in his publications), but will forward it himself. FREE through the post, to any address in any part of the United States.

Direct "DR. F. HOLLICK, Post Office Box **3606**, New York City, New York."

It may also be obtained in New York City, from his publisher, T. W. STRONG, 599 Broadway